human
sexual
expression

human
sexual
expression

benjamin a. kogan, m.d., dr.p.h.

harcourt brace jovanovich, inc.

new york   chicago   san francisco   atlanta

ISBN: 0-15-540426-1

Library of Congress Catalog Number: 73-75179

Printed in the United States of America

Cover photo: *The Kiss,* 1908 (limestone) by Constantin Brancusi. Louise and Walter Arensberg Collection, Philadelphia Museum of Art.

The following drawings are by Zena Bernstein: Figures 2-1, 2-3, 2-4, 2-6, 2-7, 2-8.
The following drawings are by Benedict Umy: Figures 3-1 and 9-1.

acknowledgments

AMERICAN SOCIAL HEALTH ASSOCIATION for Tables 2-3 and 2-4, "Primary and Secondary Syphilis and Gonorrhea," from "Today's VD Control Problem: 1972," American Social Health Association: Committee on the Joint Statement (New York, 1972). Reprinted by permission.

THE AMERICAN SOCIOLOGICAL ASSOCIATION for Table 7-1, "Marriage Stability: The Religious Factor," adapted from Judson T. Landis, "Marriages of Mixed and Non-Mixed Religious Faith," *American Sociological Review,* Vol. 14, No. 3 (June 1949). Reprinted by permission.

CALIFORNIA MEDICAL ASSOCIATION for Table 1-1, "Parent and Child Development," from David Belais Friedman, "Parent Development," *California Medicine,* Vol. 86, No. 1 (January 1957). Reprinted by permission.

JONATHAN CAPE LTD for an excerpt from *George Seferis Collected Poems, 1924–1955,* translated, edited, and introduced by Edmund Keeley and Philip Sherrard. Copyright © 1967 by Princeton University Press; Supplemented Edn., 1969. Reprinted by permission.

CENTER FOR DISEASE CONTROL, PUBLIC HEALTH SERVICE for data used in Table 2-3, "Primary and Secondary Syphilis and Gonorrhea," from "Today's VD Control Problem: 1972," American Social Health Association: Committee on the Joint Statement (New York, 1972). Reprinted by permission.

CHARLES CLAY DAHLBERG for his "Sexual Behavior in the Drug Culture," *Medical Aspects of Human Sexuality,* Vol. 5, No. 4 (April 1971). Reprinted by permission.

M. EDWARD DAVIS for Table 6-1, "Stages of Labor," from M. Edward Davis and Reva Rubin, *De Lee's Obstetrics for Nurses,* 18th ed. (Philadelphia: Saunders, 1966). Reprinted by permission.

ERIK H. ERIKSON for excerpts from "Growth and Crises of the Human Personality," in Clyde Kluckhohn, Henry A. Murray, and David Schneider, eds., *Personality in Nature, Society, and Culture* (New York: Knopf, 1953), and from "Eight Ages of Man," in G. B. Levitas, ed., *The World of Psychoanalysis,* Vol. I (New York: Braziller, 1965). Reprinted by permission.

W. H. FREEMAN AND COMPANY for Figure 5-3, "The Synthesis of Proteins," from Masayasu

continued on page 372

preface

A teacher should impart what's true
At least when they allow him to;
A college teacher should not vex
His pupils with his thoughts on sex . . .[1]

Although these wry lines were written only a generation ago, they seem quaint today. Across the country, an increasing number of college students are turning to their instructors for help in better understanding their sexuality. This has created the need for a book, based on recent and authoritative research, that is designed to aid the teacher in meeting this new and complex responsibility.

The central concept of this book, which is developed in the first chapter, is that human sexuality is an expression of the total personality. As personality development involves a search for self-esteem, it is only from a growing sense of self-esteem that competence and fulfillment in sexual expression can be achieved. Respect for oneself is a prerequisite to respect for another person. The first chapter of this book, then, considers how the concept of a worthy self may develop.

The second chapter considers first the structure and functions of those body parts involved in reproduction and sexuality. This by no means implies that sexual activity is (or should be) limited to reproductive purposes. Sexual activity, to a different degree in different people, is a manifestation of the personality long before reproductive ability begins and long after reproductive capacities or interests end. Sexual pleasures are by themselves rich contributions to the entire spectrum of life. The second part of this chapter considers the major dysfunctions resulting from sexually transmitted diseases. In a general book about health, these dysfunctions would be discussed in a chapter on communicable diseases; in a book of a more limited scope, it is more appropriate to treat functions and certain dysfunctions in the same chapter.

---

[1] Irwin Edman, "Flowers for a Professor's Garden of Verses," quoted in A. C. Spectorsky, ed., *The College Years* (New York, 1958), p. 148.

Months before external environmental influences begin to mold the personality, momentous happenings within the embryo are destined to affect the individual's sexual behavior. As the result of recent research, it is known that human embryonic tissue must undergo profound changes for maleness to occur. The embryonic tissues are originally female; if no changes occur a female develops. The fact that these changes occur primarily in the embryonic reproductive and central nervous systems within a critically brief time is significant to our thinking about the nature and origins of sexual expression. In the light of this new knowledge, the third chapter goes on to describe sexual intercourse, the various ways in which its maximal pleasures may be achieved, and the sexual similarities of and the differences between the sexes. As becomes evident in the discussion, some of the similarities and differences are cultural rather than biological. Finally, some of the more common myths about sexuality are considered.

The fourth chapter is concerned with birth control. Included with a discussion of the better known methods used are descriptions of recent studies of the "morning after" contraceptive pill, long-acting contraceptives, and the ongoing research for a safe male contraceptive. Vasectomies and abortions are also discussed at length, as these operations have been growing in number.

The fifth chapter deals with the mechanisms of genetics, as well as those problems that may result from genetic or congenital disorders. The effects of both internal and external environments on the unborn child are discussed; there is a section about the effect of drugs on the cellular organization of the embryo and fetus. The new findings in genetic research make the creation of artificial genes, the alteration of the chemical structure of DNA, or test tube fertilization followed by intrauterine implantation increasingly probable. Such capabilities can bring mankind relief from disease, but they also create a dilemma foretold by C. S. Lewis more than twenty-five years ago:

> *What we call Man's power over Nature turns out to be a power exercised by some men over other men with Nature as its instrument . . . And all long-term exercises of power, especially in breeding, must mean the power of earlier generations over later ones . . . If any age really attains, by eugenics and scientific education, the power to make its descendents what it pleases, all men who live after it are the patients of that power.*[2]

The subject of the sixth chapter is pregnancy. Among the topics discussed are such vital matters as sexual intercourse during and after pregnancy, lactation, and the too often neglected "pregnant father."

[2] Quoted in Paul Ramsey, "Shall We 'Reproduce'?" *Journal of the American Medical Association,* Vol. 220, No. 11 (June 12, 1972), p. 1483.

The chapter also describes newer methods of dealing with subfertility and ends with a consideration of adoption.

It has been said that marriages are made in heaven, and that proof of this is apparent in the divorce rates. The seventh chapter is meant to help the reader consider some down-to-earth premarital problems in a realistic way. Although the eighth chapter emphasizes sexuality in marriage, it is not restricted to that specific topic. Only too often sexual disorders among married people are merely symptoms of seemingly unrelated problems. In this chapter the sexuality of the elderly is also discussed. That sexual expression can be sheer pleasure, that its fun and fulfillment can be an enduring and joyous communication between two people, is good for both the young and the elderly to know. Moreover, an appreciation of one another's sexuality may be of some help in bridging the so-called generation gap.

The ninth chapter uses the recent work of Masters and Johnson as a framework for dealing with inadequacies of sexual expression. William H. Masters and Virginia E. Johnson have made significant contributions, not only to the treatment of sexual disorders but to their definition and classification. It should be emphasized that they vigorously reject a mechanical approach to sexual expression. They make clear that sexual expression, when removed from the total personality, can become "unstimulating" and "immaterial," in short, a bore.

Divergent sexual behavior is the subject of the tenth chapter. As is the case with all discussions of sexual psychology in this book, the use of judgmental labels such as "deviant" or "abnormal" is avoided. There is much disagreement about whether homosexual behavior is a disease or a minority's method of sexual expression. Both sides of the question are presented. And, although recent and incomplete research indicates that there is a biochemical equivalent to some homosexual behavior, the multifactorial aspects are emphasized.

The last chapter can best be understood from the viewpoint of the first. Human personalities are molded by their cultures, but they influence them too. The problems of personalities become the problems of society. "Personally," wrote Adolf Hitler from a wintry foxhole in 1915, "I would prefer attacks. Otherwise you fall mentally sick." Thirty years later he had misled his people to another disaster from which the world has yet to recover. What role did his birth out of wedlock, his bitter childhood, his alienation, and his subjugation of women play in his tragic era? Alienation and violence, women's liberation, the diminished father, the changing family, widespread drug abuse—all these are as inextricably involved with sexuality as they are with the personality. For this reason they are problems to ponder and discuss.

Some of the material appearing in this book was originally published in the author's *Health: Man in a Changing Environment* (New York: Harcourt Brace Jovanovich, 1970). However, all such material has been revised and brought up to date.

The author would like to thank Evelyn Ballard, M.D., California State University at San Francisco; Catherine Cline Pike, M.D., University of California Medical Center; and Edwin A. Schwartz, Clinical Psychologist, College of San Mateo, for reading an earlier draft of the manuscript. For his constant encouragement and thoughtful criticism, a special word of thanks is due Claude T. Cook, Chairman of the Department of Health Sciences, California State University at Northridge. Nor could this book have been written without the patient help of Mrs. Ruby Pearson, whose efficient organization of the author's work days made the time available for its completion. For errors in this book, the author must accept complete responsibility. Their correction by its readers will be welcomed.

Benjamin A. Kogan

table
of
contents

preface   v

1

personality and sexuality:
an interwoven development   1

begin at the beginning *1*   personality development: the
search for self-esteem *3*   parent development *27*

2

the reproductive system: structure, function,
dysfunction—and sexual sensitivity   30

the brain's chemical "fertility switch" *30*   the reproductive
systems *33*   the structure and function of the erogenous
zones *54*   sexually transmitted diseases *60*

3

the sexual life   79

the biological logic of mutuality *79*   the roots of sexual
behavior *82*   on the physiology of the human sexual response *84*   sexual intercourse *87*   sexual similarities
90   sexual differences *91*   some myths and misconceptions about human sexuality *100*

4

controlling human reproduction 108

birth control *108*   abortion *129*

5

the human beginning 137

"in the beginning . . ." *137*   genetics: molding a new person *137*

6

on continuing the human beginning 190

pregnancy *190*   parental anxiety *208*

7

some premarital considerations and advisements 224

courtship and conquest: animal instinct, human learning *224*
on the establishment of marital codes *225*   the lover, whom
all the world does not love *228*   premarital sexual standards *231*   promiscuity: sexual behavior without rules *242*
searching for someone to marry *244*

8

marriage: "the craft so long to lerne" 255

prologue *255*   war and marriage *256*   the campus marriage *258*   marital monotony *261*   senior citizen sexuality *270*   epilogue *276*

9

correcting problems of sexual expression 278

masters and johnson's study of human sexual inadequacy *278*
masters and johnson classify and treat sexual inadequacy *281*

10

divergent sexual behavior 297

homosexual behavior *297* transvestite behavior *316*
transsexual behavior *318* the significance of the child's
cross-dressing *321* other forms of sexual expression *322*

11

problems to ponder 330

alienation and sexuality *330* violence and sexuality *331*
rock music and sexuality *334* better sexuality through
chemistry? *335* sexual vagabondage in some communes
348 women's lib for the sexes *351* the fragile monogamous family *354*

glossary 361

index 375

personality and 1
sexuality:
an interwoven
development

And if the soul
is to know itself
it must look
into a soul:
the stranger and enemy, we've seen him in the mirror.[1]

begin at the beginning

Begin with the birth of the baby. He can suck and he can look, but not at the same time. Through eyes vacant like tiny unwashed windows, he can see only peripherally. He is aware of light and dark. He can cry and perhaps raise his head a trifle. Although six months will pass before his teeth can be seen, he has an immediate sweet tooth. He dislikes bitters. He can smell, and even before he was born he could hear. Three to ten minutes after he is born, he will turn his eyes toward a sound. He can feel pressure and warmth and cold. He can cough and sneeze. For a day or two, he will eliminate a blackish-green material called meconium from his rectum. This was formed during intrauterine life, when trial secretions of his digestive glands mixed with swallowed fluid. In a few days he will eat. Most of the time his gut will be able to push the food down. Sometimes he will spit it up. It will be months before he can suck and look at the same time.

Even before his umbilical cord is cut, the male infant is quite capable of having an erection; in her earliest moments of life, it is likely that the girl can develop vaginal lubrication.[2]

---

[1] George Seferis, *Collected Poems, 1924–1955* (Princeton, N.J., 1967), p. 9.
[2] Masters and Johnson consider the male penile erection the "neurophysiologic parallel to the human female's production of lubrication." (William H. Masters and Virginia E. Johnson, *Human Sexual Response* [Boston, 1966], p. 181.)

1

During his first day, the infant will pass between one-half and one and one-half ounces of urine. This amount will increase. His heart beats about 150 times a minute, and he breathes thirty to fifty times a minute. If his head was born first, as is ordinarily the case, he probably breathed before all of him was delivered. At about six weeks of age he smiles, not because of a colicky pain but from pleasure. Yet there is an old saying that man is expected to grieve. If he does not weep at birth, he is spanked until he does. Be that as it may, the child's first staccato cry heralds the change from aquatic to terrestrial life—an evolutionary change that required millions of years. After his first crying spell, the infant sleeps. When he awakens, he cries again. At this tender age, no other creature can howl so mightily. This second episode of weeping tells that the infant can suffer, but the infant can also be relieved of his suffering. Yet, collecting stress and distress, he often reaches adulthood only to feel like Shakespeare's Antonio in *The Merchant of Venice*.

> *In sooth, I know not why I am so sad.*
> *It wearies me, you say it wearies you;*
> *But how I caught it, found it, or came by it,*
> *What stuff 'tis made of, whereof it is born,*
> *I am to learn.*
> *And such a want-wit sadness makes of me*
> *That I have much ado to know myself.*[3]

What sadness makes Antonio feel a "want-wit"? What is the root of his anguish? In every time, in every tongue, in every lonely troubled corner on earth, this bewilderment has been uttered. It is a bewilderment that can permeate every aspect of a person's life. Only too often does it block the pleasures of human sexual expression. Why is this so? Before the work of Sigmund Freud there were few answers.

FREUD: PERSONALITY AND SEXUALITY
DEVELOP TOGETHER

It was Freud who first saw that the patterns of sexual behavior are woven into the very fabric of the personality at a very young age. Freud understood what has since been stated so clearly: "Sex is not something we do, it's something we are." Thus sexuality is "everything that has to do with your being a man or being a woman . . . education for sexuality is every experience you have had up to your particular stage of development as a male or as a female."[4] And it

[3] William Shakespeare, *The Merchant of Venice*, I.i.1-7.
[4] The Sex Information and Education Council of the United States, "An Interview with Mary Calderone, M.D.," by Harold I. Lief, *Medical Aspects of Human Sexuality*, Vol. 2, No. 8 (August 1968), p. 46.

begins "from the moment of birth when impressions of the mother and the father—who are sexual people—begin to flood in . . . without any words."[5] To understand one's own sexuality, one must first understand oneself. The maxim "Know thyself," inscribed in gold on the ancient temple of Apollo at Delphi, is attributed to the Greek philosopher Thales of Miletus (640?-546? B.C.). More than twenty centuries later, Roger Ascham, the sixteenth-century teacher of Queen Elizabeth I, expanded the maxim this way: "That wise proverbe of Appollo, *Knowe thy selfe:* that is to saye, learn to know what thou are able, fitte, and apt vnto, and folowe that."[6] At best this is not an easy task, especially when it concerns sexual behavior. There are no human equations; everybody is unique.

Thus all people develop differently. Yet as their sexualities evolve within their varying personalities, they still share common qualities of humanness. Because personality and sexuality develop together, they are here considered together.

Based on observation, Freud's concepts are ecological. He began by calling attention to the child. Within each child are basic unconscious instinctual drives. Between these drives and the surrounding environment constant and inexorable negotiations occur. From this interplay human personality (and sexuality) results. Basic personality traits are established in childhood. With severe emotional trauma and crises, childhood personality development lags. The resultant adult behaves like a child. The adult personality, then, is molded by the stress responses of childhood. "Pubescence," Freud wrote, "is an act of nature; adolescence is an act of man." In this way Freud emphasized the difference between merely growing and growing up. Sexual behavior depends on more than mere biology. Human sexual destiny is also influenced by environmental factors, such as the family and the surrounding society. Moreover, Freud taught that the stresses of childhood can be changed. Therefore, patterns of behavior that are based on reactions to stresses would change. Early responses to stress, lying deeply buried in the subconscious for long periods of time, often cause emotional problems. If these responses can be uncovered, confronted, and resolved by an individual who suffers them, cure can result.

personality development: the quest for self-esteem

Among the most influential of the psychologists who built on Freud's ideas is Erik Erikson. Like Freud, Erikson is aware that human behavior is created by and helps to create its own environment. His schema of personality development provides a useful and coherent

[5] Ibid., p. 42.
[6] Roger Ascham, *Toxophilus* (1545), p. 155.

concept of the flow of psychological happenings through which people must live to grow to emotional maturity. "How does a healthy person grow or, as it were, accrue from the successive stages of increasing capacity to master life's outer and inner tasks and dangers?" [7] This is the basic question that Erikson sets out to answer, and his explorations of human personality growth simultaneously reveal much about the maturation of sexuality.

ERIKSON'S EIGHT STAGES
OF PERSONALITY DEVELOPMENT

For Erikson, every human being's personality develops in eight stages, each of which takes place at a particular age. In each stage the developing individual is faced with a task. If the task is satisfactorily resolved, the individual enters healthily into the next stage. If it is not, the individual is ill-equipped to solve the task of the next stage. Future attempts to solve tasks are hampered by the emotional impedimenta caused by past failures. To heal these wounds to the personality, the individual needs help. Adequate help at critical times stabilizes the individual. Preparation for the next stage and the transition into it are then accomplished with a greater sense of personal competence and security. Better emotional health results. Without help, the person's inadequately resolved tasks turn into cumulative emotional scars—and personality disorders.

Each of Erikson's eight stages is named according to the task that is confronted. The name identifies both the desirable resolution of the task and the contrary development that takes place if the task is not resolved. The desirable resolution of the task of the first of the eight stages is *basic trust*. Its contrary development is *basic mistrust*. Thus the first stage is named *basic trust versus basic mistrust*. But there are no sharp dividing lines between Erikson's stages. During the later stages the resolution (or lack of resolution) of the tasks of earlier stages continues to develop.

As a result of continuous interactions with his environment during these stages, man develops a feeling of self-identity. This feeling, which Erikson calls *ego-identity,* is central to human personality development. Man's ego-identity is his awareness of himself as a distinct person with an influential past, an active present, and a controllable future. What must man live through to achieve this feeling of identity?

the infant: the first eighteen months

Basic trust versus basic mistrust is the first stage. In the first year, the infant makes a decision, based on the quality of his maternal

[7] Erik H. Erikson, "Growth and Crises of the Healthy Personality," in Clyde Kluckhohn, Henry A. Murray, and David Schneider, eds., *Personality in Nature, Society, and Culture* (New York, 1953), p. 186.

care, as to whether the world is dependable and safe or fraught with frustration and fear. It is not a decision reached as the result of one incident or a few. Erikson does not mean that this stage (or any other) is like an obstacle race in which a few missteps forever doom the participant to emotional illness. The infant decision is the product of the ripening relationship between him and his mother. Completely self-centered, yet utterly dependent, he is inevitably disappointed. No mother can always immediately meet all her baby's needs. And so, as a part of normal development, the child must learn to cope with a degree of frustration. His ability to do this depends on his overall sense of security or insecurity. If his frustrations are not excessive in amount or in frequency, he learns that, although things are not always to his liking, most of the time they are fine. A baby can adjust to that. Indeed, this lesson helps him face situations that will arise as he reaches his first year—situations that involve some degree of separation from his mother. If all that has preceded has been characterized by anxiety, he will approach this and future problems with fear and basic mistrust. But if the preponderance of his experience has taught him basic trust, he will have gained a sense of self-esteem that will stand him in good stead.

"Baby love—love is free" [8]: infant sexuality The infant's self-esteem begins with an appreciation of his own body. This is a prerequisite for a satisfying sexuality in the future. Self-love is the first step toward learning to love others. However, self-love is not spontaneous at birth. Initially, the infant is utterly passive and accepts the ministrations of his mother's love. He does not seem to differentiate between his own body and that of his mother. The infant appears to accept the mother's warmth, her caressing hands and protecting arms, her rhythmic, soothing motions as part of his own body. But within a few months the infant begins to realize that there is an outside source of his bodily gratifications, and he begins to turn to that source. As his mother approaches he strains toward her, listening to her voice, cooing when he is picked up, responding eagerly to the quality of her love. The pleasures of body contact are intensified as he sucks and feeds from a nipple. But it is not only the food that completes his contentment. Appetite is a human quality. "The infant cannot be fed by food alone," writes Dorothy V. Whipple, "he needs to dine . . . He cannot eat until the conditions of dining have been met . . . the infant relaxes and is eager to eat when picked up by gentle, warm, comfortable arms." [9] These are the observations of a pediatrician, but the emotional needs of dining have also been recorded by those who treat the aged—the geriatricians. The aged person who forgets to eat because he is alone is all too common. From the first intimacy of a mother's warmth to the last suppers of

---

[8] Dorothy V. Whipple, *Dynamics of Development: Euthenic Pediatrics* (New York, 1966), p. 420.
[9] Ibid., pp. 368–69.

the aged, humans learn this: man eats alone, but he dines with others.

The infant skin and mucous membranes are not anatomically mature. But even so early in life they are abundantly supplied with eagerly accepting nerve endings. These transmit his comfort to the higher nerve centers. The mouth is the most sensitive part of the infant's body. So crucial is the mouth in providing the infant with a pleasurable sense of security that this period of development has been called the *oral phase*. Throughout life the skin, mouth, and tongue remain among the paramount receptors of pleasure.

Curiosity is a major characteristic of the infant. This curiosity is yet another road to the self-appreciation so vital to the future appreciation of others. Hours are spent in a careful examination of the fingers. Soon the toes are discovered. They are tasted and sucked and licked and endlessly fingered. At about nine months of age the infant finds the genitalia—a pleasant discovery. Even at this sexually immature stage, the penis and clitoris contain a rich nerve supply. Both organs are extremely sensitive. As they are manipulated the infant enjoys pleasurable stimuli throughout his whole body. Toward the end of his first year, the infant usually discovers his feces. He does not then realize that they are his. However, like everything else, they are felt, fingered, tasted, and, perhaps, even harmlessly swallowed. Later he learns that it was he who produced them, that they are a part of him, and that they are an achievement to be appreciated.

All these pleasant discoveries are part of the process of learning self-love. They transpire in the milieu of parental love. The father has a contribution to make, but primarily it is the mother who is responsible for giving and withholding pleasure. But she can do more. She can share the infant's pleasure. She can show the baby that she enjoys his discoveries. His normal genital manipulations, for example, are not cause for concern. They are a signal of normal growth. Indeed, there might be cause for concern if they never occurred. Many educated mothers are aware of this aspect of normal development, but some become overanxious. Fearful of impeding the infant's emotional growth, they never interrupt his genital play. They even defer diapering him until he voluntarily stops handling his genitals. This is needless solicitude. The infant's genital manipulations should be gently interrupted in order to change his diaper, just as his thumb-sucking may be interrupted in order to wash his face. Infant genital play is no more nor less important than his snuggling in his mother's arms. Both are essential to the maturation of a competent personality and sexuality.

The same is true of the infant's fingering of his feces. The child finds his feces much more pleasant than does his mother. This is particularly true when she finds that the infant has cheerfully smeared his feces over his face, crib, linen, and blanket, as well as on the adjoining wall. There is no reason why the mother should be expected to enjoy the sight of all this. She should not feel guilty about her inner disgust with the task of cleaning up. Nor need she feel guilty about inadvertently expressing these emotions. However, insofar as possible, she will do well to avoid expressing her disgust. If the mother consistently expresses disapproval of a full diaper, if her voice always implies dismay, she may eventually impress the child wrongly. In time she may teach the infant that his body product is dirty. The child will then infer that he is, therefore, dirty and unworthy. If the mother expresses satisfaction with his body product as an accomplishment to be admired, the child will come to learn that both his body and its products are unreservedly acceptable to the most important person in his life. At this stage there can be no conditions to his mother's love. Moreover, the child must learn that he also accepts and loves himself without reservation. As the average human being matures, this infant need for unconditional mother and self-love changes. But this infant experience is essential for building an adequate personality and sexuality. Such a high degree of acceptance and love is not always achieved. But if the infant receives enough love to allow him to learn to appreciate himself, he will be off to a good start.

the toddler: eighteen to thirty-six months

No longer is the toddler crib-ridden. He is free to explore, to inspect, to feel, to satiate his curiosity. In his new world he is into everything, but some things are forbidden. The toddler quickly learns the meaning of the word *no*. Sometimes it is a kindly warning. Other times it is edged with dangerous impatience. It may even be the prelude to a gentle but insulting whack on his bottom. But the meaning of the word does not change. When he hears it, it means that, for the moment at least, he has lost a certain amount of love. No longer can he accept himself without reservation. Now there are conditions to being loved. "Love has a price." [10] He is loved when he does as he is told. When he fails in this he begins to doubt himself. And, as Erikson has written so lucidly: "Doubt is the brother of shame." [11] When these twin assaults on the developing personality—self-doubt and shame—persist, they are among the major causes of sexual inadequacy. It is during the toddler stage that these tendencies may take hold and eventually hinder not only adult sexual performance but other manifestations of the personality.

Erikson's toddler needs to achieve   This stage of growing muscle control is considered by Erikson to be the second stage in

[10] Ibid., p. 423.
[11] Erik H. Erikson, "Eight Ages of Man," in G. B. Levitas, ed., *The World of Psychoanalysis,* Vol. I (New York, 1965), p. 88.

the development of the personality: *autonomy versus shame and doubt.* "From a sense of *self-control without loss of self-esteem,*" Erikson writes, "comes a lasting sense of autonomy and pride. From a sense of muscular and anal impotence, of loss of self-control, and of parental over-control comes a lasting sense of doubt and shame." [12] The word *autonomy* is derived from the Greek *autos,* self + *nomos,* law. Together they form one word—*autonomia,* independence. The quest for independence continues throughout life. For the toddler it is marked by increasing muscle control and the beginning of control of his bladder and bowel.

Bladder and bowel control are great achievements for him. He realizes that he has made his own waste products, and they merit his close observation. The toddler may even want to play with his urine and feces. In a kind but firm manner the mother can prevent him from doing this. To his hopefully appreciative mother the toddler may bring his just-used potty. The mother can help the child by expressing her appreciation of his achievement. The toddler may express misgivings as his body's products are unceremoniously flushed down the toilet. He quickly forgets this separation if he is assured that tomorrow there will be more of his achievement. So important is the technique of toilet training to psychosexual development, that it is discussed here in more detail.

Toilet-training: a cultural demand   Until he is about eighteen months old, the toddler cannot control his bowel and bladder. Not until then have enough nervous pathways from the cerebral cortex to the external sphincters of the bowel and bladder been developed to make control possible. Toilet-training, however, does not involve teaching the toddler to control his bowel and bladder. What he is taught is where to deposit his body waste. Bowel and bladder control are the result of three distinct stages of development.[13] In the *first* stage the child is aware that he has had a bowel movement or has passed urine only after their occurrence. In the *second* stage he is aware of either event as it takes place. Finally, during the *third* stage, he knows in advance that he is about to relieve himself. As the toddler progresses through these stages, the parent should take every opportunity to help him increase his sense of self-control, self-respect, self-worth, and self-love. But the parent must also be aware of the child's limitations. A child in the first or second stage may occasionally defecate or urinate when placed on the toilet at a certain time each day. This may bring him praise. But there has been no autonomy, no gained independence—just lucky performance. Toilet-training must be undertaken in terms of the normal stages of bowel

[12] Erik H. Erikson, "Growth and Crises of the Healthy Personality," p. 199.
[13] The stages of sphincter control are discussed in Dorothy V. Whipple, *Dynamics of Development: Euthenic Pediatrics,* pp. 409-11.

and bladder control, in terms of the child's realization of his own accomplishments, and in terms of the psychological growth that is so necessary to self-esteem and future psychosexual development.

Bowel and bladder control do not occur simultaneously. The bowel is usually controlled earlier. However, the stages for each are essentially the same. During the first stage the parent should teach the child words for the stool and the urine. They should not be threatening, like *nasty* or *dirty*. It is useless to rush the child to the toilet during the first stage (after he has had a bowel movement or has urinated) or during the second stage (while he is in the process of doing either). Nor do recriminations help. During the first two stages of bladder and bowel control, the toddler has no warning. How can he impart information to his parent in advance without knowing what is to happen? When, in the third stage, the toddler knows he is about to defecate, he often tells his mother. It is then, and not before, that she may suggest that he use the potty. Control of the urinary bladder poses a special problem for the toddler. Even when bladder control begins, the child has only scant warning as he continues to feel the urge to urinate immediately. With most children, control occurs as the bladder enlarges. Between the ages of two and four-and-one-half years the toddler's bladder capacity more than doubles. Usually he is then more able to regulate himself. Bed-wetting is a special problem. Heavy-handed discipline, shaming, and parental conflict are among the anxiety-producing factors that may result in bed-wetting, even after a dry bed has already been achieved. The average child stops wetting the bed between the ages of three and five years. Some children continue into their early teens; in such cases a physician's help should be sought.

During the entire period of toilet-training, the parents will do well to make allowances for occasional accidents. These should be treated as such. The child should not be made to feel guilty. Moreover, as the child learns bowel control he also learns that he can attract attention by withholding. If a baby competitor seems to have replaced him, he may attempt to regain attention by withholding on the potty and letting go on the carpet. A fussing mother only teaches him that this method works. In sum, then, intelligent toilet-training is a beginning step toward learning self-control and self-esteem. Without these, the chances for adult psychosexual competence are indeed diminished.

Toddler sexuality   The infant's interest in his genitalia continues into the toddler stage, and, indeed, intensifies. Often this increased interest begins at about two years of age, but it may be delayed until the toddler passes into the preschooler stage at about four years. Masturbation to orgasm has been commonly observed among children during this period. During the second year the toddler usually discovers whether he is a boy or she is a girl. This identity of gender is culturally learned (see pages 82–84). From the first days in the child's life the parents teach gender identity in many subtle ways. The growing interest in the genitalia along with the knowledge of gender identity stimulate the child to ask a torrent of questions about sexual matters. Truthful answers to the toddler's questions are essential, but they need not be detailed. A brief unemotional answer usually satisfies the child. There is the anecdote about the child who asked his mother perhaps the most common of all questions during this time: "Where do I come from?" The overanxious mother wanted to impart the total truth to her offspring. The puzzled youngster listened to a twenty-minute dissertation on the anatomy and physiology of reproduction. "Oh," the little boy finally said in a disappointed way, "I thought I came from Philadelphia."

Many parents are concerned with what they consider to be their child's obsession with sexual (and toilet) matters. Their relaxed approach to this stage of human development is critical to the child's future sexual competence. Regrettably some parents express disgust with the child who plays with his genitals. They begin this error during the child's infancy and carry it into his toddler and preschool phases. They answer the toddler's endless questions about sex in a brusque or shaming manner. The sensitive child then feels that his genitals are dirty, his questions are bad, and his whole self is unworthy of love. He stops asking questions as a means of self-defense. He handles his genitals in private. Even though he thus escapes reprimand, he feels guilty and deserving of punishment. He is lonely. Moreover, he loses confidence in his self-mastery. In later years the adult may not clearly remember the parental condemnation of childhood sexuality, but these memories are merely buried in the subconscious. Years later they will often affect his behavior and hinder his ability to have satisfactory sexual relationships. The understanding parent can help the future adult to avoid these emotional handicaps. Patient explanation can lessen childhood anxiety about his sexuality.

the preschooler: three to six years

During the preschool years, the child, armed with the accumulated security of his first stage and the independent body control of the second, seeks to discover more about himself. Erikson calls this stage *initiative versus guilt*.

> *Being firmly convinced that he is a person, the child must now find out what kind of person he is going to be. And here he hitches his wagon to nothing less than a star: he wants to*

be like his parents, who to him appear very powerful and very
beautiful, although quite unreasonably dangerous.[14]

Of Oedipal complexity

For many a man hath seen himself in dreams
His mother's mate, but he who gives no heed
To such like matters bears the easier fate.[15]

I want a girl, just like the girl
Who married dear old dad . . .[16]

Perhaps it is the preschooler's ardent desire to be like the powerful
parents that results in the so-called *Oedipus complex.* In this stage,
it is thought that the child develops a love relationship with the
parent of the opposite sex. Some students of childhood do not consider the Oedipus complex a necessary prerequisite of childhood
development; others believe it to be so common in the life of the
preschooler that it may be regarded as an expected phase of development. It is named after Oedipus, who, in the Sophoclean tragedy
Oedipus Tyrannus, kills his father and marries his mother. After
discovering the true relationship, Oedipus blinds himself. An unwise
parental approach to this transient childhood episode can have
grievous consequences. This is illustrated by the following case
history:

A young man of twenty-two visited a psychiatrist. His chief
complaint was that he feared to be alone. Whenever he was by
himself, he would become aware of a "creeping" uneasiness. Then
slowly terror welled up in him and spread through him "like a stain."
He quickly volunteered that he had, for two years, been engaged in
homosexual behavior.[17] He had never been able to relate well to
women. But it was not the sexual orientation that disturbed him. It
was the loneliness.

Months of psychoanalysis passed. Finally the following story was
pieced together. At five, he had worshipped his mother. Now he
described her dispassionately. She had been a graceful, beautiful
woman, almost childlike. She was fond of picking him up and stroking
his hair until he fell asleep. His father was stern and gruff. Sometimes
he would grumble, "Be a big boy. Get off your mother's lap." His
mother would blush and kiss the child or smooth his hair.

[14] Erik H. Erikson, "Growth and Crises of the Healthy Personality," p. 205.
[15] Sophocles, *Oedipus Tyrannus,* lines 981–83.
[16] "I Want a Girl (Just Like the Girl Who Married Dear Old Dad") by Harry Von Tilzer and Will
Dillon. Copyright © 1911 by Harry Von Tilzer Music Publishing Co., Inc. U.S. copyright renewed
1938 and assigned to Harry Von Tilzer Music Publishing Co. (a division of Teleklew Productions,
Inc.). Reprinted by permission of the publisher, Harry Von Tilzer Music Publishing Company (a
division of T. B. Harms Company).
[17] For a further discussion of homosexual behavior, see pages 297–316.

Early one morning his father was ill. The young man remembered every stark detail—the ashen face, the rasping breath, the ambulance, the small clot of onlookers, his own fleeting fright. His mother was inconsolable. All that day she wept. That night he crawled into her bed. "Don't worry, mommie," he said. "I'll be here and keep care of you. He will die. He'll never come back." She slapped him so hard he became confused. She hit him again and again. Then she sent him to his room. In his room he heard her raging at him. Four days later, at his father's funeral, his mother barely spoke to him.

From a five-year-old's innocent emotion, a traumatic situation had resulted. The child's guilt about wanting to rid himself of his father (a common desire at that stage) was heightened by both his mother's immature coquetry and his father's disapproval. He was later unable to identify with a father he had never learned to admire. The father's illness intensified the boy's anxiety. But it was the mother's violent renunciation of him that tore him loose from his most urgently needed moorings.

She might have told him the simple truth: she needed both him and his father. Instead, she lost them both. Instead, she sent the boy to a lonely room from which he never emerged.[18]

As "he hitches his wagon to nothing less than a star,"[19] the little boy imagines that he is as big and strong as his father. He imitates his grown-up voice and his way of walking. He controls a car, makes an electric razor buzz, and operates a camera. He owns a house like his father. And, like his father, he has a woman too. With all his heart the little boy wants his father's woman. In a burst of childish bravado the little boy may propose marriage to his mother. Despite all this, the child does not lose his sense of reality. With childhood's devastating logic, the four- or five-year-old boy reaches two irreducible conclusions. First, his genitals do not compare with his father's. Second, no matter how much he loves his mother, he cannot replace his father in her affections. The five-year-old cannot control these emotions, nor are his thoughts associated with sexual intercourse. True, he may crawl into his mother's bed to seek her body's warm comfort. But like the infant and the toddler, the preschooler's idea of love is one of receiving, not giving. The little daughter may experience similar feelings. She tries her mother's perfume and cosmetics, hat and shoes. She crawls onto her father's lap, nestles in his arms, and gazes adoringly into his face. Only he can bathe her, put her to bed, dress her, and care for her. The mother is rejected. But the little girl still needs the mother. And the little boy still needs the father, no matter how much they wish to be rid of them. It will not

[18]Problems with parents are by no means the only cause of homosexual behavior. However, in this authentic case there was a definite relationship. Moreover, although a sense of loneliness was part of this person's problems, it is by no means an invariable experience of people whose behavior is homosexual.

[19]Erik H. Erikson, "Growth and Crises of the Healthy Personality," p. 205.

be the child's last experience with emotional ambivalence (see pages 25-27).

Three hundred years ago, the philosopher Spinoza clearly defined emotional ambivalence as a "vacillation of the soul." The child wavers between loving the competing parent and wishing to be rid of him. Understanding parents can alleviate the child's guilt by showing that they love him despite his feelings. The parent will also help by not being coy. The immature mother who appears unduly flattered with her little boy's attentions, or who sensuously encourages them will merely increase his guilt. The father may help by explaining that he loves both his wife and his small daughter and that he needs them both. Parental maturity and skill in handling these transient emotions, in preventing the humiliation of the searching child, will augment the child's sense of a worthy self.

The fear of castration   The preschooler, having known his gender for some time, knowing the pleasure of handling his genitals, and still intensely curious about sex, may develop the belief that he deserves a fearful punishment. The relaxed, accepting parent teaches the child that he is worthy and that his worthiness includes his genitalia. The shocked, forbidding parent does the opposite. It is during this phase or in late toddlerhood that the child who feels unworthy fears that the genitalia will be (with boys) or have been (with girls) cut off. This has been somewhat inaccurately called the *castration fear*. (Castration refers to removal of the gonads—the testicles or ovaries.) To compensate for this fear the little boy may become unduly aggressive; the little girl, resentful.[20]

Not all children experience these fears to the same degree, nor are these fears necessarily based on something the parent may have done or said. Some children fear that they will be or have been deprived of their genitalia without any apparent cause. Understanding parents can help the child to conquer these fears. Excessive and belittling discipline may entrench these fears and thus may well hamper the development of adequate adult heterosexuality.

The amputation of a body member that gives comfort and pleasure

[20]These concepts have led to much confusion about so-called penis envy. Like "womb envy" or "breast envy" or "woman envy," penis envy is a culturally learned phenomenon. "The presence or absence of a penis may be regarded by the developing child as an asset *or* a deficit depending on the nature of the cues that he or she is getting from the environment. When a society places greater value on the birth of a son than on that of a daughter, children in the family become aware of this in a myriad subtle ways; the same is true when little boys are accorded greater freedom of movement and play, and when fathers are accorded greater respect and deference than mothers. In such a society little girls, and later women, will inevitably manifest many indications of penis envy, while indications of woman envy in men will be relatively rare. On the other hand, when these conditions no longer hold true, or become reversed (as has begun to happen in Western society in recent decades), *then we can expect to find that unconscious manifestations of penis envy will begin to diminish, and those of woman envy will begin to increase.*" (Judd Marmor, "Changing Patterns of Femininity," in Arlene S. Skolnick and Jerome H. Skolnick, *Family in Transition* [Boston, 1971], pp. 216-16, and Judd Marmor, "Changing Patterns of Femininity: Psychoanalytic Implications," in S. Rosenbaum and S. Alger, eds., *The Marriage Relationship: Psychoanalytic Perspectives* [New York, 1968], pp. 31-44.)

is not a new threat. In the pre-Hitler and Hitler eras thousands of German schoolchildren were required to memorize this verse about Conrad.

> *THE STORY OF LITTLE SUCK-A-THUMB*
> *One day, mamma said: "Conrad dear,*
> *I must go out and leave you here.*
> *But mind now, Conrad, what I say,*
> *Don't suck your thumb while I'm away.*
> *The great tall tailor always comes*
> *To little boys that suck their thumbs;*
> *And ere they dream what he's about,*
> *He takes his great sharp scissors out*
> *And cuts their thumbs clean off,—and then,*
> *You know, they never grow again."* [21]

Thumb-sucking usually begins within the uterus, and parents need not be concerned about it until the child is about four years of age.[22]

the school-age child: six to twelve years

By the time the child enters school he is in what Freud called the "latency period." Freud considered the child's sexual interest to have abated at this stage. Today this view is widely questioned. There is considerable opinion that sexual interest does not seem so intense at this time because the child is diverted by a myriad of new interests. But his sexual interest does not disappear. If the child's curiosity and ability to learn are restricted, his sexual interest will resurge. This is the fourth stage of Erikson's schema of personality development, *industry versus inferiority.*

"Personality at the first stage crystallizes around the conviction 'I am what I am given,' and that of the second, 'I am what I will.' The third can be characterized by 'I am what I can imagine I will be . . . ' The fourth: 'I am what I learn.'" [23]

No other creature has as long a period of dependency as the human, for no other creature has as much to learn before he can become self-sufficient. The child must learn skills, use tools, and do something he considers useful. Returning from school to his parents, he will hold out the result of his labor. "Look," he will say hopefully. If he is met with appreciation, he will attempt to do still better. If

---

[21] Heinrich Hoffman, quoted in Burton Egbert Stevenson, ed., *The Home Book of Verse* (New York, 1922), p. 123. These two stanzas tell only part of the grim story. Poor Conrad does suck his thumb, and the terrible tailor snips off both of his thumbs. The poem ends:

> "Ah!" said mamma, "I knew he'd come
> To naughty little Suck-a-thumb."

[22] After that age, teeth may be displaced, and the family dentist should be consulted.
[23] Erik H. Erikson, "Growth and Crises of the Healthy Personality," p. 211.

parental indifference is his lot, a deep sense of inadequacy and inferiority will overwhelm him. It is essential that the child develop a continuing sense of competence. But praise must be merited. Should he receive commendation for an effort he knows is inferior, he will lose respect for the person praising him.

Schoolchild friendship: the other I   Before the school years the child's love life is largely a matter of receiving love. The child is not yet really interested in giving love. His expressions of affection, his attempts to conform and satisfy his parents are primarily means of reinforcing his own sense of worthiness. It is in the school years that a sense of sharing the self dawns on the child. No longer is love mere acceptance. Now it is a matter of giving and returning love and of accepting some responsibility for someone else.

In school the child is exposed to many other children. From among these he chooses playmates and, importantly, a best friend. The memory of that best friend may never be lost. The ancient Greek philosopher Zeno the Stoic (334?-261? B.C.) wrote that "A friend is another I."[24] In his *Meditations of a Parish Priest* Joseph Roux wrote: "What is love? two souls and one flesh; friendship? two bodies and one soul." Friendship between schoolchildren is a momentous experience, a prevision of one of the most profound capacities of the future personality. From this love will grow more than the ability to love a member of the opposite sex, more than sexual competence. From this kind of love may grow the inner need to care about a hungry child on the other side of the world. From it can come the love of humanity.

adolescence

> *Each youth sustains within his breast*
> *a vague and infinite unrest.*
> *He goes about in still alarm,*
> *With shrouded future at his arm,*
> *With longings that can find no tongue.*
> *I see him thus, for I am young.*[25]

"I felt myself isolated, helpless and always shut up in myself: I do not complain of it, for I believe that my early meditations developed and strengthened my thinking powers."[26] So did that celebrated political magician Talleyrand describe his twelfth year. His was a

---

[24] Diogenes Laertius, *Zeno,* Book VII, section 23.
[25] An Oklahoma high school boy, quoted in Evelyn Millis Duvall, *Family Development,* 2nd ed. (Philadelphia, 1962), p. 297.
[26] From *Memoirs of the Prince of Talleyrand,* quoted in Saul K. Padover, ed., *Confessions and Self-Portraits* (New York, 1957), p. 152.

lonely adolescence. Adolescence generally is. Erikson terms this fifth stage *identity versus self-diffusion.*

Some teen-age anxieties may, if they remain unresolved, adversely affect the individual's entire personality structure, and, with it, its sexuality. To help the teen-ager handle the difficulties inherent in these critical years, a sensitive and sympathetic understanding of the sources of anxiety is essential. Teen-age anxieties begin with the onset of *puberty* and *adolescence.*

Puberty and adolescence   These two terms are not synonymous. Puberty is a biological event. Adolescence is cultural. Puberty begins with the spurt in development of the reproductive organs. In girls this occurs earlier (at about eleven years) than in boys (at about thirteen years). In the male, puberty ends with the beginning of *spermatogenesis,* the formation of spermatozoa (see pages 33–35). In the female, puberty ends with the beginning of *oögenesis* (the formation of mature ova) and ovulation (see pages 39–44).[27] Puberty and adolescence begin together but they do not end together. Adolescence continues beyond the onset of spermatogenesis and ovulation. In a gradual way it leads the individual to adulthood.

Because each individual is unique the variances in the age at which puberty is attained may be considerable. For some girls puberty begins before ten years of age, for some boys not before fifteen years or even later. This results in widely varying degrees of maturity among young people of approximately the same age. One boy regards his scanty pubic hair with embarrassment, even alarm. All his friends, he tells himself anxiously, have more. A slowly maturing girl despairs over her budding breasts as she compares them with those of her more developed friends. It is difficult for her to understand that there is no real reason for concern.

The adolescent's increased body-awareness makes this an opportune time in which to teach about the body and its development. No age group is more receptive to information than the teen-age. Pubescence is marked by a tremendous increase in appetite; this presents a rare opportunity to explain nutrition. By the same token adolescence presents a splendid opportunity for education about sexuality.[28]

The adolescent, often tormented by inconsistent emotions and thoughts, has a great need for patient help. Few writers have described the adolescent's turmoil with such consummate understanding as has the distinguished child psychologist Anna Freud, daughter of Sigmund Freud. Adolescents, she writes, are

---

[27] For a discussion of female adolescent sterility, see page 91.
[28] For a discussion of the differences in the development of male and female adolescent sexuality, see pages 91-92.

excessively egoistic, regarding themselves as the center of the universe and the sole object of interest, and yet at no time in later life are they capable of so much self-sacrifice and devotion. They form the most passionate love-relations, only to break them off as abruptly as they began them. On the one hand they throw themselves enthusiastically into the life of the community and, on the other, they have an overpowering longing for solitude. They oscillate between blind submission to some self-chosen leader and defiant rebellion against any and every authority. They are selfish and materially-minded and at the same time full of lofty idealism. They are aesthetic but will suddenly plunge into instinctual indulgence of the most primitive character. At times their behavior to other people is rough and inconsiderate, yet they themselves are extremely touchy. Their moods veer between light-hearted optimism and the blackest pessimism. Sometimes they will work with indefagitable enthusiasm and, at other times, they are sluggish and apathetic.[29]

So many changes happen to the adolescent that he needs to become reacquainted with himself. Powerful new sexual urges send him soaring into confused dream worlds. These frighten him and make him feel vaguely guilty. Added to these disturbances are the "inability to settle on an occupational identity" and "the inexorable standardization of American adolescence."[30] Erikson has further described this stage:

There is a "natural" period of uprootedness in human life: adolescence. Like a trapeze artist, the young person in the middle of vigorous emotion must let go of his safe hold on childhood and reach out for a firm grasp on adulthood, dependent for a breathless interval on his training, his luck, and the reliability of the "receiving and confirming" adults.[31]

Without reasonably satisfactory resolutions in the previous four stages—without basic trust, for example—adolescence can be a tribulation. Not identity but identity diffusion may result. In this culture this diffusion is common. Temporary identity may be found by some in a gang. With others, self-identity is interminably slow in coming. From his elders, the adolescent hears apprehensive criticism. Parents have been known to say, "Grow up. Stop hanging around the public

[29] Rudolf Ekstein, "Psychotic Adolescents and Their Quest for Goals," in Charlotte Bühler and Fred Massarik, *The Course of Human Life* (New York, 1968), p. 202, citing Anna Freud, *The Ego and the Mechanisms of Defense* (London, 1948).
[30] Erik H. Erikson, "Growth and Crises of the Healthy Personality," p. 218.
[31] Erik H. Erikson, "Identity and Uprootedness in Our Time," in H. M. Ruitenbeek, ed., *Varieties of Modern Social Theory* (New York, 1963), pp. 55–68.

square and wandering up and down the street. Go to school. Night and day you torture me. Night and day you waste your time having fun." [32] These words are translated from a Sumerian clay tablet four thousand years old. But the confusion of adolescence is no easier to endure today than it ever was before. Emotional illness still may result.

Masturbation

When I was a schoolboy I thought a fair woman a pure Goddess; my mind was a soft nest in which some one of them slept, though she knew it not.[33]

"For most males of every social level masturbation provides the chief source of sexual outlet in early adolescence. It is in that period that the activity reaches its highest frequencies." [34] For this reason a discussion of masturbation is included in the consideration of adolescence. However, masturbatory activity does not reach its peak during the same age-group for both sexes. The frequency of male masturbation usually declines after the teen years. With women, the frequency of masturbation increases up to middle age. After that time the activity becomes more regular.

Cultural attitudes in regard to childhood masturbation vary from total permissiveness to complete prohibition. As is to be expected, education about sexual matters is common in permissive societies and ignored in those that are restrictive. In some societies the parents may teach masturbation to their young. In New Guinea, young Trobriand children of both sexes freely amuse themselves by means of manual and oral stimulation of the genitalia.[35] But among another people of New Guinea, the Kwomas, children are permitted little or no sexual expression. A woman who sees a Kwoma boy with an erection will beat his penis with a stick.[36] It is not unlikely that human masturbatory activity is rooted in evolutionary development. Among mammals much genital handling occurs as a part of grooming and cleaning. However, it is hardly limited to these purposes. "For many male monkeys and apes and for some female chimpanzees masturbation constitutes a supplement to or a substitute for coitus." [37]

At about two or three, the child explores and stimulates his genitalia. He thereby initiates pleasure in himself and perhaps anxiety

[32] From Samuel Noah Kramer, *Everyday Life in Bible Times,* quoted in Jerome Beatty, Jr., "Trade Winds," *Saturday Review* (March 16, 1968), p. 18.
[33] John Keats, from a letter dated July 18, 1818.
[34] Alfred C. Kinsey, Wardell B. Pomeroy, and Clyde E. Martin, *Sexual Behavior in the Human Male* (Philadelphia, 1948), p. 506.
[35] Clellan S. Ford and Frank A. Beach, *Patterns of Sexual Behavior* (New York, 1951), p. 196.
[36] Ibid., p. 187.
[37] Ibid., p. 170.

in his parents. The parental anxiety originates in conditioning and culture.

The stigma attached to masturbation has ancient beginnings. Early Hebrews and Christians believed children should be seen and sexless. In that period of constant external threat to both groups, it was thought necessary to forbid any practice that might become an internal threat. To strengthen the authority of the family and community, practical controls by adults, including strict sexual repression of the young, were thus deemed essential.

During the Dark Ages, fear of disease was added to sin as a deterrent to masturbation. This attitude died slowly. On August 10, 1897, Michael McCormick of San Francisco was granted patent number 587,994 for a male chastity belt. Fathers were to fit them on their adolescent sons to keep them from masturbating. It was a cruel device, but at least it was an improvement over those manufactured by Victorian engineers. In those days a padlock locked a metal cage that was fitted over the boy's genitals at bedtime. To make certain that he did not disturb himself while resting, the cage was outfitted with sharp spikes. In those days the young were led to believe that masturbation would visit upon them every malady from sterility to stuttering. Even today, there are unfortunates who believe this. Others, who are fully aware that masturbation does not cause disease, still feel ashamed of masturbating. Thus, an aura of anxiety envelops practically all the males and more than half the females in this culture.

"Don't do that!" This admonition, punctuated with a sharp slap, too often is the two-year-old's introduction to his parent's lack of understanding about sexual development. The child is taught a crippling lesson: part of him is bad. What is worse, it is a part that feels good. He may never unlearn this. Faced with the catastrophe of losing parental love, he learns early that masturbation is one pleasure that he must enjoy in guilty loneliness. At age two, that is a harsh discovery, especially since he loves his parent with all his dependent heart. Filled with a mournful sense of guilt, he represses his feelings. Years later, they may rise, cloaked in anxiety.

The mother who is overly conscious of these possibilities has already been mentioned (see page 6). She certainly need not exercise excessive care to avoid disturbing her toddler during his genital manipulations. The child should be interrupted if his diaper needs changing or for any other sensible reason. Some three- or four-year-olds masturbate publicly. They should be firmly but gently told not to do this. A mother's instruction is better than a stranger's taunt. Ginott writes:

The solution lies in so involving the infant with our love, and the child with our affection and interest in the outside world,

*that self-gratification will not remain his only means of satis-
faction. The child's main satisfactions should come from personal relationships and achievements. When this is so, occasional self-gratification is not a problem. It is just an additional
solution.*[38]

Why is it often more difficult for the male adolescent to divert
his thoughts from masturbation than it is for the older male or the
adolescent female? The aged Sophocles thanked the gods that he was
no longer ruled by the tyranny of sexual desire. In our society some
believe that the repressed male adolescent lives with that tyranny.
They consider it a major cause of his anxiety. As will be explained
on page 91, sex play, kissing, petting—all stimulate sperm production. Pressures are built up. The trapped sperm must be released.
Ejaculation occurs. In the boy this is a local experience. Without
direct stimulation, the adolescent girl does not respond locally to
petting. What is a local experience for the boy is a romantic experience for the girl. Ova are not produced in great numbers. Unlike
spermatozoa they are not imprisoned to cause pressures that must
be released. With the girl there is no ejaculatory reflex stimulation.
In the adolescent girl, therefore, sexual stimulation does not necessarily result in an overpowering desire for release by sexual intercourse. Many students of the subject suggest that, for the adolescent
boy, sexual stimulation does have this result.

This difference between the adolescent sexes is also manifested
by what they want and need to know. Secrecy about sexuality is
not conducive to emotional serenity. Many an adolescent girl wants
to know about menstruation and pregnancy and delivery, and she
wants to know if sexual intercourse hurts. If she sees a magazine
double-page spread of children with fins instead of arms, she wants
to know all about that, too. She wants to know what kind of sexual
activity boys have. And she should know that at least half of all girls
masturbate.

"Diseases of the mind impair the powers of the body," wrote the
Roman poet Ovid (43 B.C.-17? A.D.). So it is with the needless
emotional distress that some girls and women endure because they
masturbate. Some females develop pruritis (itching) of the vulva
as a consequence of their masturbatory activity. This is not due
to the irritation of the area from the mechanical friction but is a
result of utterly futile feelings of guilt that are associated with
masturbation. "Itching of the vulva then is an indirect form of masturbation."[39]

Before "wet dreams" occur, the boy should know about these

[38] Haim G. Ginott, *Between Parent and Child* (New York, 1965), pp. 161–62.
[39] Michael J. Daly, "The Clitoris as Related to Human Sexuality," *Medical Aspects of Human
Sexuality,* Vol. 5, No. 2 (February 1971), p. 85.

entirely normal nocturnal emissions; he will then realize that they are not dirty. Many authorities suggest that, for the boy, sex and love are quite unrelated. Unlike the girl, he usually does not romanticize his sexual tensions. Almost all adolescent boys (over 95 percent) masturbate. The frequency varies from once or twice to several dozen times a month. This the boy needs to know, and he should be told. The realization that virtually all boys masturbate at his age dilutes his sense of guilt.

The senseless guilt and anxiety to which adolescents have been subjected because of masturbation has abated somewhat. There is considerable opinion among psychiatrists that masturbation is a valuable transition to mature sexual relations. One thing is certain. In this culture, no other activity indulged in by over 95 percent of all males and 50 percent of females is looked upon with such intolerance.

Boys or girls who masturbate privately and without guilt or a sense of moral unworthiness will be able to give the best of themselves to a mate. Since they look upon themselves as people of worth, they give something valuable and good.

Those who find in masturbation their only source of gratification and consolation need help. But so does any disturbed person obsessed with one activity to the virtual exclusion of all else in a rich and varied world. From the point of view of body function, however, there is no scientific evidence whatsoever that masturbation can be excessively frequent.

adulthood

Discussion concerning various aspects of adult sexuality will be continued throughout this book. The remaining three stages of Erikson's schema of personality development, which comprise adulthood, will be considered below.

The first stage   In the first stage the individual truly seeks to give and to receive love. The necessary self-love of childhood and adolescence has begun to expand, to widen, as it were, to the mutuality so characteristic of the capacity to love others. The young adult has emerged from the anxious quest for identity. Now (in Erikson's words) he "is eager and willing to fuse his identity with that of others." In these lovely lines Walt Whitman celebrates this passage from the constrictions of self-searching to the freer searching for others:

Henceforth I ask not good-fortune, I myself am good-fortune,
Henceforth I whimper no more, postpone no more, need nothing . . .
Strong and content I travel the open road.[40]

[40] Walt Whitman, "Song of the Open Road," lines 4-7.

Erikson calls this stage *intimacy* (the task) *versus isolation* (the consequence of the failure to achieve the task of intimacy). True intimacy requires commitment. With the adequate resolution of previous tasks, the developing personality is able to fulfill its commitments. But intimacy and commitment may be hampered by the fear of losing the conscious self, the "I", the *ego*. The ego is the conscious part of the emotional structure that maintains self-identity. To commit oneself, to be intimate with another person, may involve a high degree of selflessness. In extreme circumstances there may even be a sense of self-abandonment. The orgasm, for example, is a physical and emotional peak of self-abandonment. Indeed, while lost within the arms of another person, the individual may experience a temporary loss of consciousness. Paradoxically, the orgasm may be a sublime expression of the self. On a lesser scale of emotional response intimacy still requires concern for another person, rather than total concern for the self. The person who is capable of intimacy does not fear the loss of ego. Sexual union is by no means the only emotional relationship that involves intimacy and commitment. They may occur with the loyalties of profound friendship and in other experiences in which the self is shared. The capacity for intimacy, then, is a hallmark of earned humanness.

It is in this stage that "true genitality" can develop. In explaining this important term Erikson refers to Freud:

> *Freud was once asked what he thought a normal person should be able to do well. The questioner probably expected a complicated answer. But Freud, in the curt way of his old days, is reported to have said: "Lieben und arbeiten" (to love and to work). It pays to ponder on this simple formula; it gets deeper as you think about it. For when Freud said "love" he meant genital love, and genital love;[41] when he said love and work, he meant a general work-productiveness which would not preoccupy the individual to the extent that he loses his right or capacity to be a genital and loving being. Thus we may ponder, but we cannot improve on "the professor's" formula.*

> . . .

> *The total fact of finding, via the climactic turmoil of the orgasm, a supreme experience of the mutual regulation of two beings in some way takes the edge off the hostilities and potential rages caused by the oppositeness of male and female, of fact and fancy, of love and hate. Satisfactory sex relations thus make sex less obsessive, overcompensation less necessary, sadistic controls superfluous.*

> . . .

[41] Erikson's shift of emphasis indicates that appreciation of the genitals is a means of expressing love (*genital* love) and that love is expressed via the genitals (genital *love*). Human sexuality, then, is more than mere physiological relief.

In more complex societies ... a human being should be potentially able to accomplish mutuality of genital orgasm, but he should also be so constituted as to bear a certain amount of frustration in the matter without undue regression wherever emotional preference or considerations of duty and loyalty call for it.

.   .   .

In order to be of lasting social significance, the utopia of genitality should include:
1. *mutuality of orgasm*[42]
2. *with a loved partner*
3. *of the other sex*
4. *with whom one is able and willing to share a mutual trust*
5. *and with whom one is able and willing to regulate the cycles of*
   a. *work*
   b. *procreation*
   c. *recreation*
6. *so as to secure to the offspring, too, all the stages of a satisfactory development.*[43]

The key to this definition of true genitality is the concept of love. But what is love?

"There is a land of the living and a land of the dead and the bridge is love, the only survival, the only meaning."[44]

Life begins and ends with separation. Both are inevitable. Each has its own poignancy.

There is separation at birth. Filling the gulf is love. Without mothering, without embracing love, the infant suffers. Yet, mothering is not smothering. True mother love teaches further separation. The constancy of the mother's love, even after her child's departure, is mirrored by the child's ability to learn to love others in later life.

As the normally learning child explores his body, he learns the glories of self-love. This self-love is not necessarily selfish. The child was born selfish. He will remain selfish only if he learns to hate himself. But if he learns self-worth, he will love this worthy self. And, by giving of a worthy self, he will be able wholeheartedly to enter into the long learning process of loving others. He must, for example, learn to love his neighbor. Were he born with the ability, he would not have had to be commanded.

But how may the child learn to hate himself? He can be taught that he is evil. He can be told a thousand times that he is naughty, that he is bad, that he should be ashamed of himself. A devaluated

---

[42] This should not be construed to mean "simultaneous orgasm." It indicates, rather, the desire to share an orgasmic experience.

[43] Erik H. Erikson, "Eight Ages of Man," pp. 97–99.

[44] Thornton Wilder, *The Bridge of San Luis Rey* (New York, 1927), p. 235.

child devaluates himself still further. And such a child has been cruelly robbed of life's paramount need—the need to give a worthy love. When it is necessary, the child should be corrected, even punished, briefly and to the point, but never heartlessly. He must never feel unloved.

Love is not lust. Love gives. Lust takes. True, both find expression through coitus. Yet, coitus satiates lust, but continues love. With neither animals nor man is love a prerequisite for coitus. However, the profound need of love is characteristic only of man. Sexual desire may result from loneliness, vanity, a desire to conquer or be conquered, a need for social status, a desire to hurt or destroy someone. Any strong emotion (of which love is but one) can stimulate sexual desire.[45] After that desire is satiated, the individual may experience physiological relief. But the deeply significant mutuality, the need to do for another without direct reward, so characteristic of human love, has evaded him. He has given the least of himself. He has not given tenderness nor given up greed. He remains separate, alone.

In Chapter 3 there is some discussion of the techniques of sexual intercourse. These are important. However, the techniques of sexual intercourse do not replace the art of loving. Both may be learned. But, as food without love leaves the infant emotionally starved, so does sexual intercourse without love leave the adult still hungering. Only love can solve the anxiety of separation.

Entering adolescence with self-esteem unshaken, convinced of a wholesome personal value, the young person can further develop the vital enrichments of his humanness. Since he has self-respect, he respects. For a few years, a "best friend" occupies the interest, then members of the opposite sex. In these years, slowly, now clearly, then beclouded, but ever recurring, there comes to the youth a new perception. Love is the art of giving. And part of the art of giving love lies in taking it without exploitation. When he has learned to give and to take love, the young person is ready for adulthood. Prepared to exchange separation for union, he seeks a mate.

The second stage   In this stage, *generativity versus stagnation,* the mature person is prepared to share creatively. He understands that taking can be a way of giving, but that there is a difference between taking and exploiting. Generativity includes a mutual desire for parenthood, for creating the next generation. But it is more than mere reproduction. It is the ability to help another person gain those constructive strengths necessary for effective living. So generativity can come to those who are childless, yet whose desires and talents are involved with the welfare of younger generations.

The third stage: toward the great experience   This stage is called *integrity versus despair and disgust.* The first Earl of Balfour

[45] Erich Fromm, *The Art of Loving* (New York, 1951), p. 54.

(1840–1930) was a gentle man and a gentleman. His had been a good and exciting life in the service of his country. His last words were, "This is going to be a great experience."

An originator and leader, he had met life with courage and verve. The last stages of his life were a continuum of doing. He even died with anticipation. The final stages of his life had given him integrity. His life was a full circle. It excluded despair and disgust. The rich fruits of old age do not grow from arid soil. Those whose beginnings were permeated by a sense of basic trust are more likely to end their lives in full circle—with a sense of basic trust.

Albert Einstein once said that "Every kind of peaceful cooperation among men is primarily based on mutual trust and only secondarily on institutions such as courts of justice and police." Without the basic trust of infancy there cannot be the mutual trust of adulthood.

So it is with the remaining tasks that are encountered in the various stages of life. Those who are so unfortunate as to fail to adequately resolve the tasks of the developing personality will, unlike Balfour, fear death. Why? Because they cannot completely accept the life they have lived. Their despair and disgust is rooted in regret. To them comes the realization that "the time is now short, too short for the attempt to start another life and to try out alternate roads to integrity."[46]

EPILOGUE: THE AMBIVALENT STRUGGLE FOR INDEPENDENCE

Months before birth the first human heartbeat pumps not mother's but fetal blood independently produced. Intrauterine life is not mere unremembered slumber. Unborn, the child sucks, preparing for later oral pleasures of feeding and sexuality. Within the womb, jerky movements prelude the initial tottering independence from the mother. Sometime after birth—in body exploration and use, in later creative curiosities at school—the child seeks freedom from dependency. He is dependent, and seeks independence, longer than any other creature. His prolonged dependency gives him the time he needs to learn the behavior expected of him by his culture. But this dependency can also produce frustration, insecurity, hate, guilt, anxiety.

The childhood struggle for freedom takes place in a milieu of love and hate. He loves the breast that gratifies him; he hates it when it frustrates him. He loves his parents when they comfort him; he hates them when they control him. This love-hate ambivalence is carried into later years. It is a major cause of anxiety. The frustrations of dependency continue, as hostility, into adulthood. The adult loves his child. He hates his child. He loves his mate. He hates his mate. This emotional paradox is not a predicament peculiar to modern man.

[46]Erik H. Erikson, "Eight Ages of Man," p. 101.

personality and sexuality: an interwoven development

Twenty centuries ago the Roman lyric poet Catullus wrote these perplexed lines:

> *At once I love and hate*
> *You ask why this should be,*
> *I know not, 'tis my fate*
> *A fate of Agony!*[47]

When the universality of this ambivalence is recognized, man will not be so governed by the anxiety it creates. The paths to independence are obstructed by parent-child conflict. But the child will travel those paths nevertheless. The loving parent can help. Should help not come, the child will struggle on alone, unaided. Should the parent impede the child in the quest for independence, the child will retaliate with hate, and suffer guilt and anxiety because of it. All people have dependent needs. Yet a degree of independence is essential for maturity.

During each stage of personality development, the child collects problems. Usually he learns from them. They do not necessarily become serious impedimenta. Problems vary. Should the heart form imperfectly and leak, it will, nonetheless, beat as long as possible. Should the child's oral needs in the first year be thwarted too often, those needs may well be manifested in later life by constant emotional overeating. But the child will, to repeat, develop nonetheless. Well equipped or not, he will seek independence. This, then, the wise parent will accept.

As he strives for independence, the developing child needs to understand discipline, not continuously suffer from it. The more the child clearly comprehends what his parents expect of him, and why, the less will he need discipline and the less will he suffer when disciplined. The mother who literally screams her emotional responses to the child's behavior is more successful, at least in this respect, than the parent who is sanctimoniously silent and ends by being mysterious. Mysterious parents frighten their children. There may be room for mystery in love of God or love between the sexes. There is no room for it in parent-child love. The child who never really knows how his parent feels has problems with discipline.

One day, the little girl pulls the pots and pans from the cupboard. She is kissed and told she is cute. The next day, repeating the same performance, she turns happily to her mother. But a previous marital tiff has angered the mother. The child is scolded and spanked. The child is hurt, not corrected. One day the father answers his little girl's proposal of marriage with a "sure, honey, aren't you my best girl?" (a lying answer to an honest question). The next week, the little girl repeats her proposal. It is met with cold indifference or even harsh

[47] Quoted from *Catullus*, translated into English verse by T. Hart-Davies (London, 1879), p. 122.

hostility (adding injury to error). Or the little girl, living with her divorced mother, must listen to a constant rehearsal of her father's faults. From her father there is nothing but tenderness. She is confused, then angry. The mother retaliates with discipline. The child retaliates with sullen obedience. Children are not miniature adults. They do not spring into adulthood. They do not develop suddenly after a long quiescence. Neither do their anxieties. They need constancy, not confusion. That is why children love peek-a-boo games. That is why they never tire of hearing the same bedtime story. They know what will happen. They can count on it. Discipline of children works best when it arises from constant love, not intermittent hate.

parent development

Parents develop too. They pass through stages related to the stages of their child's development (see Table 1-1). Parents and child develop together, experiencing singular, yet interwoven, problems. And, like the child, the parent in the throes of one stage may still be occupied with unsolved problems of a past stage.

It takes time for parents to learn how to interpret the howl of the child. What is the baby trying to tell them? He is dry, fed, fondled. No diaper pin pierces his bottom. Why, then, does he weep? Is it still another gas bubble? Or is it because his bed was accidentally moved six inches from the window and he misses the usual shaft of bright light from an adjacent window?

When the recliner becomes a sitter and suddenly a toddler, he is into everything. Again the parents need time. It is not always easy to wholeheartedly accept the child who seems to be winning an all-day footrace with his mother. No sooner may this acceptance come about than the third stage of parental development—separation—is reached.

The pain of separation is not limited to children. The child's first day at school, punctuated by the peremptory command, "Mommie, g'wan home," is a trauma that mothers (and grandmothers) are not prone to forget. Nor is the fourth stage, manifested by the child's independence, any easier for the parent. Their child's "declaration of independence" hurts some parents and angers others. It is almost as difficult for the rejected parent to remember that he is still desperately needed as it is for him to understand the rejection. The fifth stage of parental personality development is marked by an opportunity for the parents to rebuild their lives, not around the child, but with themselves more in mind.

Parental development begins with the parents' own childhood. Parents need help. Almost every parent comes to realize that the child is trying to give that help. This effort, in turn, helps the child to

TABLE 1-1 parent and child development

STAGE ONE: INFANT	STAGE TWO: TODDLER
Parent Development: Learning the *cues*. **Erikson:** Trust. **Spock:** Physically helpless; emotionally agreeable. **Ogden Nash:** *Many an infant that screams like a calliope* *Could be soothed by a little attention to his diope.*	**Parent Development:** Learning to *accept growth and development*. **Erikson:** Autonomy. **Spock:** A sense of his own individuality and will power; vacillates between dependence and independence. **Ogden Nash:** *The trouble with a kitten is that* *Eventually it becomes a cat.*
STAGE THREE: PRESCHOOLER	STAGE FOUR: SCHOOL-AGER
Parent Development: Learning to *separate*. **Erikson:** Initiative. **Spock:** Imitation through admiration; learns about friends; preliminary interest in sexuality. **Ogden Nash:** *But joy in heaping measure comes* *To children whose parents are under their thumbs.*	**Parent Development:** Learning to *accept rejection*—without deserting. **Erikson:** Industry. **Spock:** Fitting into outside group; independence of parents and standards; developing conscience; need to control and make moral judgments. **Ogden Nash:** *Children aren't happy with nothing to ignore* *And that's what parents were created for.*
STAGE: FIVE: TEEN-AGER	
Parent Development: Learning to *build a new life,* having been thoroughly discredited by one's teen-ager. **Erikson:** Identity. **Redl:** Conflict to be confined to specific and major issues at hand; peer orientation and fair play. **Ogden Nash:** *O adolescence!* *I'd like to be present I must confess* *When thine own adolescents adolesce!*	

Source: David Belais Friedman, "Parent Development," *California Medicine*, Vol. 86, No. 1 (January 1957), pp. 25–28.

identify with his parents and to grow with them. Their effort is mutually beneficial.

THE CHILD'S DEVELOPMENT:
WHOSE RESPONSIBILITY?

The parent has become the scapegoat of modern times. "Look at how badly you raised me," is the accusation and excuse of many an emotionally distressed young person. The parents' sense of guilt is deep. But "the fact is that children, too, possess freedom of choice.

It appears at an early age and develops with the intelligence and other capacities of the youthful personality. Children, then, share the responsibility for their behavior and emerging characters with their parents, relatives, teachers and friends." [48] It was once observed that someone who points the finger of blame at another person will find three fingers of his hand pointing at himself.

Freedom of choice is a durable freedom that may remain when all other freedoms are gone. Frankl writes:

> *We who lived in concentration camps can remember the men who walked through the huts comforting others, giving away their last piece of bread. They may have been few in number, but they offer sufficient proof* that everything can be taken from a man but one thing: the last of the human freedoms—to choose one's attitude in any given circumstances, to choose one's own way.[49]

Undeniably, parents need improving, but the child must share in the responsibility for his own development. It is an opportunity. Again, he can help not only himself but also his parents.

[48] Corliss Lamont, *Freedom of Choice Affirmed* (New York, 1967), p. 32.
[49] Victor E. Frankl, *Man's Search for Meaning* (New York, 1959), p. 112.

the reproductive 2 system: structure, function, dysfunction— and sexual sensitivity

the brain's chemical "fertility switch"[1]

Attached to the base of the brain by its short stem, and snugly encased in its bony fortress, is the *pituitary gland.* This ductless, endocrine gland weighs no more than two baby-dose aspirins. It is no larger than a cherry. It has a front (anterior) lobe and a back (posterior) lobe. The posterior lobe stores and releases several hormones; one stimulates contraction of the uterus at the beginning of childbirth. The anterior lobe produces and releases hormones. These both activate and control other endocrine glands—the thyroid, adrenals, and ovaries and testes. The anterior lobe of the pituitary has long been called "the master gland." It is not. Its relationship to the other endocrine glands is as much reciprocal as it is controlling.

Moreover, recent research has shown it to be controlled by chemicals from that part of the base of the brain that is nearest to it—the *hypothalamus.* The brain chemicals are called *releasing hormones* (or *factors*). Via tiny blood vessels they leave the hypothalamus to reach the anterior lobe of the pituitary. There they trigger the release of hormones that influence the other endocrine glands. The releasing hormones from the hypothalamus that are of present concern are those stimulating the anterior lobe of the pituitary to, in turn, produce and release the hormones that control the sex glands—the ovaries and testes.

[1] Graham Chedd, "The Switch of Fertility," *New Scientist and Science Journal,* Vol. 51, No. 758 (July 1, 1971), pp. 11-13.

the brain's chemical "fertility switch"

On a late midsummer afternoon in 1971, Andrew V. Schally, of Tulane University's School of Medicine, rose to deliver a paper at a meeting of the American Endocrine Society. What he had to say made worldwide scientific headlines. In the laboratory, his group had successfully synthesized the ultimate control in the reproductive hormone network. That control is in the form of a releasing factor (or hormone) generated in the brain's hypothalamus. This factor is now known as the *luteinizing hormone-releasing hormone* (*LH-RH*). It has not yet been shown that the follicle-stimulating hormone has its own releasing factor. However, it is known that the hypothalamic hormone LH-RH induces not only the release of luteinizing hormone (LH) but of follicle-stimulating hormone (FSH) as well.

Specific signals from the central nervous system are decoded and the hypothalamus produces the releasing factor. Upon reaching the anterior lobe of the pituitary, LH-RH effects the release of luteinizing hormone and, probably, also follicle-stimulating hormone. In the female, FSH stimulates the growth and maturation of the follicles in the ovaries (see page 42). But of the two to thirty-two follicles that begin to mature in each cycle only one will usually come to complete maturity. LH, helped by FSH, promotes the maturation of that single follicle and, following its maturation, LH causes the rupture of the follicular wall and the release of the ovum (*ovulation,* see page 43). Moreover, in the human being, LH also stimulates the corpus luteum to release progesterone (see page 46). The male hypothalamus generates the same releasing factor as that of the female; in addition, the anterior lobe of his pituitary gland releases the same follicle-stimulating and luteinizing hormones. In the pubescent male, however, FSH acts to open the testicular tubules, to enlarge the testes, and to initiate the production of spermatozoa (*spermatogenesis*). Male LH stimulates testosterone (a male sex hormone) production. Thus, the differences between the male and female, in these respects, is not in the chemical structure of the factors generated by the hypothalamus or the hormones produced and released by the anterior lobe of the pituitary. The difference lies in their action and in their timing. In the female the hormonal production and action is cyclic. In the male, it is not (see pages 94-95).

Research begets research. Schally's announcement of the synthesis of the chemicals generated and used by the hypothalamus of the brain to communicate with the anterior lobe of the pituitary, and by means of which the elaborate reproductive system is controlled, paves the way for a better understanding of conception and contraception. As examples: it is known that there is a mechanism whereby estrogens and progesterone feed back to the hypothalamus to control the production of FSH and LH by the anterior lobe of the pituitary gland. This feedback mechanism accounts for the periodicity of ovulation and the efficacy of the more recent contraceptive pill. A basic component of the contraceptive pill is estrogen. Whether both FSH and LH are suppressed depends on the level of estrogen in the blood. This has been useful in determining the dosage of estrogen in the new contraceptive pill. Twenty micrograms of estrogen suppress only FSH; a dosage of fifty micrograms (.05 milligrams) suppresses both FSH and LH and is also relatively safe (see page 109). Furthermore, it has been learned that FSH and LH peaks indicate that a woman will ovulate within forty-eight hours. This correlation may some day lead to a single pill (or only a few) that will suppress FSH and LH only during the established period of ovulation. Or better still, rather than depend on the presently practiced risky rhythm method, the woman may be able to abstain from sexual intercourse during an ovulatory period that is based on scientifically precise laboratory measurements.

It has also been discovered that there is a feedback mechanism between anterior pituitary LH and FSH and the male hormone testosterone. Thus, the level of testosterone in the male seems to be monitored by the amounts of LH and FSH in the anterior lobe of the pituitary. That the subfertility of some men may be due to inadequate levels of the executive hormones in the anterior pituitary is further demonstrated by the discovery that, via an unknown substance, there is also a feedback mechanism between sperm maturation and FSH. It is possible to measure FSH levels in human beings; these may now be correlated with a type of subfertility that occurs because there is something amiss in one of the stages of spermatogenesis. Finally, the work of Schally and his group may yet lead to fertility and subfertility controls at the hypothalamic level, rather than at the level of the pituitary, or at the target ovaries, or even at the testes.[2] Contraception is further discussed on pages 108-29; subfertility is considered on pages 214-16.

THE PINEAL GLAND

Increasing knowledge suggests that the single pea-sized *pineal gland* may play an important role in the activities controlling sexual function and reproduction. Buried near the center of the brain, and attached to its cerebellar portion by a slender stalk, this organ was

[2] Joan Arehart-Treichel, "Sperm and Eggs on the Go," *Science News*, Vol. 102, No. 7 (August 12, 1972), pp. 108-09. In the future LH-RH may also be used as a contraceptive. By inducing ovulation, the hormone could make the rhythm method of contraception more reliable. Use of the drug could establish the exact date of ovulation, and the woman could have sexual intercourse accordingly. ("Giving Reason to Rhythm: Inducing Ovulation," *Science News*, Vol. 100, No. 19 [November 6, 1971], p. 310.) In addition, the development of an LH-RH antagonist is imminent. "The antagonist, which could be given to block the release of luteinizing hormone [and consequent ovulation], could be the first contraceptive free of side effects . . . It might someday be used as a long term 'inoculation' against conception." ("Synthetic Hormone Could Improve Fertility Control," *Journal of the American Medical Association*, Vol. 217, No. 6 [August 9, 1971], p. 757.)

thought by the ancients to be the seat of the soul. Today, some scientists regard the pineal gland as a sort of relay station, sending messages to the nervous system that influence the body's "biological clock." This still mysterious timing system within the body synchronizes with the external cosmic clock that determines day and night. (Temperature, for example, is lower in the morning than in the late afternoon.)

The pineal gland is rich in chemicals, some of which are secreted in synchronization with the ebb and flow of daylight. *Melatonin,* a chemical that acts as a hormone, is found in the pineal gland. In lower animals it appears that melatonin has an inhibiting effect on the sexual function. Moreover, it has been found, by animal experimentation, that light can effect the sexual cycle by controlling the synthesis of melatonin in the pineal gland. This may account for the seasonal mating periods of many animals. Human beings are almost unique in that they do not mate according to season. If and how light generates nervous activity into pineal gland function in human beings is being investigated.

the reproductive systems

THE MALE REPRODUCTIVE SYSTEM

This system consists of a pair of male gonads (testes) and excretory ducts (the epididymis, vas deferens, and ejaculatory ducts). The accessory structures are the seminal vesicles, prostate gland, Cowper's glands (also called the bulbo-urethral glands), and penis.

the male reproductive organs

About two months before birth, the *testes* usually descend from the abdomen into the external sac, the *scrotum*. It is crucial that this occur before adolescence. Only at a temperature cooler than that of the abdominal cavity can the development of spermatozoa in the testes occur. Should both testes fail to descend, sterility results. Should only one testicle reach the scrotum, there would probably be enough normal spermatozoa to insure fertility. In some males only one testicle descends and years may elapse before the other descends. In many cases, surgery and hormones have been successful in the treatment of undescended testicles.

A basic purpose of the testes is to produce *spermatozoa* (Greek *sperma,* seed). This first function is carried on by germinal cells of the *seminiferous tubules*. These coiled little tubules (straightened out

the reproductive system: structure, function, dysfunction—and sexual sensitivity

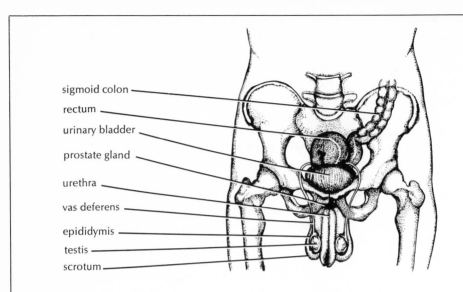

sigmoid colon
rectum
urinary bladder
prostate gland
urethra
vas deferens
epididymis
testis
scrotum

2-1   the male reproductive system

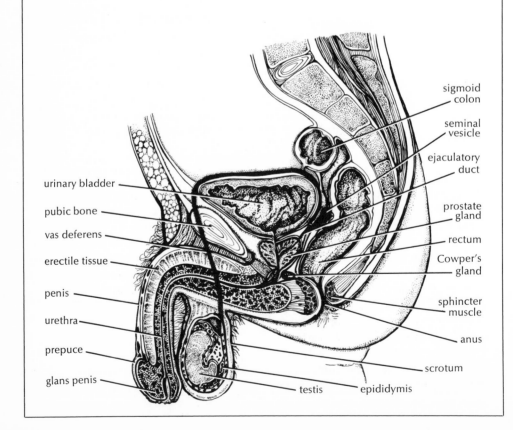

sigmoid colon
seminal vesicle
ejaculatory duct
prostate gland
rectum
Cowper's gland
sphincter muscle
anus
scrotum
epididymis
testis

urinary bladder
pubic bone
vas deferens
erectile tissue
penis
urethra
prepuce
glans penis

in both testes they would be a mile long) are supported by connective tissue in which special cells carry out the second basic function of the testes—the production of the hormone *testosterone*. The same hormone of the anterior pituitary that maintains the corpus luteum (see page 45) in the female is responsible for the production of testosterone in the male. It is the testosterone that causes the male genitalia to develop, the voice to deepen, the bones to increase in size, the beard to appear, and the psyche to change. The growth of the external genitalia is the first sign of puberty in the boy.[3]

Eventually, the seminiferous tubules unite into a single convoluted tube at the back of each testis called the *epididymis*. Mature spermatozoa leave the seminiferous tubules and are temporarily stored in the epididymis. At maturity, enough spermatozoa have accumulated in the epididymis for ejaculation.

The *vas deferens* (or spermatic cord) is a continuation of the epididymis. It goes upward along the back of the testes and, by way of a canal in the groin, into the abdomen. Eventually the vas deferens joins the duct of the *seminal vesicle* of its side of the body. The two seminal vesicles are located between the bladder and rectum and produce a secretion that adds to the volume of the seminal fluid. The seminal vesicles empty their secretions into the *ejaculatory ducts* which, in turn, empty into the *urethra*. The urethra is the canal of the male organ for sexual intercourse, the *penis*. Through the penis,

---

[3] *Androgens* are substances capable of producing masculine body characteristics. Thus *testosterone* and *androsterone* are among the androgens. Testosterone is the predominant androgen produced by the testes; it is, therefore, the major hormone of male sexual development. Its functions are both numerous and profound. It is essential in the fetus for male internal and external genital differentiation (see pages 79-80). After puberty, it contributes to spermatogenesis. In addition, testosterone stimulates the development of the seminal vesicle and prostate, is necessary for the contribution of the seminal vesicle and prostate to semen and ejaculation, and matures the secondary sex characteristics of the adult male, such as the deepening voice, penile enlargement, muscularity, and facial hair. (Daniel D. Federman, "The Assessment of Organ Function—The Testis," *The New England Journal of Medicine*, Vol. 285, No. 16 [October 14, 1971], p. 901.) The subtle interrelationships of androgens to sexual activity were recently demonstrated in a unique way by a curious scientist. He studied the effect of his sexual activity on his beard growth. For two years he had to spend periods of several weeks in comparative isolation on a remote island. By collecting his beard shavings from the head of an electric razor and weighing them, he found that his increased beard growth was related not only to resumption but also to anticipation of sexual activity. He suggests that this, in turn, caused an increased testosterone secretion, which induced a subsequent speed-up in beard growth. "Even the presence of particular female company in the absence of intercourse, after a period of separation, usually caused an obvious increase in beard growth." (Anon., "Effects of Sexual Activity on Beard Growth in Man," *Nature*, Vol. 226, No. 5240 [May 30, 1970], p. 869.)

By their action on the *sebaceous glands* of the skin, androgens predispose teen-agers to acne. The intense self-concern characteristic of the pubescent person does not make acne easy to bear. This disease of the sebaceous glands in the skin occurs in some 75 percent of children at puberty. Usually it is mild. The normal sebaceous glands produce an oily substance called *sebum*. In acne an abnormal amount of sebum blocks the outlet of the gland. It enlarges. The outer part of the lesion turns black, not from dirt, but because of chemical changes. These are the "blackheads." Infection may occur and spread deep into the skin. Washing several times daily with a disinfectant soap is wise. However, there is no evidence whatsoever that the initial lesion of acne begins because of uncleanliness. Moreover, the prevalent belief that acne is caused by masturbation is utterly untrue. Even mild cases of acne are often best seen by the family physician. He may refer severe cases to a skin specialist (dermatologist). Many physicians forbid their acne patients to partake of chocolates, nuts (peanut butter), and soft drinks. The understandable emotional distress caused by severe acne makes professional counsel desirable.

the reproductive system: structure, function, dysfunction—and sexual sensitivity

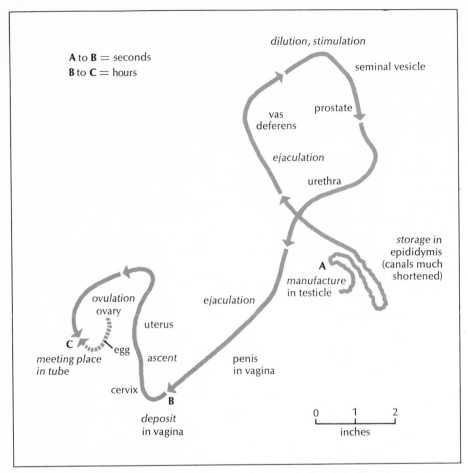

2-2 The route of a spermatozoon from its origin to its fertilization of an ovum.

the semen is discharged and urine is passed from the bladder. Through a remarkable engineering mechanism (see page 38), urine and semen never pass at the same time.

The first one-and-one-half inches of the urethra, as it leaves the bladder, is surrounded by the chestnut-sized *prostate gland,* which also contains many muscle fibers. The gland part secretes a thin fluid that helps carry the semen and provides it with a necessary alkaline medium. The muscle part of the prostate helps eject the semen out of the penis. On each side of the prostate glands is one of the two *Cowper's glands.* They look like peas and secrete the thick material characteristic of seminal fluid.

The penis hangs in front of the scrotum. At the tip of its head (*glans*) is the slitlike opening of the urethra. The thin skin of its body is loose. At the neck of the penis, the skin folds upon itself to form the *prepuce* (foreskin). This is the portion of the skin of which part is removed at circumcision. Circumcision is associated with a decrease in the incidence of cancer of the penis. There is, moreover, some evidence that cancer of the cervix is more common among wives of uncircumcised men. However, there is considerable opinion that both cervical and penile cancers are more closely associated with poor personal hygiene than with the presence of the prepuce. Not all physicians agree that routine circumcision is essential.

The belief, moreover, that the uncircumcised male has more control over his ejaculations than the man who is circumcised is a fallacy. It doubtless arose from the mistaken notion that since the glans of the uncircumcised male is largely covered by the prepuce it would be less exposed to friction during coitus. The fact is that the prepuce of the uncircumcised male is significantly retracted during sexual intercourse (it may not be when he masturbates). He is, therefore, no more likely to be able to control his ejaculations than is a circumcised male.[4]

Another fallacy is the belief that a larger penis is more effective during a coital connection than a smaller one. This misconception is discussed on pages 105-06.

mechanism of erection of the penis and ejaculation

Not every penile erection is due to increased sexual stimulation. For example, partial erection may result from lifting heavy loads or from straining while having a bowel movement. This is due to stress on the muscles of the perineum. Newborn males may have a penile erection; this is probably related to the infant's increased muscle and nerve irritability, such as may be caused by crying. When a penile erection is due to sexual excitement, its stimuli begin in the higher

[4]William H. Masters and Virginia E. Johnson, *Human Sexual Response* (Boston, 1966), pp. 189-91.

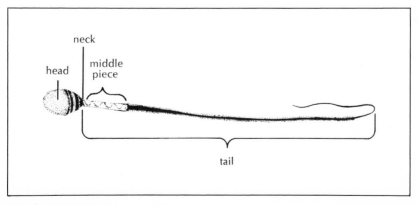

2-3 A spermatozoon.

brain centers; the erection itself is the result of a spinal reflex. Cerebral influence is apparently not always necessary for an erection; indeed, it may inhibit penile erection. Man does not have voluntary control of an erection; he cannot will it. To understand how the spinal nerve reflex cause erection, consider first some of the internal structure of the penis.

The penis contains three cylindrical bodies of erectile tissue (see Figure 2-1). They run the length of the penis to its head. These cylindrical bodies contain many small vascular spaces; they are thus a spongy erectile tissue. For an erection to occur, nerve stimuli cause dilatation of the little penile arteries (arterioles). At the places where the arterioles and the vascular spaces join are valvelike structures. When the penis is flaccid these structures (called *polsters*) cause blood to be shunted away from the vascular spaces and directly into the veins. With adequate nerve stimuli these polsters relax. This permits rapid inflow of blood into the spaces of the cylindrical erectile tissue of the penis. The rate of the inflow of blood from the arterioles is then temporarily greater than the rate of the outflow from the veins. This causes an increase of blood volume in the penis. When a steady state is reached, in which blood inflow equals outflow, penile enlargement ceases, and the penis is stiff. The veins of the penis are also equipped with valvelike structures, which some investigators think slow down the return of blood from that organ. Others disagree with this.

Before ejaculating, the male frequently has an emission of a few drops (or more) of fluid that may contain active spermatozoa. (This accounts for pregnancies that may result despite the practice of coitus interruptus [see page 108].) The ejaculatory process begins with contractions of the ducts leading away from the seminiferous tubules in the testes. These contractions continue along the epididymis to the vas deferens. The vas deferens then contracts along with the seminal vesicles. The contents of the vas deferens, as well as those of the seminal vesicles, are expelled into the part of the urethra that passes through the prostate. The prostate has also been contracting rhythmically to add fluid to the ejaculatory content. At the onset of the ejaculatory process, the ringlike band of muscle fibers (the sphincter) surrounding the exit from the urinary bladder contracts. Semen is thus prevented from entering the urinary bladder; semen and urine are not ordinarily expelled together. After ejaculation, nerve stimuli cause constriction of the penile arterioles, and the erection is gradually lost.

semen

The ejaculated fluid containing the sperm is a thick, whitish material. It is about a teaspoonful in amount. However, the consistency and amount of the seminal fluid may vary, for example, with the age of the male. In healthy men, the ejaculatory amount is reestablished in about twenty-four hours or less. During ejaculation, the entire transit from testes to vagina occupies but a few seconds. Although sperm can remain motile in the vagina for as long as two hours, some can reach the cervix in seconds. Indeed, ejaculation may well take place directly on the cervix. However, hours may be required for ascent of the sperm through the uterus and part of the Fallopian tube in order to fertilize an ovum (a distance of about six inches). On an average, the journey probably requires about an hour (see Figure 2-2). Each spermatozoon has a bulbous head. Its long mobile tail propels it to its destination (see Figure 2-3). When one compares the size of a spermatozoon with the relatively enormous distance it must travel to fertilize an ovum, one cannot help but be struck by its vigor. Yet, of the millions of spermatozoa emitted in each ejaculum, usually only one manages the task of fertilization. Why? It may be that the destiny of a spermatozoon is determined by differences in the structure of the membrane surrounding it.[5]

THE FEMALE REPRODUCTIVE SYSTEM

The essential glands of this system are the pair of female gonads (ovaries). The female reproductive *duct* system is composed of the Fallopian tubes (named after the Italian anatomist Gabriello Fallopio [1523–62], the structures are also called the oviducts or uterine tubes), the uterus (womb), and vagina, and the associated structures—the external genitalia. The mammary glands (breasts) may also be considered as part of the female reproductive duct system (see Figure 2-8).

the ovaries and ova

The two *ovaries* (egg containers) are the fundamental organs of femininity. About the size and shape of a shelled almond, each ovary is situated on one side of the *uterus* and is attached to it by ligaments. Just as the organs of masculinity (the testes) produce male sperm, so do the ovaries produce mature *ova* in the female. When the female child is born, each of her ovaries contains about two hundred thousand tiny sacs or follicles.[6] In each follicle lies a microscopically small primordial sex cell (or *oögonium*). Each woman is born with all the primordial sex cells she will ever have. At this primitive, unripened stage, no sex cell is capable of fertilization. The ripening process whereby a primordial sex cell becomes an ovum must await puberty. This usually occurs between the ninth and seventeenth year

[5] Garth L. Nicolson and Ryuzo Yanagimachi, "Terminal Saccharides on Sperm Plasma Membranes: Identification by Specific Agglutinins," *Science*, Vol. 177, No. 4045 (July 21, 1972), pp. 276–78.
[6] Estimates of the number vary enormously. Some students believe that, at birth, there are as many as half a million follicles in each ovary.

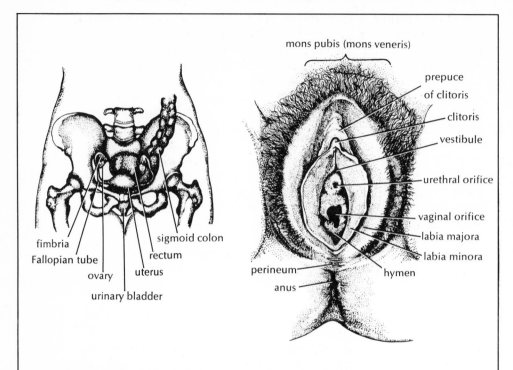

mons pubis (mons veneris)

prepuce of clitoris

clitoris

vestibule

urethral orifice

vaginal orifice

labia majora

labia minora

perineum

hymen

anus

fimbria

Fallopian tube

ovary

urinary bladder

uterus

rectum

sigmoid colon

2-4 the female reproductive system

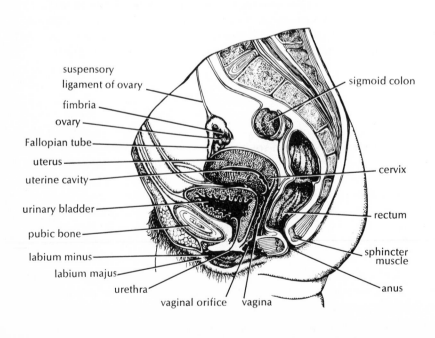

suspensory ligament of ovary

fimbria

ovary

Fallopian tube

uterus

uterine cavity

urinary bladder

pubic bone

labium minus

labium majus

urethra

vaginal orifice

vagina

sigmoid colon

cervix

rectum

sphincter muscle

anus

(twelve-and-one-half years is the average). During a woman's lifetime, only about 400 (perhaps 1 in 1,000) ova leave either of the ovaries.

Every month the mature human female experiences a series of changes basically involving the hypothalamus in the brain, the anterior lobe of the pituitary gland, the ovaries, and the *endometrium* (the lining of the uterus). The purpose of these changes is to prepare for possible pregnancy. For pregnancy to occur, an egg must leave the ovary, be fertilized, and then be firmly implanted in the endometrium of the prepared uterus.[7]

What happens to the ovary (ovarian cycle) is related to what happens to the uterus (menstrual cycle). *Menstruation* and *ovulation* are different events, happening at different times, to different organs. But each intimately affects the other.

Ovulation To follow the events leading to the release of a mature egg from the ovary (1-8 below), start with a landmark—day one, the beginning of the menstrual period. Why day one? Because the woman can observe the first day of her period more easily than her last. She can thus count from that day more reliably. Also assume that every twenty-eight days the average female menstruates five days. With different people these time periods vary normally. They are used here only as examples. Note, however, that the ovarian and menstrual cycles are correlated here.

1. Menstruation begins on day one and continues through day five (see Figures 2-5 and 2-6). Chemicals from the hypothalamus stimulate the anterior lobe of the pituitary gland to release the follicle-stimulating hormone (FSH) directly into the venous blood stream.

[7]The Roman Catholic church teaches that conception occurs with fertilization. Others, such as the American College of Obstetrics and Gynecology, consider biological life to begin with implantation.

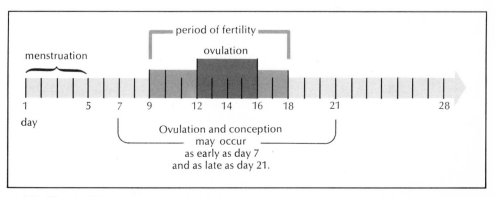

2-5 The menstrual cycle.

the reproductive system: structure, function, dysfunction—and sexual sensitivity

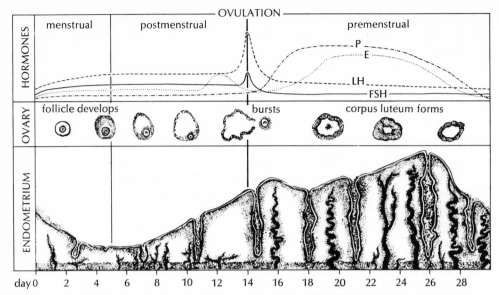

2-6 The menstrual and ovulatory cycles. (FSH = the follicle-stimulating hormone; E = estrogen; LH = the luteinizing hormone; P = progesterone.) Note that the progesterone level is detectably higher within twenty-four hours after ovulation occurs.

2. The FSH reaches and activates the ovaries. Not one but several (of the many thousands) of immature ovarian follicles in one or both ovaries respond to the FSH and begin to ripen. Which ovary is more affected is unpredictable. Estimates of the number of immature follicles that respond to the FSH usually vary from two to thirty-two.

3. The cells of those ovarian follicles that are ripening multiply greatly and the single maturing ovum within each follicle increases in size. The increased layers of follicular cells secrete a *follicular fluid.* This fluid forms tiny pools, which first separate groups of cells but which then run together to form a little lake within each follicle (see Figure 2-6). The follicles mature at different rates of speed, so some are at earlier stages of development than others. By about day ten, a few of the most mature follicles look like fluid-filled rounded sacks. The developing ovum is in the wall of the sack and is surrounded by follicular cells, which separate it from the lake. The follicle is now called a *Graafian follicle,* after a seventeenth-century Dutch anatomist, Regner de Graaf, who first described it.

4. As they ripen, the cells of maturing follicles also produce a hormone of their own called *estrogen.* Its function at this stage is to begin the preparation of the uterus for implantation of a fertilized ovum.

5. On about day ten, one (very rarely two) of the follicles undergoes a sudden spurt of growth. In three or four days it is completely mature. As a rule only one follicle and ovum matures and only one ovum leaves the ovary. (If a woman has a tendency for multiple births there may be more than one.) No one knows what determines which follicle (and ovum) will be selected. The other follicles, and their contained ova that are not destined to leave the ovary, develop to varying extents, only to regress, die, and be replaced by small scars. No other trace of them remains.

6. A few hours before the ovum is ready to leave, the follicle that contains it migrates to the surface of the ovary. By day thirteen or fourteen the ovum is ready to go. It has been seen at surgery as a tiny blisterlike protrusion from the ovarian surface.

7. A few days before, the anterior lobe of the pituitary gland had begun the release of a second hormone, the luteinizing hormone (LH), directly into the venous blood. Like the FSH, the release of LH is governed by hypothalamic chemicals from the brain.

8. The LH causes the follicle to rupture, and the ovum is released. This is *ovulation*. On the average, ovulation occurs on day fourteen. Ovulation, then, occurs at about the middle of the menstrual cycle. In 1972, it was reported that the ovary contracts slightly to gently squeeze the ovum loose and send it on its way.[8] Presumably, just a few ennervated muscle cells are responsible for one of the most significant squeezes in biology.

To this point it has been seen that, influenced by releasing chemicals from the brain's hypothalamus, the anterior lobe of the pituitary gland has produced and released two hormones. One, FSH, stimulated the growth of follicles that, as they developed, produced estrogen. The second pituitary hormone, LH, caused rupture of the follicle, releasing the egg.

Three parenthetical observations will be made here. First, *conception,* the fertilization of an ovum by a sperm, cannot occur unless both mature sex cells are viable. Upon being released from the ovary, the ovum usually survives from twenty-four to thirty-six hours. For the ovum, assume a maximal survival time of two days. Upon being deposited in the vagina, sperm usually survive one to three days. This would include the several hours of survival in the vagina and the two or three days in the cervix and above. For sperm, assume a maximum survival time of three days. Usually ovulation occurs, in the average woman, about fourteen days before the onset of the next menstrual period, give or take two days. Keeping in mind the average maximum survival times of the ovum and of sperm, as well as the average day of occurrence of ovulation (with its two-day leeway),

[8]"The Gentle Squeeze that Sent You on Your Way," *New Scientist,* Vol. 53, No. 783 (February 17, 1972), p. 366.

refer to Figure 2-5 for an illustration of the average period of fertility of the woman who menstruates every twenty-eight days. Counting from day one of the menstrual period, she will ovulate between day twelve and day sixteen. However, her ovum will survive about two days. A viable ovum may thus be available for fertilization until approximately day eighteen of the menstrual cycle. The woman may have ovulated as early as day twelve. For about three days a sperm can survive to fertilize an ovum. It then follows that conception can occur if a sperm is deposited in the vagina as early as three days before ovulation. If the woman menstruates regularly every twenty-eight days (and many do not), she will, on the average, be most likely to become pregnant if sperm are deposited in the vagina between day nine and day eighteen of her menstrual cycle. Throughout this book human individuality is stressed. Menstruation and ovulation are hardly exceptions. Some women flow every twenty-one days. Others menstruate every thirty-five days. They should calculate their periods of maximum fertility accordingly. For example, the woman who menstruates every twenty-one days can set an ovulation date on day seven of the menstrual cycle. If she menstruates every thirty-fifth day she will usually ovulate on day twenty-one. In either case her calculations of maximum fertility must make allowances for a two-day leeway for ovulation and the viability of both ovum and sperm. There are women whose menstrual cycles from month to month are irregular. Without obtaining a reliable average over a year, they cannot calculate a reasonably reliable period of maximum fertility.

Second, when ovulation occurs, the rupture is accompanied by a small amount of ovarian bleeding. This blood may be irritating and may cause brief abdominal discomfort. With right-side middle-of-the-month pain, the woman may worry that she has appendicitis. Only the physician is equipped to differentiate between the two.

Third, as the follicle develops, its estrogen (step 4 above) affects the uterus. In preparation for implantation of the developing product of the fertilized egg (the embryo), the lining (endometrium) of this organ thickens, as does the muscle layer. Estrogen also affects the cervical secretions, making them more receptive for the sperm if it is there. It also causes the Fallopian tubes to contract more rapidly. (Estrogen, the basic female sex hormone, is responsible for many of the female sex characteristics, such as the growth of breast tissue.)

The destiny of the released ovum   Where does the ovum go? It enters the *Fallopian tube* (see Figure 2-7)[9] nearest the ovary from

[9]Obstruction of these tubes by inflammation is one of the most common causes of sterility, for the egg cannot reach the uterus. Sometimes, with a partially blocked tube, the sperm does reach the egg to fertilize it. But then the larger fertilized egg cannot get through the tubes to the uterus. A tubal pregnancy results, which can be terminated surgically.

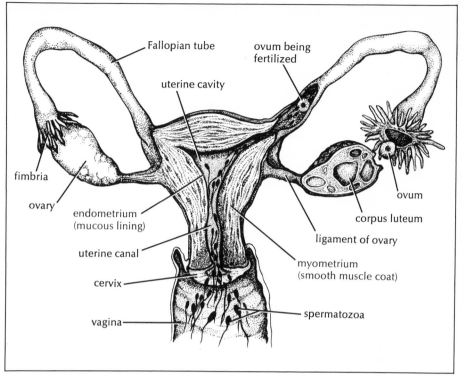

2-7 An ovum is shown leaving the ovary. The same ovum is shown later being fertilized in the upper Fallopian tube. The fertilized ovum (zygote) will cleave daily as it continues down the Fallopian tube to the uterus. After floating in the uterus for several days, it will be implanted in the uterine wall. It should be noted that this is a highly schematic representation.

which the egg came. At its lower end, each of these three- to five-inch tubes opens into the upper uterine cavity. At its upper end, each Fallopian tube lies close but not directly attached to its corresponding ovary. This free end of the Fallopian tube ends in fingerlike projections called *fimbria*. And it is the fimbria that draw the escaped ovum into the Fallopian tube. Now the ovum is ready to be fertilized, to make the journey to the uterus. Unlike the male sperm, however, it cannot move alone. By the gentle sweeping motions of hairlike cilia lining the Fallopian tube, and by waves of contractions passing along the tube itself, the ovum is helped along its way.

As the ovum begins its journey down the Fallopian tube, what goes on in the emptied follicle that remains behind in the ovary? Under the influence of LH it closes, grows to the size of a lima bean, and takes on a yellowish tint. Now it is called the *corpus luteum* (Latin *corporis,* body + *luteum,* yellow). Its future function depends on whether or not the ovum is fertilized.

If the ovum is not fertilized within forty-eight hours, it continues down the Fallopian tube to the uterus. There it disintegrates. Any remnant of it is eliminated through the vagina with the menstrual flow. The time period of ovum viability (its ability to be fertilized) has not been exactly determined. It is somewhere between twenty-four hours and about two days. In the ovary, triggered by LH, the corpus luteum produces the hormone *progesterone,* which means "to promote pregnancy." Indeed, this is its function. Acting upon the uterine endometrium, progesterone causes it to mature in preparation for a fertilized ovum. In the absence of fertilization, the corpus luteum continues to produce progesterone until late in the menstrual cycle. Not until about day twenty-five does the corpus luteum begin to degenerate to become a small depressed scar in the ovarian tissue. Progesterone is then diminished. Fragments of the uterine endometrium and mucus from the uterine glands slough off with an average of one to three ounces of menstrual blood. A new ovarian cycle is ready to begin.

If the ovum is fertilized (usually this happens in the upper portion of a Fallopian tube), the sequence of events is entirely different. Between two to four days are required for the trip of the fertilized ovum (the *zygote*) down the tube to the uterus. Once there, it is not immediately implanted. Several days may go by before the uterine endometrium is entirely ready. So it is about five to seven days following ovulation that implantation occurs. The elaborately prepared uterine endometrium receives the new life. The zygote is now an embryo. Implantation usually happens between day eighteen and day twenty-two. It may, however, occur as late as day twenty-three of the menstrual cycle.[10] After implantation, the membranes of the embryo produce a *gonadotropic hormone.* This hormone, like LH, stimulates the corpus luteum to produce progesterone.[11]

Indeed, with pregnancy the corpus luteum in the ovary continues its activity for twelve weeks before some of its functions are taken over by the *placenta* (afterbirth). By its timely continued production of estrogen and progesterone, it promotes persistent endometrial growth, so essential in sustaining the intrauterine being. It also prevents the maturation of new follicles. And this last fact makes

[10] This assumes ovulation occurs on about day fourteen. Add approximately two to four days in the Fallopian tube, and about another two to four days in the uterus. The subsequent history of the embryo is described in Chapter 6.

[11] Rarely, in about 1 in 350 pregnancies, implantation occurs outside the uterus. These are ectopic pregnancies (Greek *ektopos,* displaced). The extrauterine implantation most commonly occurs within a Fallopian tube, but it can take place in an ovary or even within the abdomen. Within the abdomen the developing embryo may be attached to the large intestine. Severe pain is usually the pregnant woman's first warning that her pregnancy is ectopic. With a pregnancy in the Fallopian tube, this pain usually occurs at about the sixth week. The cure is surgical. Almost all ectopic pregnancies fail to survive. Very rarely, an ectopic pregnancy results in a healthy baby. Perhaps the most unusual of all instances of misplaced pregnancies was reported from Hong Kong. "A three-month-old boy . . . had three fetuses removed from his abdominal cavity after his mother became suspicious of his swelling condition. Of the three fetuses one was 2 inches long and well formed." (Anthony Smith, *The Body* [New York, 1968], p. 109.)

possible the contraceptive "pill"—a synthetic chemical combination of progesterone and estrogen. Properly taken, the pill prevents ovulation (see Table 4-1).

the uterus and menstruation

The hollow uterus, about the size and shape of a pear, is a muscular pelvic organ. Nourished and sheltered in this abode, the developing child is an *embryo* for two months, then a *fetus,* and, upon birth, an *infant.* The upper part of the uterus, its *body,* is mostly muscle. During pregnancy, the uterus enlarges to about sixteen times its normal size. Its muscle enlarges enough to produce contractions adequate to help expel the baby. The smaller lower end of the uterus, the *cervix,* points downward and tilts slightly toward the back into the vagina. It can be felt by the woman and has the consistency of the tip of the nose. Its identification is important to the woman who uses a diaphragm for birth control. The physician can both see and feel the cervix with ease. This is fortunate, for it affords early diagnosis of cancer of the womb, which most commonly begins at this site. There are small mucous glands in the cervix that may become infected. Sometimes they become clogged, causing a mucoid discharge.

The uterus is loosely moored to the bony pelvis by tough fibrous bands called *ligaments.* It is thus suspended in the pelvic cavity between the bladder, in front, and the rectum, behind. The stretching of these ligaments during pregnancy may cause a pulling sensation in the groin. The enlarging pregnant uterus diminishes space for the bladder and rectum (see Figure 2-4). This explains the frequent urinary dribbling that occurs during late pregnancy and the importance of emptying both bladder and rectum to facilitate delivery of the child.

As has been mentioned, the endometrium (the lining of the uterine cavity) is elaborately prepared in anticipation of a viable fertilized egg. Hospitality for the fertilized egg is the basic function of the uterus. Under the influence of estrogen from the maturing ovarian follicle, the endometrium thickens. Fluid accumulates. Blood engorges the tissue. When, however, these preparations are met with naught but an unfertilized and, therefore, degenerating egg, the uterus bleeds. With *menstruation,* the excess endometrium loosens and is discharged, with the mucus from the uterine glands, through the cervical opening and vagina as blood-filled tissue.

Some untruths about menstruation   The Greeks, wrongly considering menstruation to be a cleansing process, called it *kathar-sis.* In the first century, Pliny the Elder wrote that menstrual blood dulled razors, and Aristotle thought menstruating women ruined mirrors. The early Hebrews punished those who had intercourse during menstruation (Leviticus 20:18). During medieval times, menstruating women were excluded from churches and wine cellars alike. In the latter case it was believed they would spoil the wine. Menstruating women are still segregated in "blood huts" by some African tribes. Child marriage developed among the Hindus because they incorrectly believed that the menstrual blood is essential for the embryo. To lose menstrual blood before pregnancy is still considered irreligious by many Hindus. Not long ago, in rural Russia, menstrual blood was collected in flasks by unmarried girls from as many village women as possible. It was then used by the village witch to determine fertility. Elsewhere in Europe a drop of menstrual blood used to be placed in a swain's wine to help him win the love of its owner.

Some truths about menstruation   During menstruation an absorbent pad is used to absorb the *menses,* or menstrual flow. It may be worn externally, although many women prefer an internal tampon. There is no reason whatsoever to limit physical activity during menstruation. Some couples have sexual intercourse during menstruation and there is usually no contraindication to this. The mild abdominal cramping that sometimes occurs during menstruation may require an aspirin or two, but usually even this is not necessary. Douching at the end of menstruation is neither necessary nor recommended. The action of normal vaginal bacteria maintains vaginal cleanliness and health. Because of fluid retention some women may gain a pound or two during the week before the onset of menstruation. This does not call for a change in diet; with the onset the weight is lost, as is an occasional heavy feeling in the pelvis and legs. *Premenstrual tension,* manifested by increased moodiness and irritability, even mild depression, is not uncommonly experienced during the few days prior to the onset of menstruation. These are not usually significant symptoms. In the case of a very few women, the mild physical discomfort and increased emotional sensitivity combine to make her a trial both to herself and to others. An occasional woman will even use this situation to gain sympathy. But such instances are quite rare. The very rare personality change associated with menstruation usually indicates other deeply rooted problems. The vast majority of young women handle their monthly menstrual periods as what they are—an entirely normal indication of femininity during the reproductive years.

   Dysmenorrhea, or painful menstruation, does not refer to the ordinary discomfort mentioned above; it is more severe. It may have a wide variety of causes, either physical, psychological, or both. *Menorrhagia* refers to excessive and usually prolonged uterine bleeding occurring at regular intervals. *Metrorrhagia* is uterine bleeding at completely irregular intervals. The amount may be normal; the flow may be prolonged. *Amenorrhea* refers to the cessation of menstruation before the menopause. Sudden changes in climate or emotional distress are among the variables that may cause a change in the amount of menstrual flow; a period may be delayed or may even be skipped because of such factors. Amenorrhea of longer duration is, of course, most commonly due to pregnancy. However, endocrine disorders or severe malnutrition and anemia may cause amenorrhea. Dysmenorrhea, menorrhagia, metrorrhagia, and prolonged amenorrhea all indicate prompt consultation with the family physician.

Normal differences among women   Women who desire to be different from other women surely accomplish this with their menstrual histories. The onset of menstruation (*menarche*) varies. On the average, as noted above, it occurs at about twelve-and-one-half years. First menstruations are usually irregular. They may not be associated with ovulation. Some girls menstruate for months or even years without ovulating; so the onset of menstruation does not always mean fertility has begun (see page 91). Abnormally early onsets of menstruation and ovulation are rare. Lena Medina, a classic case in medical history, was delivered of a healthy child when she was only five years and nine months old. An ovarian tumor accelerated her sexual maturity. Lena's pregnancy had been caused by rape.

Women normally differ as to the duration (one to six days, with an average of four or five days) and the amount (one to eight ounces, with an average of about two or three ounces) of menstrual bleeding. Individual women also vary from month to month in their onsets of bleeding. For women who calculate "safe periods" based on the first day of menstruation, it is essential to keep an accurate record of monthly onsets for at least a year.

An important note: *it is vital for a particular individual to know what is ordinary for her. Any marked departure is the signal for an immediate visit to a physician.* A gross change in menstruation, such as excessive bleeding or spotting between periods, may be of minor significance. It may, however, signify disease such as cancer that, treated early, is easily curable. The diagnosis of such cancers by means of the Papanicolaou test is a painless procedure.

The menopause   The age of the cessation of menstruation (*menopause*) varies widely. The U.S. average is about forty-nine. Some women may cease menstruating even before forty, though this is not common. Many women menstruate in their fifties. Although both ovulation and menstruation may stop abruptly, the menopause is usually not a sudden event. With most women, ovulation and menstruation taper off gradually; failure to realize this may result in pregnancy. Just as puberty is accompanied by body changes and the beginning of menstruation so is the menopause accompanied by body changes and the cessation of the function. The period in the woman's life that is begun by the menopause and during which she enters her postreproductive years is called the *climacteric*. (The diminution of male sexual activity is also called the climacteric.)

Two grossly cruel and senseless untruths about the menopause should be dismissed. First, the menopause does not herald old age. Second, it is not a common cause of insanity. Most menopausal women need no medical treatment. As a rule, sexual life continues. Frequently it improves. For many women, hot flashes and sweating are merely annoyances. With a considerable number, they do not occur. For a few, the symptoms, which occasionally include headaches and depression, do require some medical attention. Results of treatment are generally excellent. Her brood raised, her fear of pregnancy gone, relieved of some of her pressures, the postmenopausal woman can anticipate thirty or more happy, productive years.

A second important note: *the "flooding" of the menopause is not normal. To repeat: excessive bleeding and bleeding between periods (regardless of the time of life) always indicate immediate consultation with a physician. Delay has cost many a woman her life.*

the vagina

The *vagina* is a tube about three-and-one-half inches long. The vaginal walls are composed of muscle. The inner surface of the vagina is lined with transverse folds. During childbirth both muscle and folds expand tremendously. Cells from vaginal fluid are useful in determining not only the time of ovulation but also cancer of the uterus. In both instances the cells characteristically reflect these changes. In the virgin, the external opening of the vagina may be partially closed by a fold of mucous membrane called the *hymen* (see Figure 2-4). The hymen is frequently absent in females who have never had sexual intercourse. Rarely, the hymen interferes with the passage of menstrual blood. This is easily corrected by the physician. The normal reaction of the vagina is acid. A bacillus is involved in maintaining this normal reaction. If this acid reaction is not maintained, the vagina is prone to infection. Douching may be advised by a physician to encourage the acidity of the vagina. A woman should not douche unless so directed by her physician. Some popular douches not only harm delicate tissues but remove beneficial bacteria (see page 285).

the external genitalia (see Figure 2-4)

The *mons pubis* is a rounded fatty pad above the labia majora and over the front pubic region. The *pubes* refer to the hair growing over the pubic region.[12] The *labia majora* are skin folds that pass back-

---

[12] *Pubes* is also the plural of *pubis*, which refers to the pubic bone.

ward from the mons pubis. Like the mons they are fatty pads covered, in the adult, with hair. The *clitoris,* at the upper end of the labia minora, is extremely sensitive. Its sole purpose is to stimulate sexual desire. The *labia minora* are about as thick as a large rubber band. They arise from the clitoris and then pass backward and enclose an area called the *vestibule.* The *urethra* (leading from the urinary bladder) and vagina open into the vestibule, as do the *Bartholin's glands (vulvovaginal glands).* During more prolonged sexual excitement, the Bartholin's glands secrete a small amount of lubricating material; it should not be confused with the vaginal lubrication that occurs early (within seconds) in the woman's sexual response (see page 85). On either side of the opening of the female urethra are the several small *Skene's ducts.* These and the Bartholin's glands may easily become infected, particularly by the gonococcus.

the mammary glands

Before puberty there is little difference between the male and female breasts. In adult males they remain rudimentary. However, with the onset of puberty in the girl and the production of certain hormones by the ovaries, the breasts begin to develop. With each menstrual cycle the breasts enlarge slightly; they feel heavier, and the nipples are more sensitive. Just below the center of the adult female mammary gland is the raised *nipple,* surrounded by the circular pigmented *areola* (see Figure 2-8). Small openings on the surface of the nipple mark the openings of the ducts of the underlying glandular elements. With pregnancy, these are quite visible during the secretion of milk (*lactation*). The numerous small elevations on the areolar area are due to sebaceous glands. The breast structure is composed of about twenty distinct tubular glands or *lobes,* which, in turn, are composed of many *lobules.* The lobes are embedded in loose connective tissue and fat, which give the breast its shape. Each lobe eventually drains into the *lactiferous duct* of the nipple. Just before the duct terminates into the nipple it is dilated as a *lactiferous sinus.*

During pregnancy the nipples and areolae darken. Around the areola a secondary, lighter areola usually develops. The sebaceous glands of the areola enlarge. They are then called *Montgomery's glands.* They secrete an oily material that keeps the nipple supple and prevents the skin from cracking. Early in pregnancy a thin, scanty, yellow-white precursor of milk is secreted. This continues throughout the entire pregnant period. This secretion is called *colostrum.* During the first days of the baby's life, colostrum is a good food. Before the milk is produced, colostrum may be drawn off to stimulate milk flow. The sense of fullness and the tingling of the breasts, sometimes felt in the early months of pregnancy, soon abates.

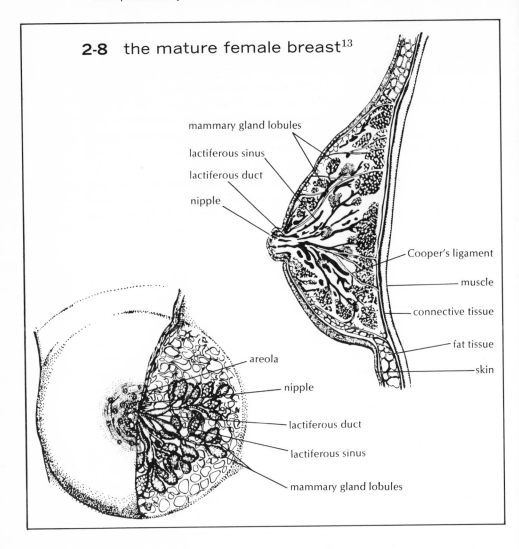

2-8 the mature female breast[13]

mammary gland lobules

lactiferous sinus

lactiferous duct

nipple

Cooper's ligament

muscle

connective tissue

fat tissue

skin

areola

nipple

lactiferous duct

lactiferous sinus

mammary gland lobules

Lactation: milk secretion   At times the lactating woman's provision of milk takes on economic overtones. Even today primitive women, such as the Papuans, suckle an infant at one breast as they suckle a wolf cub or a piglet at the other. In more civilized but stricken societies breast milk has been used to feed the starving adult.

[13]The significance of Cooper's ligaments has recently been reemphasized by two consultant surgeons. These fibrous attachments help to support the breasts. Without adequate brassiere support, the ligaments stretch as does the intrinsic connective tissue. This causes the breasts to droop. No amount of exercise will restore the ligaments. However, exercise may embellish breast contour (sagging or otherwise) by improving posture and increasing the thickness of the underlying pectoral muscle. Modern surgery can restore severely pendulous breasts. Patients who have had such surgery may find that they do not need brassieres as consistently as do other women. (John H. Wulsin and Milton T. Edgerton, "Cooper's Droop: Mystique of the Bra-Less Mamma Maligned," *Journal of the American Medical Association,* Vol. 219, No. 5 [January 31, 1972], p. 625. The term "Cooper's Droop" is credited to Dr. Carl Manion of the University of Kansas Medical Center.)

In John Steinbeck's *Grapes of Wrath,* Rose of Sharon smiles mysteriously as she feeds a starving migrant. Wet nurses have long profited from the prime value of their product. During two lactating periods, one woman not long ago expressed thirty thousand ounces of surplus milk that brought her $3,717.00. Another woman earned $2,020.00 for her twenty thousand ounces of surplus milk produced during only one lactation. Yet another wet nurse maintained seven babies at one time with her daily product.[14] The buyers are mothers who desire to feed their babies breast milk, but are unable to produce it in adequate amounts.

However, such mass-production and -distribution is not ordinarily desired or needed by the average mother who wishes to breast-feed her baby. Breast milk has been called the ideal food. Some of its advantages include its freedom from contamination, its immunity-imparting qualities, its cheapness, and its superior protein balance. In areas where sanitation is poor, such as the tropics, milk that does not come from the mother's breast may be so contaminated as to imperil the baby's life. Moreover, the colostrum of mother's milk contains antibodies that provide the child with immunity to various ailments. Breast-fed babies endure fewer respiratory infections. Among breast-fed babies, allergies are less common as is the likelihood of soreness about the anus. The protein balance of mother's milk is superior for the baby's growth to the protein balance of cow's milk, but there is little evidence that, in the long run, bottle-fed babies suffer as a result of this nutritional difference. Cow's milk contains more protein, thiamin, riboflavin, and calcium, but less iron and vitamin C. In the more affluent countries, the nutritional deficiencies of cow's milk are easily corrected with supplements. Also, although difficult to prove by controlled studies, many psychiatrists feel that, to a varying extent, bottle-feeding deprives both the child and mother of some psychological advantage that is gained by intimacy. But it is doubtless just as true that the mother who unhappily breast-feeds her baby has and gives a more harmful experience than the mother who happily bottle-feeds her baby.

Although the lactating mother must eat more to have an adequate milk supply, breast-feeding is probably cheaper. Breast-feeding may mean less work for the mother. True, the stools of bottle-fed babies are firm, and the looser stools of breast-fed babies make diapers more difficult to clean. But these days this advantage is negated by the use of disposable diapers. And breast-feeding obviates sterilization of bottles as well as measuring and mixing and warming the feed.

There are also some disadvantages to breast-feeding that should be considered. Not uncommonly, breast-fed babies are underfed, a fact that may never occur to the willing mother. This may be due to an inadequate milk supply. The drugs and chemicals to which the

[14]Ronald S. Illingsworth, *The Normal Child* (Boston, 1968), p. 13.

mother is exposed and that then pass into her milk constitute a serious modern problem. The nursing mother should be extremely careful about drug use, for her milk may become dangerously contaminated. The toxicity of a drug depends, in part, on body weight. A safe dose for the mother may be an unsafe dose for her breast-fed baby. Among those drugs that should be used with caution or not at all are alcohol, tobacco, oral contraceptives, and marijuana. A daily cocktail or two is not a contraindication to breast-feeding. More alcohol may be. Mothers who drink excessively rarely want to breast-feed their babies anyway. The woman who smokes heavily should not breast-feed her baby because of the toxicity of the nicotine. Oral contraceptives interfere with the production of milk and should not be used by nursing mothers. The effects of marijuana on a baby are unknown—reason enough to contraindicate its use by the mother who desires to breast-feed her child. Although in the future contamination of the mother's milk by DDT or radiation may become a problem, there is not enough evidence to indicate that present levels of DDT or radiation in the environment are high enough to make mother's milk dangerous to the child.

"Do you perhaps think," mused the ancient Greek physician Favorinus, "that nature gave women nipples as a kind of beauty spot, not for the purpose of nourishing their children?" [15] The venerable doctor had dry wit. He doubtless knew that the female nipples and breasts provide nourishment for both sexuality and the baby belly. The male's nipples are also sexually sensitive to stimulation. (For a discussion of the function of the female and male breasts in human eroticism, see page 59.)

the structure and function of the erogenous zones

> Without shame the man I like knows and avows the
>   deliciousness of his sex,
> Without shame the woman I like knows and avows hers. [16]

In Chapter 1 it was pointed out that by resolving the tasks of life the human personality grows in adequacy and competency. A sense of adequacy and competence lends confidence to the striving individual. So it is with sexual expression. To achieve a feeling of adequacy, to enjoy competence and confidence in one's sexual life, requires creative learning. This does not mean that every sexual encounter becomes a test of competence. It does mean that sexual expression can become infinitely more satisfying when one approaches the encounter with a confidence based on a growing

---

[15] Aulus Gellius, *Noctes Attica,* Book XII, Chapter 5, section 7.
[16] Walt Whitman, "A Woman Waits for Me," lines 9-10.

knowledge of what to do. Self-esteem is a primary goal of personality development. Sexual competence, a belief in one's own sexuality, grows from a sense of self-esteem—and adds to it, too.

From the earliest moments of life the human infant gains the pleasures of love via the nervous system. Touch, pressure, and body contact stimulate nerve endings called the *end organs of touch.* These nerve endings are distributed throughout the skin and some of the body's deeper organs. Certain of these nerve endings are organized in a unique way. Some parts of the adult body are so richly supplied with these uniquely structured end organs of touch that, under certain circumstances, their stimulation leads to sexual excitement. These are the *erogenous zones.* However, the human being can learn to be sexually excited as a result of the stimulation of a wide variety of end organs of touch that are not strictly within the erogenous zones. The sensitivity of the erogenous zones varies greatly with different people, but touch is part of the language of love. As two lovers seek to discover one another's erogenous zones, they embark on an adventure in intimacy. The explorations and discoveries, the givings and takings of love can bring about a transcendent and mystical enthrallment in which (as the poet John Milton wrote) two people are "Imparadis'd in one anothers arms."[17]

THE SKIN OF THE PENIS

Not all parts of the penile skin are equally sensitive to the touch. The skin of the head of the penis (*glans*) is far more sensitive than that of the body (*shaft*). The under surface of the glans penis is especially sensitive to stimulation. Gently holding the penile shaft, the woman may stroke the penile head. This is a sexually exciting stimulus for almost all men. Despite the lesser sensitivity of the shaft, it may also be caressed and stroked if the man so desires. For those individuals who enjoy oral-genital contact, stimulation may, of course, be carried out with the lips, tongue, and mouth.

THE CLITORIS

The latest edition of the *Oxford English Dictionary* defines the *clitoris* as a "homologue of the male penis [which is correct] present, as a rudimentary organ, in the females of many of the higher vertebrata [which is incorrect]." The female clitoris is the anatomic *homologue* of the male penis in that it is an organ that is similar in structure,

---

[17] John Milton, *Paradise Lost,* Book IV, line 506.

For some people, the sheer pleasure of being held is paramount. "For some at times and for a small number always, being held is the major sexual aim." For great numbers of people it is a source of warmth, comfort, and security that is a prelude to coitus. (Marc H. Hollender, "Women's Wish to be Held: Sexual and Nonsexual Aspects," *Medical Aspects of Human Sexuality,* Vol. 5, No. 10 [October 1971], p. 26.)

position, and embryologic origin to the penis. It is not a rudiment of the penis. The penis develops from the same embryonic cells as the clitoris (see page 80). The clitoris is functionally unique. No male organ has the single purpose of initiating and increasing sexual desire.

Like the penis, the clitoris is made up of a head (glans) and a body (shaft). There is considerable difference among women in the size and shape of both the head and the body of the clitoris. Again like the penis, the clitoral body contains considerable vascular tissue, but the head is more lavishly supplied with sensitive nerve endings. However, clitoral response to sexual stimulation does not occur as rapidly as does penile erection. With stimulation, vaginal lubrication precedes the clitoral reaction. The first male response to sexual stimulation is penile erection; in the woman the first response is vaginal lubrication. Covering the clitoris is the prepuce (see Figure 2-4), which is formed by the highly sensitive merging labia minora and is also richly supplied with nerve endings.

The clitoris may be stimulated either directly or indirectly. Direct clitoral stimulation occurs when the head or shaft of the clitoris is manipulated. Indirect stimulation, which results in a slower clitoral response, may occur when, for instance, the breasts and vagina are stimulated or when the woman engages in sexual fantasies. During coitus, direct stimulation occurs easily only with the female-superior or with the face-to-face positions. Direct stimulation of the clitoris does not occur with the male-superior position; in this position satisfactory clitoral stimulation is achieved in an indirect fashion by the traction caused by the thrusting penis. Moreover, it has been observed that masturbating women actively continue to manipulate the clitoral shaft or mons area throughout the entire orgasm. Such continued stimulation is also sought by the woman during coitus. In this the average male differs; during the latter part of his orgasmic experience (see page 87), he usually discontinues his rapid thrusting.

In order to determine how the clitoris should be stimulated to increase female sexual tension, and how much, Masters and Johnson studied the masturbatory techniques of hundreds of women.[18] Those women who employed direct clitoral manipulation as a masturbatory technique usually concentrated on the shaft. Rarely did they manipulate the head of the clitoris; the few women who did usually applied a lubricant first and limited their manipulations to the excitement phase. Most women, however, avoided direct clitoral manipulation when they masturbated; instead, they preferred to stimulate the general mons area. The orgasm resulting from mons area stimulation is brought about more slowly than that occurring from clitoral manipulation, but it is just as satisfying. So sensitive is the clitoral

[18]William H. Masters and Virginia E. Johnson, *Human Sexual Response*, pp. 63-64.

head immediately after an orgasm that the woman who desires re-stimulation is careful to avoid touching it. It is, therefore, not true that the clitoris must be directly stimulated in order to bring all women to orgasm. Indeed, there are women who have undergone necessary surgical procedures that involve removal of the clitoris and who are still able to achieve orgasm. The stimulation of a wide variety of areas can induce orgasm in either sex. Many women find direct clitoral stimulation distinctly unpleasant. Moreover, "many well-adjusted women enjoy a minimum of three or four orgasmic experiences before they reach apparent satiation."[19] An understanding of clitoral structure, function, and sensitivity is essential for the sexual fulfillment of both sexes. Misconceptions concerning the clitoris are as common as those about the penis. Some of these are discussed on pages 102–05.

THE LABIA AND THE SCROTUM AND TESTES

Part of the skin of the penile shaft is homologous to the female labia minora. Both the inside and outside of the labia minora are extremely sensitive to stimulation; indeed, manipulation of the labia is often included in the woman's masturbatory activities. The outer thicker lips of the female genitalia, the labia majora, are homologous to the scrotum of the human male. Neither the skin of the male scrotum nor the female labia majora are markedly sensitive to sexual stimuli. (The testes within the scrotum may respond to erotic stimuli; however, manipulation of the testes should be gentle—for many men the difference between pain and pleasure in this area is indeed slight.)

THE VAGINAL VESTIBULE AND THE WOMAN'S MOST EROGENOUS ZONE

The woman also finds the vaginal vestibule singularly receptive to stimulation. One may delineate a small and contiguous area of the female genitalia that is almost always sensitive to erotic stimuli. This area is composed of the vaginal vestibule into which the vagina opens; the labia minora, which on both sides continue inwardly into the vaginal vestibule; and the clitoris, above. Also included in this sensitive area is the prepuce, which partly covers the clitoris. The prepuce is formed by the merging labia minora. Including the mons with this area would delineate those parts of the female body that are ordinarily most sensitive to sexual stimuli.

The various ways by which these zones may be effectively stimulated are entirely a matter for the couple to decide. Most women are aroused by a gentle finger stroking the area. A great number find intense pleasure when the clitoris or clitoral area is kissed and

[19] Ibid., p. 65.

licked (*cunnilinction,* see page 89). It should be remembered that, as the woman nears the height of her sexual pleasure, the clitoris withdraws under its hood (prepuce). Direct contact with it is then impossible (see page 85).

OTHER EROGENOUS AREAS NEAR THE GENITALIA

However, with a considerable number of women, the sexual sensitivity of the genitalia is hardly limited to these specific locations. Some women also find the upper walls of the vagina, just inside the vaginal entrance, sensitive. When this is the case, the woman may insert a finger into the vagina and press into that area to heighten her sexual pleasure. Moreover, also just beyond the vaginal entrance, and at the base of the clitoris, lies a ring of powerful muscles. Most women find pressure on these muscles sexually pleasurable. The muscles may also be used to heighten the man's pleasure. The woman can learn to rhythmically contract and relax them about the thrusting penis. This erotic signal by an intensely participating partner can do much to bring about masculine satisfaction.

So bereft of sensory nerves is most of the human vagina that the surgeon can often operate on its surface without the use of anesthesia. However, some women experience pleasure as a result of deep vaginal penetration by the penis. Moreover, this pleasure is unlike that provided by the stimulated clitoris or labia minora. Between the anus and the genitalia of both sexes lies the *perineal area.* In both sexes the perineal surface skin is sensitive to stimulation. Beneath the perineal surface skin and fat is a mass of muscle and nerve. When the penis is thrust deeply and vigorously into the vagina, it may press against this mass. The woman is thus erotically stimulated. (For the same anatomic reason, such perineal pleasure can be obtained by some men as a result of pressure applied at a point midway between the scrotum and anus.) Within the vagina, the protruding cervix has few or no sensory nerves on its surface. Like the deeper vaginal walls, the cervical surface may be operated on without anesthesia. It is, therefore, usually totally uninvolved in erotic feeling.

Since the anus and the genitalia share the same muscles, stimulation of one affects the other. Some people find anal stimulation erotically gratifying. Anal intercourse is common among men whose behavior is homosexual. Because the anus is closed off by muscular sphincters, anal intercourse may be painful. It also results in the above-mentioned stimulating pressure on the pelvic muscles and nerves. Sometimes anal intercourse is practiced as a variety of heterosexual intercourse. Some people induce orgasms via the anus using an enema. It has been noted that an increasing number of people seem to be "investigating the rectum as a sexual equivalent."[20] Re-

[20] Gerald Mason Feigen, "Erotic Potential of Enemas," *Medical Aspects of Human Sexuality,* Vol. 4, No. 4 (April 1972), p. 199.

portedly, King Louis XIV had two thousand enemas during his lifetime. Since he was provided with many alternatives, it is doubtful that this was his single source of erotic stimulation.[21]

THE EROTICALLY SENSITIVE BREASTS

The Kinsey group noted that "there is reason to believe that more males in our culture are psychically aroused by contemplation of the female breast than by the sight of the genitalia"[22]—a fact noted with immense profit by the publishers of girlie magazines. Both the female and male nipples may be sensitive to manual and oral manipulation. Indeed the woman may occasionally experience erotic pleasure, even orgasm, as she breast-feeds her baby. This is not an uncommon reaction. For many people in this culture manual and oral stimulation of the breast is an important part of foreplay. The breasts and nipples may be kissed, sucked, or titillated with the tongue. A very small percentage of women are able to be brought to orgasm in this way without genital contact. Some women are not erotically stimulated by breast manipulation, and most are only moderately aroused.[23]

ORAL AND OTHER EROTIC AREAS

The mouth—lips, tongue, and interior—ranks with the genital area as one of the two most erotic zones of the human body. This is true of all mammals and other vertebrates as well. That deep-kissing, oral-breast, and oral-genital contact are so commonly a part of human sexual expression is hardly surprising. People who purposely limit their oral sexuality are responding to their cultural conditioning—not to their biology.[24]

During sexual excitement the ear lobes become engorged with blood. Some people respond erotically to stimulation of the ear lobe or the rest of the external ear, and of the external part of the auditory canal. Excitation of the lobes by sucking or by lingual stimulation can bring a few people of either sex to orgasm.

[21] Felix Marti-Ibañez, "Two Windows on Medical History," *M.D., Medical Newsmagazine*, Vol. 14, No. 2 (February 1970), p. 16.
[22] Alfred C. Kinsey, Wardell B. Pomeroy, and Clyde E. Martin, *Sexual Behavior in the Human Male*, (Philadelphia, 1948), p. 575.
[23] Alfred C. Kinsey, Wardell B. Pomeroy, Clyde E. Martin, and Paul H. Gebhard, *Sexual Behavior in the Human Female* (Philadelphia, 1953), pp. 587, 592.
[24] Kissing has been called a "salute by tasting . . . Just to distinguish it from salute by touching which involves such advances as handshaking, and 'salute by smelling' which is where the Eskimoes come in." The adult Japanese do not kiss, at least not publicly, and the Chinese "regard a kiss as suggestive of cannibalism." The world's record of eighteen hours of continuous kissing was recently broken by four Australian student teachers. During their twenty-four-hour kiss they danced, ate chocolate, and managed to clean their (each other's?) teeth. (Patrick Ryan, "And the Last Word . . . on Kissing," *New Scientist and Science Journal*, Vol. 50, No. 757 [June 24, 1971], p. 730.)

Always depending on who is being stimulated, how, by whom, and under what conditions, a wide variety of other body areas are known to be sexually sensitive. The sensitivity of these areas is not due to any special characteristics of the nerves; it is usually a learned phenomenon. Stimulation of the skin of the buttocks, thighs (particularly the inner surfaces), legs, feet, soles, abdomen, navel area, armpits, arms—all may bring about sexual arousal in both men and women. Many people enjoy having their hands and fingers kissed and sucked. Kinsey and his group, who were among the first to make a thorough study of the erogenous zones, have reported erotic stimulation involving the hair and the teeth—both of which have nerve endings at their roots. Some women have been brought to orgasm "by having their eyebrows stroked, or by having the hairs on some other part of their bodies gently blown, or by having pressures applied on the teeth alone. This may be a factor in the biting which often accompanies sexual activities."[25] As is to be expected, such stimuli are most effective when accompanied by others that are of a psychological and physical nature. Some women have certain nerve reflexes that are so highly sensitive that lingual stimulation of the external ear canal or the nape of the neck brings about orgasm. Breast and nipple stimulation alone may induce orgasms in some women. So rich may be the stimulus of a favorite musical composition to a woman that she may enjoy an orgasm while listening to it.

Orgasmic reactions may thus be stimulated in a wide variety of ways.[26] All lend possible enrichments to human sexual expression.

sexually transmitted diseases

THE MAJOR VENEREAL DISEASES

historical notes

"Because the daughters of Zion, . . . walk with stretched forth necks, and wanton eyes . . . the Lord will smite with a scab the crown of the head . . . and . . . will discover their secret parts" (Isaiah 3:16-17). Long ago, then, the ancient Hebrews considered venereal disease (probably syphilis) a divine punishment for sexual trans-

---

[25] Alfred C. Kinsey et al., *Sexual Behavior in the Human Female,* p. 590.

[26] Recent brain research at Tulane University has revealed some interesting information in this respect. In certain patients, electrodes were implanted and left in a selected area of the brain. These electrodes were connected to levers so that the patients could stimulate different brain structures. "One of these patients would have a most pleasant feeling when he stimulated the septal region. It made him feel as if he were building up to a sexual orgasm. He was unable to achieve the orgastic end point, however, and explained that his frequent, sometimes frantic, pushing at the septal button was an attempt to reach a 'climax' although at times this was frustrating and produced a 'nervous feeling.' Another patient also found that stimulation in this region made him 'feel wonderful'; it gave him sexual thoughts." (Peter Nathan, *The Nervous System* [Philadelphia and New York, 1969], p. 243.)

gression. "Thy bones are hollow," wrote Shakespeare, somewhat piously, many centuries later, "impiety has made a feast of thee."[27] In the bard's bawdy day, the houses of prostitution were located in London's theater district. Elizabethan plays made frequent mention of syphilis. The "French pox," it was often called. French writers preferred the word *venereal* (Latin *venereus,* pertaining to Venus, the goddess of love). But they were outnumbered. Outside of France, the "Gallic Disease" was perhaps the most common medical reference to the malady.

Syphilis gives still more evidence that microbes know no borders. Two years after Columbus discovered America, Charles VIII of France (1470-98), seeking a Byzantine Empire, invaded Italy and laid siege to Naples. At that time the port city was being defended by Spaniards. Like all armies of that era, the Spanish army was accompanied by a host of harlots. Many of these women, it was thought, had been infected by sailors formerly with Columbus. If the account of the sixteenth-century anatomist Fallopius is to be believed (and it is not by everyone), the Spanish deliberately sent their infected women to meet the French army. This unmilitary maneuver succeeded. The soldiers of the French army lost no time in meeting the harlots. They caught syphilis.[28]

Too diseased to fight, the French army retreated. In dispersing, they spread their disease throughout Europe. The Italians and Spanish called the affliction the "French disease." To the French, it was, at first, the "Neapolitan disease" and then the "Spanish sickness." The Germans named the malady the "Polish pocks." The Poles retaliated with "German pox." Bitterly remembering the Crusades, the unforgiving Turks called it the "disease of the Christians." To others, it could only be the "Persian fire." Finally, in 1530, an Italian medical man and poet, Girolamo Fracastorius, wrote of a shepherd, Syphilus, who aroused the ire of the sun god by worshiping at an altar of his king. In jealous anger, the sun god sent a plague to earth. Syphilus was its first victim. The disease was thus named, if not claimed.

Often contracted together, syphilis and gonorrhea were, at first, incorrectly thought to be different manifestations of one disease. An eccentric eighteenth-century Scottish surgeon, John Hunter, did not help matters. Deliberately, he infected himself. "Two punctures were made on the penis with a lancet dipped in venereal matter from a gonorrhea."[29] Apparently he got more than he experimented for. Developing both gonorrhea and syphilis, he carefully and wrongly described them as one disease. Another—less heroic—Scottish physician, Benjamin Bell, inoculated his students and learned from them

---

[27] William Shakespeare, *Measure for Measure,* I.ii.60-61.
[28] Gabriel Fallopius, *On Gallic Disease,* quoted in Herbert Silvette, *The Doctor on the Stage* (Knoxville, Tenn., 1967), p. 196.
[29] Greer Williams, *Virus Hunters* (New York, 1959), p. 18.

the reproductive system: structure, function, dysfunction—and sexual sensitivity

TABLE 2-1 natural history of acquired syphilis

DISEASE	RESERVOIR FOR AGENT	CAUSATIVE AGENT	INCUBATION PERIOD	MODE OF TRANSMISSION	IMMUNITY
Syphilis	Man	*Treponema pallidum* (a spirochete)	10–90 days, usually 21 days following exposure.	Direct physical contact, usually during sexual relations	A vaccine to prevent syphilis recently proved successful in rabbits. Hopes are high that a successful vaccine to prevent human syphilis will soon be available.

the disease process

Syphilis The first sign of *primary syphilis* is usually a single, painless sore called a *chancre*. Most often it appears at the place where the germs enter the body—the genital area. Sometimes this chancre does not appear or is overlooked, especially in women. If it does appear, it disappears without treatment in about two weeks. In a short time, which may vary from a few weeks to six months, *secondary syphilis* signs appear. The disease is then no longer local. The entire body is infected. Although different people have different symptoms, the most common are lesions, which may be few or many, large or small, and which may appear on various body areas. There may be a widespread rash. This is not common; frequently it is absent. This rash, and the chancre that preceded it, teems with spirochetes. Whitish patches in the mouth or throat, "moth eaten" or "patchy" falling hair, low fever, painless swelling of lymph glands, and pain in bones and joints may

all be signs of secondary syphilis. While the *primary* and *secondary* manifestations persist, the disease is highly contagious. Lesions in moist body areas, such as the mouth, anus, or genitals are most contagious. Without treatment, the secondary symptoms often disappear in less than a month although they may persist for a longer period.* The disease then enters a period of *early latency*. The degree of communicability associated with *early latent syphilis* is governed by the recurrence of secondary lesions. Because of such a possibility, the disease is considered communicable for approximately two years following initial infection. The final category, *noncommunicable late latent syphilis,* may eventually cause heart disease, insanity, paralysis, blindness, or death. These end results of untreated syphilis may not take place until ten to thirty years after the primary infection. Often they do not occur.

* The chancre of primary syphilis and the signs and symptoms of secondary syphilis disappear by themselves without treatment. This accounts for the "success" of the quack. His phony treatments "cure" these signs and symptoms. But the patient is left with the destructive living spirochetes in his body.

Source: Gerald A. Heidbreder, Health Officer, County of Los Angeles Health Department.

that the diseases were clinically different. In Dublin, William Wallace inoculated healthy patients to prove that the rash of syphilis was contagious.[30] Not until the gonococcus was identified (in 1879) and the *Treponema pallidum* discovered (in 1905) were gonorrhea and syphilis proved to be diseases caused by different microorganisms.

syphilis and gonorrhea

There are five different venereal diseases. In this country, the most important are syphilis and gonorrhea. They are described in Tables 2-1 and 2-2. The other three—chancroid, lymphogranuloma venereum, and granuloma inguinale—are infrequently seen in this country.

[30] R. S. Morton, *Venereal Diseases* (Harmondsworth, Eng., 1966), p. 21.

TABLE 2-2 natural history of acquired gonorrhea

DISEASE	RESERVOIR FOR AGENT	CAUSATIVE AGENT	INCUBATION PERIOD	MODE OF TRANSMISSION	IMMUNITY
Gonorrhea	Man	*Neisseria gonorrheae,* the gonococcus (a bacterium)	Within 3–8 days (often less) following exposure for 85% of males; 2–8 days for females when symptoms occur.	Usually sexual intercourse. Practically never from toilet seats, towels, or other objects.	Meaningful results of field trials of a vaccine against gonorrhea will not be available until at least mid-1973.

the disease process

Gonorrhea is a local disease of the body parts affected. Unlike syphilis, it is usually not a body-wide or systemic disease. In the male, the disease manifests itself as a burning on urination and a discharge of pus. The disease is quite painful. Discomfort may force the male patient to seek medical attention. A man may have gonorrhea without symptoms. Although not very common, *chronic* male gonorrhea may lead to involvement of other portions of the body, particularly the urinary or generative system and may, if not treated early, produce sterility. In the female, the early symptoms of gonorrhea are usually absent or very mild. For this reason, the infected female rarely seeks early treatment. Progression of the disease often leads to infection of the Fallopian tubes, ovaries, and lower abdomen. In this event, pain is severe. Due to scarring and closure of the tubes, or to emergency surgery, sterility often results. Rectal infection can occur in both sexes. This occurs more commonly among men whose sexual behavior is homosexual. It is seldom recognized because its symptoms consist only of a sensation of wetness or itching around the anus (see page 67).

Source: Gerald A. Heidbreder, Health Officer, County of Los Angeles Health Department.

the v.d. problem: extent and causes

The estimated total number of people with infectious syphilis and gonorrhea in the world today roughly equals the population of the United States. Worldwide, about 50 million people have infectious syphilis, 150 million gonorrhea. The risk of acquiring venereal disease seems to be taken rather casually in general. "In a series of 20,000 cases of gonorrhea seen at Paris' St. Louis Hospital, the youngest patient was 12 years old. He had been taken to a Paris brothel by his father for initiation, caught gonorrhea, and his father paid the hospital bill. The oldest patient was an 84-year-old man who had been taken to the brothel by his son. He contracted gonorrhea and his son paid for him."[31]

In the United States, the problem does not seem to be regarded any more seriously. The major reason for this attitude is the discovery, in 1943, that a single massive dose of penicillin cured most early syphilis as well as gonorrhea. This led to a deemphasis of previously energetic venereal disease control programs. Contact tracing, the search for those people who were sources of new infections, was no longer considered of paramount importance. This policy turned out to be a grievous error. People came to believe that penicillin was

[31] "The Last Word—It Could Happen Only in Paris," *Family Health,* Vol. 4, No. 2 (February 1972), p. 64.

the reproductive system: structure, function, dysfunction—and sexual sensitivity

TABLE 2-3

primary and secondary syphilis and gonorrhea

Reported Cases and Rates per 100,000 Population
United States, Fiscal Years 1957, 1963–1971

| | Primary and Secondary Syphilis | | |
YEAR	NUMBER OF REPORTED CASES	RATE PER 100,000 POPULATION	PERCENT CHANGE FROM PREVIOUS YEAR
1957	6,251	3.8	—
1963	22,045	11.9	+ 9.8
1964	22,733	12.1	+ 3.1
1965	23,250	12.3	+ 2.3
1966	22,473	11.6	− 3.3
1967	21,090	10.8	− 6.1
1968	20,182	10.3	− 4.3
1969	18,679	9.3	− 7.4
1970	20,186	10.0	+ 8.1
1971	23,336	11.5	+15.6

| | Gonorrhea | | |
YEAR	NUMBER OF REPORTED CASES	RATE PER 100,000 POPULATION	PERCENT CHANGE FROM PREVIOUS YEAR
1957	216,476	129.8	—
1963	270,076	145.7	+ 3.7
1964	290,603	154.5	+ 7.6
1965	310,155	163.8	+ 6.7
1966	334,949	173.6	+ 8.0
1967	375,606	193.0	+12.1
1968	431,380	219.2	+14.8
1969	494,227	245.9	+14.6
1970	573,200	285.2	+16.0
1971	624,371	307.5	+ 8.9

Source: "Today's VD Control Problem: 1972," American Social Health Association: Committee on the Joint Statement (New York, 1972), p. 11. Data from USDHEW, Public Health Service, HSMHA, Center for Disease Control, Atlanta, Georgia.

insurance against venereal disease. For some years in the United States there was a downward trend in syphilis cases, but in 1970 the number of cases began to rise. In the case of gonorrhea in the United States, the downward trend reversed itself in 1959, and the rates have climbed steadily since that time. Major urban areas experienced an increased rate of infectious cases of both syphilis and gonorrhea in 1971, as compared with 1970 (see Table 2-4). The late autumn months of 1972 still saw no decline in the epidemic of gonorrhea in the United States, and the rate of infectious syphilis was still rising. Yet the alarming rates do not tell the whole story. The data refer to reported cases. A 1968 survey indicated that private physicians were treating 80 percent of all syphilis and gonorrhea cases diagnosed,

TABLE 2-4

primary and secondary syphilis and gonorrhea

Reported Cases and Percent
Increase or Decrease
Selected Metropolitan Areas, Fiscal Years 1970 & 1971

Primary and Secondary Syphilis

CITIES	REPORTED 1970	CASES 1971	PERCENT CHANGE
Baltimore	270	330	+ 22.2
Las Vegas	89	127	+ 42.7
Los Angeles	942	1,411	+ 49.8
Louisville	58	193	+232.8
Memphis	60	136	+126.7
Miami	263	520	+ 97.7
Newark	367	485	+ 32.2
New York	3,124	3,940	+ 26.1
Oakland	88	120	+ 36.4
San Francisco	386	575	+ 47.7
United States	20,186	23,336	+ 15.6

Gonorrhea

CITIES	REPORTED 1970	CASES 1971	PERCENT CHANGE
Birmingham	2,871	3,685	+ 28.4
Chicago	44,367	39,354	− 11.3
Dallas	12,259	14,761	+ 20.4
Dayton	1,530	2,158	+ 41.0
Denver	2,678	3,202	+ 19.6
Indianapolis	4,136	3,866	− 6.5
Kansas City	4,951	6,032	+ 21.8
Los Angeles	41,639	39,987	− 4.0
Memphis	8,706	11,293	+ 29.7
New Haven	1,468	1,895	+ 29.1
New York	37,399	36,562	− 2.2
Oklahoma City	1,739	2,608	+ 50.0
Richmond, Va.	1,928	2,981	+ 54.6
San Diego	3,347	4,396	+ 31.3
San Francisco	15,362	14,592	− 5.0
Washington, D.C.	13,569	11,197	− 17.5
United States	573,200	624,371	+ 8.9

Source: "Today's VD Control Problem: 1972," American Social Health Association: Committee on the Joint Statement (New York, 1972), p. 12.

but were reporting less than one-fifth of them.[32] Thus, the reported cases show only the tip of the iceberg that is the problem.

[32]"International Venereal Disease Symposium," *Modern Medicine*, Vol. 39, No. 12 (June 14, 1971), p. 61.

A basic reason for the physicians' reluctance to report their venereal disease cases to the health department for contact tracing is their unwarranted concern that the traditional physician-patient confidence will thus be abrogated.

Venereal disease is particularly frequent among the young. In 1971, the majority of cases were reported in persons under twenty-five years of age. In the County of Los Angeles, for example (where the rate of gonorrhea has increased some four-and-one-half times the rate of population increase), gonorrhea is increasing among teen-agers at twice the rate of other age groups. The repeat-rate of gonorrheal infection is striking. Two, three, four, and even more gonorrheal infections per year in one person are common. Alexander Fleming, who discovered penicillin, is reported to have remarked "We have made it possible to catch gonorrhea three times a week."[33]

Several interrelated factors seem to be responsible for the epidemic. Changes in sexual behavior, the greater availability of contraceptives, and homosexual behavior are among the causes that relate to the individual who contracts venereal diseases. It is of interest to note that the average V.D. patient whose behavior is homosexual names ten contacts, while the average patient whose behavior is heterosexual names only four. The environment has also changed; societal factors influencing the rise of venereal disease include increased population mobility, widespread employment of women accompanied by their increased financial and sexual independence, the drug culture, and increased sexual permissiveness as evidenced by the diminution of restraints formerly exercised by religion, the family, and public opinion. Added to these societal factors is a shift from public clinics as the major treatment centers of venereal disease to private physicians, who do not have adequate facilities to engage in contact tracing. One of the microbial agents has also changed; the microbe that causes gonorrhea is increasingly resistant to antibiotics, especially penicillin.[34]

homosexual behavior and venereal disease[35]

Among people whose behavior is homosexual, venereal disease is much more commonly spread between men than women. Although many men with a homosexual orientation are sexually indiscriminate, the majority are not and so are seldom exposed to venereal disease. The rate of venereal disease infection among homosexually oriented men is roughly proportional to their incidence in the population. As is the case with individuals whose behavior is heterosexual, the ways that syphilis is transmitted among those whose behavior is homosexual depends on the anatomic site of the infectious lesions. The untreated primary and secondary lesions of syphilis teem with spiro-

[33]Arthur S. Wigfield, "Attitudes to Venereal Disease in a Permissive Society," *British Medical Journal,* Vol. 4, No. 5783 (November 6, 1971), p. 343.
[34]Nicholas J. Fiumara, "Factors in VD Increase," *Medical Aspects of Human Sexuality,* Vol. 5, No. 3 (March 1971), pp. 216, 220.
[35]Warren A. Ketterer, "Homosexuality and Venereal Disease," *Medical Aspects of Human Sexuality,* Vol. 5, No. 3 (March 1971), pp. 114, 118-21, 126-29.

chetes. Among males "the insertion with primary or secondary lesions of the penis, tongue, or perhaps the finger, can infect the mouth, genitalia or rectum of the recipient insertee. Conversely, syphilitic lesions of the insertee can infect the probing organ of the insertor."[36] The symptoms of syphilis have been described above (see Table 2-1).

Gonorrhea among homosexually oriented males has more limited methods of transmission than among males whose behavior is heterosexual. Gonorrhea due to oral-genital contact is infrequent (see pages 76-77). The major mode of transmission among homosexually oriented men is anal intercourse. The signs and symptoms of gonorrhea of the penile urethra have been described above (see Table 2-2). As is the case with gonorrheal infection of the female reproductive organs, gonorrhea of the male rectum is usually without symptoms for several months. During that time, the infected male is an inadvertent source of the disease. When symptoms do appear, they vary considerably. Some men experience a feeling of moistness about the rectum and anus. Others have some discomfort with bowel movements. Less frequently there is pain about the rectum, and a discharge of pus and even blood from the rectum accompanied by varying degrees of pain, diarrhea, and a burning sensation.

a silent epidemic

Both syphilis and gonorrhea are more commonly reported in males. Although the primary sore, or chancre, of syphilis neither hurts nor generally itches, the man can usually see it. Very often, however, the primary chancre may be absent or be so insignificant as to be missed. The male, moreover, most often sees a gonorrheal discharge, and his pain on urination may drive him to a physician. By no means, however, is this always true. In one study of 124 males brought to treatment by contact tracing, 61 percent had symptoms but had not sought medical advice.[37] Nor do all males with gonorrhea have symptoms; investigators report asymptomatic gonorrhea in 12 to 30 percent of men examined.[38] Not only do these men spread their disease, but they risk serious complications, such as gonorrheal inflammation of the joints, heart, and meninges.

For the female, syphilis and gonorrhea are a special risk. Because of her anatomy, the woman may more readily miss a syphilitic infection than the male. Her external genitalia are not as visible to her; much of the vagina and the cervical surface are without nerves. Her infection is most often located in the opening of the womb—the

[36] Ibid., p. 118.

[37] "Many Males with Symptoms of GC do not Seek Therapy, CDC States," *VD Clinical News,* Vol. 2, No. 1 (January-February 1972), p. 4.

[38] Ibid., p. 4, and "Beware Male Asymptomatic Gonorrhea," *Medical World News,* Vol. 13, No. 16 (April 21, 1972), pp. 4, 5.

cervix. A painless, invisible syphilitic lesion can hardly give the woman any warning of her infection. Gonorrheal infection gives her even less warning. The female urinary system is not usually involved so that pain on urination is uncommon. Between 70 and 90 percent of women who have gonorrhea do not know it.[39] Unless found and treated, such women may remain a reservoir of infection for months. Approximately 10 to 15 percent of women who have gonorrheal organisms in the cervix develop serious complications from their silent infection. These may be manifested as an arthritis, gonorrheal blood poisoning, or an inflammation of one or both Fallopian tubes and ovaries.[40] Without early treatment, sterility often results. The need for surgery to cure illness due to an old gonorrheal infection is not uncommon. It should be noted that rectal gonorrhea in women may result from anal intercourse; most such infections, however, are due to drainage from the vaginal tract.[41] Since the symptoms may be mild or absent the woman may be a source of infection for a long time.

One clinician emphasizes that "in terms of frequencies and consequences of gonorrheal complications the most important is pelvic inflammatory disease (PID) or salpingitis [inflammation of the Fallopian tube]. Eighty percent of patients with gonococcal arthritis and other forms of disseminated gonococcal infection are women." He estimates that almost 12 percent of asymptomatic patients with gonorrhea develop pelvic inflammatory disease. The symptoms are acute lower abdominal pain, fever, and occasionally a gastrointestinal disturbance. "Abscesses," he continues

> *may occur as early as five to ten days after infection in the untreated or inadequately treated cases. Scarring of the inner walls may lead to sterility. Damage from previous gonococcal salpingitis is considered the No. 1 predisposing factor in the occurrence of ectopic or tubal pregnancy [see page 46, footnote 11]. Probably the most important of all sequelae of acute PID is chronic or recurrent infection. Often, less virulent organisms invade the pelvic tissue previously devitalized by gonococcal infection . . . Rupture of an ectopic pregnancy is a surgical emergency that always necessitates the removal of the Fallopian tube that is involved . . . 6% to 7% of maternal deaths are due to rupture of ectopic pregnancy . . . the fetus can never survive.*

He reports the case of the twenty-three-year-old woman with a gonorrheal peritonitis whose pelvic abscess was adherent to the

[39] "In the Norfolk Venereal Disease Clinic, 90% of the women found to have gonorrhea were asymptomatic." ("International Venereal Disease Symposium," *Modern Medicine*, p. 64.)

[40] R. H. Kampmeier, "The Matter of Venereal Diseases in 1971," *Annals of Internal Medicine*, Vol. 75, No. 5 (November 1971), p. 794, and "What to do About Rampant Gonorrhea," *Medical World News*, Vol. 12, No. 24 (June 18, 1971), p. 20.

[41] Nicholas J. Fiumara, "Gonococcal Pharyngitis," *Medical Aspects of Human Sexuality*, Vol. 5, No. 5 (May 1971), p. 199.

bowel. Only hysterectomy and surgical castration helped save her life.[42] Had she been found, diagnosed, and treated early, this could have been avoided.

"It's no worse than a cold," one young man was heard to scoff.

There are an increasing number of young people who are finding it difficult to believe him.

For women the problem is complicated by yet another factor. Birth control pills reduce the acidity of the vaginal environment, thus encouraging the growth of the gonorrhea-causing microbes. The birth control pill may be responsible for other problems. By mid-summer 1971, for example, Boston physicians were examining two to four patients a week who had gonorrheal microbes in the blood stream—a much rarer event before the use of the pill became widespread.

In 1969, 1970, and 1971, routine screening of women for gonorrheal infection was carried out in thirty-six towns and cities in twenty-two states. In those three years, 740,446 women were tested; 8.9 percent had gonorrhea. Of these, 620,060 were tested in settings other than a venereal disease clinic; 5.2 percent had gonorrhea. Eighty percent of those who had gonorrhea had no symptoms. In May 1971, 640,000 women in the United States were estimated to have gonorrhea without knowing it. The highest incidence of positive tests (30 percent) were among women attending venereal disease clinics. Manpower training agencies, jails, and neighborhood health centers reported 10 to 12 percent of the cases, public and private hospital outpatient clinics and family planning clinics, 4 to 6 percent. Private physicians reported only 2 percent positives of the patients they tested.[43]

prevention of syphilis and gonorrhea

The condom is an effective mechanical barrier to the organisms that cause both syphilis and gonorrhea. Although the condom can hardly prevent occasional adult gonococcal infection of the eye and the pharynx, it can prevent gonorrheal infection of the penile urethra. The condom prevents gonorrhea more efficiently than it does syphilis. The infectious primary chancre of syphilis is most frequently found on the genitalia, but it may be on the lip, anus, finger, or elsewhere. Both the secondary skin lesions of syphilis and the mucous patches teem with infection. Urination after exposure and thorough washing of the genitals with soapy water may prevent infection in the man. Careful washing of the genital area after intercourse is also wise for

[42] "You Pay and Pay for 'Hidden' Gonorrhea," *Medical World News,* Vol. 13, No. 23 (June 9, 1972), pp. 15-16.
[43] "Gonorrhea Culture—Screening Summary, United States FY Fiscal Year 1969-71," U.S. Department of Health, Education, and Welfare, Public Health Service, Health Services and Mental Health Administration, Center for Disease Control, *Morbidity and Mortality Weekly Report for the Week Ending December 11, 1972,* Vol. 20, No. 49, pp. 1, 2.

the woman. Although douching following coitus has been suggested, there is much doubt as to its effectiveness; most physicians do not advise routine douching after sexual intercourse (see page 285). Some clinicians recommend the use of large doses of antibiotics, such as penicillin, several hours before, or immediately after, exposure. Undoubtedly, this would reduce the individual risk of infection, but as a program of prevention it presents problems, such as the development of patient allergic reactions to the antibiotics as well as the growing resistance to antibiotics of the microbe that causes gonorrhea.

In Nevada, an old drug called progonasyl is being tried.[44] This iodine preparation has been used in the effective treatment of vaginal inflammation and as a killer of spermatozoa.[45] It is now being used on a trial basis by a group of Nevada's legal prostitutes; they are examined weekly for venereal disease and possible impairment of vital body functions. The prostitutes who cannot use the drug because of sensitivity to iodine are used as controls.[46] Initial reports indicate that a daily vaginal instillation of progonasyl reduced the rate of gonococci found by laboratory examinations of the Nevada prostitutes. Since blood tests for syphilis were negative for two years before the study, the negative blood tests during the study could not be considered significant.[47] Some women experienced a drying of the vaginal mucous membrane after using progonasyl; there were no serious side effects.

Also being studied is the preventive action of the presently lesser used contraceptives, such as the jellies, foams, and powders. Unlike the contraceptive pill, these produce an acidic vaginal environment; this is believed to inhibit the survival of several venereal disease-causing bacteria. Furthermore, some vaginal contraceptives contain a chemical called phenylmercuric acid; mercury was effective in the treatment of syphilis in preantibiotic days. Other contraceptives contain nonoxynol and additional chemicals that may be found to be effective against venereal disease.[48]

A word of caution for the man treated for gonorrhea

Having been treated, some male patients who are recovering from gonorrhea strip or "milk" the penis to see if there is still a discharge. This is inadvisable; the inflamed mucous membrane does not toler-

[44]Horace H. Porter, Robert B. Witcher, and Cecil Knoblock, "Social Diseases at the Crossroads," *Journal of the Oklahoma State Medical Association,* Vol. 32, No. 2 (February 1939), pp. 54-61.
[45]Virginia E. Johnson and William H. Masters, "A Product of Dual Import: Intravaginal Infection Control and Conception Control," *Pacific Medicine and Surgery,* Vol. 73, No. 4 (July–August 1965), pp. 267-71.
[46]"Progonasyl Study Gets Red . . . Er . . . Green Light," *Medical World News,* Vol. 12, No. 31 (August 20, 1971), pp. 4, 5.
[47]"Venereal Disease Symposium," *M.D., Medical Newsmagazine,* Vol. 16, No. 5 (May 1972), p. 92.
[48]"Vaginal Contraceptives Declared Anti VD," *VD Clinical News,* Vol. 2, No. 1 (January–February 1972), pp. 1, 2.

ate rough handling. The practice may delay healing and worsen the inflammation of the urethra.[49] For the same reason, the patient should not masturbate while he has, or is recovering from, gonorrhea.

venereal disease infection transmitted from mother to child

The child born of a gonorrhea-infected woman, in passing through the cervix and vagina, may contract the disease. His eyes may become infected. For this reason, forty-seven states make it mandatory to apply a preventive 1 percent solution of silver nitrate to the newborn infant's eyes. It has recently been discovered that the gonococcus may pass up into a pregnant woman's uterus, causing the gonococcal amniotic infection syndrome.[50] Premature birth, umbilical cord inflammation, and maternal fever are among the complications of this syndrome. It has yet to be proved that the gonorrhea-causing microbe is the exclusive agent of the condition; other organisms may be involved.

After the seventeenth week of pregnancy, the syphilitic woman can transmit her infection to her unborn child. Before that time, the woman's spirochetes cannot pass through the insufficiently developed placenta. After a few years, an untreated person with syphilis does not spread the disease because the microbes settle deep in the tissues. Occasionally, however, spirochetes do appear in the blood stream; thus an untreated woman with syphilis can transmit the disease to her unborn child for six to eight years. However, even late in pregnancy, adequate treatment of the woman can prevent syphilitic infection of her unborn child. It is wise to have blood tests done several times during pregnancy. Several states still lack adequate laws requiring premarital and prenatal blood tests for syphilis.

on helping to find those who need help

People who have a venereal disease almost always got it from someone. And frequently they give it to others. The sick must be immediately and adequately treated. In addition, public protection demands a thorough investigation of the source and spread of every new case. Without active contact tracing, the reservoir of the venereally infected in a community grows; and with it, a spreading sea of chronic sickness and despair. The venereally infected individual who refuses to name his contacts is not being chivalrous. He is refusing information (held, both by law and practice, in absolute confidence) that will spare others endless pain. "Fools alone their

[49]Walter H. Smartt, "Aggravating Urethritis," *Medical Aspects of Human Sexuality,* Vol. 6, No. 4 (April 1972), p. 10.
[50]"Gonococcal Infection Can Blight Newborn," *Medical World News,* Vol. 13, No. 8 (February 25, 1972), p. 19.

ulcered ills conceal," wrote Horace. This ancient thought of the Roman poet might well be applied to modern venereal disease control.

OTHER COMMON SEXUALLY TRANSMITTED DISEASES

trichomoniasis

Trichomoniasis is a very common infestation of the female genitourinary tract; it is caused by a unicellular member of the lowest division of the animal kingdom—the protozoa. The protozoon that causes trichomoniasis, the *Trichomonas vaginalis,* is readily visible under the microscope. In females it may live in great numbers on the vaginal surface as well as on the cervix; in about 20 percent of the cases the urinary tract is also affected. The Bartholin's glands and Skene's ducts may also become involved (see page 51). However, it rarely spreads to the upper female tract. In males, trichomonads usually inhabit the urethra, bladder, and seminal vesicles, and, rarely, the prostate and upper urinary tract are involved (see page 36). Trichomoniasis is most commonly spread as a result of heterosexual intercourse, although it can be spread between women whose behavior is homosexual. There are two other types of trichomonads that inhabit the human body; one lives in the mouth, the other in the pouch situated between the small and large intestines. Neither inhabits the genital tract. Therefore, it is doubtful that trichomonas infections are transmitted by men whose behavior is homosexual, and who practice oral and anal intercourse.[51] Treatment of both sexual partners is mandatory. Otherwise one partner is treated only to be reinfected by the untreated partner (a situation that is also common in gonorrheal infections).

Sometimes the woman is accidentally infected as a result of using borrowed clothing or towels. As has been pointed out above, trichomonads found in bowel material are not necessarily the same as those found in the vagina.

Trichomonads may inhabit the vagina for years without producing any symptoms. In some women the infection may be so mild as to cause only minor itching. This annoyance is often aggravated by the soiling of underclothes due to vaginal discharge. Frequently symptoms are exacerbated during pregnancy and before and after menstruation. Many women develop more severe symptoms. Itching, burning, and soreness of the vulva and even the thighs plague the more severely infected women. The profuse and frothy yellowish-white vaginal discharge has a musty, foul odor. Pain during sexual intercourse (dyspareunia) and urination are common symptoms.

[51] Warren A. Ketterer, "Homosexual Transmission of Trichomonas and Monilia," *Medical Aspects of Human Sexuality,* Vol. 5, No. 6 (June 1971), p. 144.

In the male the signs and symptoms are much milder. Often they are absent. The male may experience limited itching. He may also feel a burning sensation while urinating, and there may be mild or profuse discharge. During the period of treatment, sexual intercourse should be avoided. Recently developed drugs that are taken by mouth have proved effective in the great majority of cases. These are curative for both sexes.

moniliasis

Another infection that may be sexually transmitted is variously known as moniliasis, candidiasis, thrush, and candidosis. This condition is usually caused by the fungus *Monilia albicans (Candida albicans)*. Most often the disease has a nonsexual basis. In both sexes, oral and skin moniliasis may occur in babies and debilitated elderly people. Sometimes ill-fitting dentures promote the disease.

The fungus can live in the female genital tract without causing symptoms. But there are conditions under which the monilia may increase in number to produce symptoms.[52] Among these are pregnancy, an excess of sugar in the urine, and the prolonged use of antibiotics. An antibiotic may kill the microbes that check the growth of the fungus; the resultant overgorwth of the fungus causes illness. Oral, penile, and anal monilial infection may occur in the male; there is thus the possibility of spread among homosexually oriented males.

Since vaginal thrush in the pregnant woman can be transmitted to the newborn, it is particularly important to treat it early in the pregnancy. The disease may be transmitted by contact with excretions from the mouth, skin, vagina, and feces of people who carry the fungus. Thus it is commonly contracted as a result of sexual intercourse. The principal symptoms in the woman are vulval itching associated with a white vaginal discharge. The anus may also itch. The skin of the external genitalia may become red and fissured. In the male, discomfort may be due to inflammation of the urethra, penis, scrotum, or thighs. Medicated vaginal pessaries have proved effective in the treatment of the female. Certain ointments help to cure the disease in both sexes. As yet there is no routinely effective drug. Both moniliasis and trichomoniasis may often exist together in the same individual. Both can be successfully treated.

---

[52] "Investigators have recently discounted the belief that the incidence of moniliasis (candidiasis) is increased among users of either sequential or combined oral contraceptives." (George E. Tagatz and Richard B. McHugh, "Oral Contraceptives—A Continuing Appraisal," *Postgraduate Medicine,* Vol. 50, No. 2 [August 1971], p. 124, citing B. Lapan, "Is 'The Pill' a Cause of Vaginal Candidiasis? Culture Study," *New York State Journal of Medicine,* Vol. 70 [1970], p. 949; B. A. Davis, "Vaginal Moniliasis in Private Practice," *Obstetrics and Gynecology,* Vol. 34 [1969], p. 40; and C. A. Morris and D. F. Morris, "'Normal' Vaginal Microbiology of Women of Childbearing Age in Relation to the Use of Oral Contraceptives and Vaginal Tampons," *Journal of Clinical Pathology,* Vol. 20 [1967], p. 636.)

genital herpes

Herpes simplex is the common "cold sore." It is caused by a virus. Genital herpes results from a different virus than herpes simplex. Both infections, however, cause blisters. In the woman groups of blisters occur on the vulva and the surrounding skin. They may also appear on the cervix. The blisters break down to become ulcers, which in turn become infected. An odorous discharge results. Infection around the opening through which urine must pass can cause pain on urination. The same is true of the male. In recent years treatment for this condition has been more successful than formerly. However, it can be an infection that stubbornly resists treatment and, for long periods, tends to recur rather than to taper off. There is an increased frequency of cancer of the cervix in women with genital herpes. Although a causal relationship between herpes virus and cervical cancer has not been proved, a woman with genital herpes should have frequent Papanicolaou tests. Until the viral-cancer association is clarified, a possibly effective West German vaccine against genital herpes will not be used in this country. Should a pregnant woman have the active infection at the time of delivery, a Caesarean section is advisable. This is true even though the unborn child would have had antibodies delivered to him via the placenta.[53]

genital warts

Another virus transmitted by genital contact causes genital warts. The wart is one of the only two human tumors believed to be caused by a virus. Neither is malignant. In the female, genital warts usually begin their growth on the mucous membrane of the vulva. They can extend to the vaginal wall, the cervix, and about the anus. Any vaginal discharge worsens genital warts. Trichomoniasis and, less frequently, gonorrhea exacerbates them. In the male, genital warts usually begin about the base of the glans penis. They may also become extensive. Various applications and, sometimes, electrocautery, are useful in curing the condition.

scabies

The mite causing scabies ("the itch") invades only the outer skin. It may be distributed over most of the body or (more uncommonly) be somewhat limited to the genital area. In both instances sexual intercourse is one way in which the mite is transmitted from one person to another. The male scabies mite is difficult to see; the female

[53] Andre J. Nahmias, "Herpes Genitalis: Treatment, Effect on Pregnancy," and "Herpes Genitalis: Risk to Newborn," *Journal of the American Medical Association,* Vol. 217, No. 9 (August 30, 1971), p. 1250.

is twice as large and can be seen. The female burrows into the superficial skin to deposit her eggs. The resultant itching is worse at night than in the daytime. Treatment involves the use of an ointment or lotion that contains a chemical that kills the mite. Scrupulous body cleanliness and attention to linens, which are also infested, are essential. The details of the treatment and hygiene must be carefully followed by the affected person. All close contacts of the patient, both sexual and nonsexual, must also be treated to avoid reinfection.

The cause of scabies has been known since 1687; indeed it was the first disease of man for which the cause was known.[54] Present-day treatments are effective, yet, since 1963, the prevalence of the disease has been increasing in many parts of the world. It is now being seen with greater frequency in venereal disease clinics in London and San Francisco. Occasionally the chancre of syphilis is seen in a skin lesion of scabies.[55]

genital lice

In his "To a Louse" the great eighteenth-century Scottish poet Robert Burns wrote indignantly:

> *Ye ugly, creepin', blastit wonner,*
> *Detested, shunn'd by saunt an' sinner!*
> *How dare ye set your fit upon her,*
> *   Sae fine a lady?*
> *Gae somewhere else, and seek your dinner*
> *   On some poor body.*

Shakespeare had been more tolerant. In *The Merry Wives of Windsor* the Welsh parson refers to the louse as "a familiar beast to man, and signifies love."[56] Inadvertently, he differentiated between the head louse, the body louse, and the crab (genital) louse. The crab louse is a distant relative of the other two; it is the one that is most often transmitted as a result of sexual intercourse. From the pubic region in which they multiply, these stubborn travelers spread to the other hairy parts of the body except the scalp. The lice can be seen anchored at the hair roots and can be removed for examination. The nits (eggs) can also be removed for examination. Treatment is easy, but, again, all close contacts must be found and treated. Without early treatment the itching and skin irritation may become most distressing. Genital lice may also be contracted from unclean beds or toilet seats.

[54] Milton Orkin, "Resurgence of Scabies," *Journal of the American Medical Association,* Vol. 217, No. 5 (August 2, 1971), p. 593, citing R. Friedman, *The Story of Scabies,* Vol. 1 (New York, 1947).
[55] Ibid., p. 595, citing C. H. Beek and K. Mellanby, "Scabies," in R. D. G. P. Simon, ed., *Handbook of Tropical Dermatology and Medical Mycology* (Amsterdam, 1953), pp. 875–88.
[56] William Shakespeare, *The Merry Wives of Windsor,* I.i.21.

NONSPECIFIC VENEREAL DISEASE

There have been recent reports of a common, sexually communicable disease caused by an as yet unspecified microbe. A variety of organisms, among them staphylococci and streptococci, have been incriminated, but the cause remains uncertain. More than one microbe may be involved. Symptoms begin seven to twenty-one days after exposure; there may be a mild mucous discharge, although some cases resemble gonorrhea or an infection with trichomonas. The disease has a tendency to persist and recur. An antibiotic is the most effective treatment of what may be a stubborn condition.[57]

ABOUT ORAL-GENITAL TRANSMISSION
OF VENEREAL INFECTION

The oral area is much more resistant to gonorrheal infection than it is to infection by the microbe causing syphilis. By far the greatest number of gonococcal infections are of the urinary tract. Nevertheless, a gonococcal sore throat (pharyngitis) is now being increasingly seen. In the United States this condition has yet to be reported to result from lip-kissing or cunnilinction; it has only been diagnosed following fellatio. The person with gonococcal pharyngitis cannot spread his infection to the genitals of a male or female partner. This is because the gonococci that enter the body via the mouth can only survive in the tonsillar area where some lymphoid tissue is present even in those individuals who have had a tonsillectomy. The patient with gonococcal pharyngitis develops a sore throat within a day or two after oral exposure; there may be some redness and swelling of the tonsillar area and some fever. Sometimes lymph nodes in the neck may be enlarged. Patients with gonococcal pharyngitis commonly have gonorrheal signs and symptoms in other areas such as the rectum, urethra, or cervix.[58]

Two Danish physicians associated with a Copenhagen municipal hospital suggest that a considerable number of cases of gonococcal tonsillitis are being missed. This may be due to the possibility that many sore throats are treated without first obtaining a complete bacteriologic diagnosis from a laboratory. People with sore throats do not customarily go to venereal disease specialists. Nor are the Danish physicians prepared to eliminate the likelihood that there are a variety of ways in which the disease may be transmitted. "The high incidence of gonococcal tonsillar infections, their resistance to treatment, the lack of any characteristic signs and symptoms, and the possibility of innocent acquirement of the disease by kissing are

[57] "Venereal Disease Symposium," *M.D., Medical Newsmagazine*, p. 92.
[58] Nicholas J. Fiumara, "Gonococcal Pharyngitis," pp. 177, 195, 199, 204, 209.

factors which presumably may result in a rather high prevalence of this hitherto disregarded gonococcal infection."[59]

Syphilis of the oral area occurs during the secondary stage of the disease. A common manifestation of secondary infectious syphilis is the mouth lesion (patch). Since they teem with *Spirocheta pallida,* these oral patches are ready sources of infection. Of course, the primary chancre of syphilis is also extremely infectious; although most frequently located on the genital area, it may be in numerous other places on the body. Also infectious is the rash of secondary syphilis, which is less commonly seen nowadays. Infection results from direct transmission of the disease, such as occurs, for example, with lip-kissing or oral-genital contact.

Infections other than those caused by syphilis or gonorrhea microbes could occur as a result of oral-genital sexual contact, although these are very rarely reported. Oral thrush (moniliasis, see page 73), might conceivably be transmitted as a result of cunnilinction. Some physicians believe that genital herpes may also be spread as a result of oral-genital contact. Infections may occur more easily when the skin and mucous membrane are broken. A cut in the skin or a break in the mucous membrane provides an open wound in which infecting agents easily flourish.

PELVIC PAIN FROM PETTING AND CONGESTION

Many men between twenty and forty-five years of age who think they have prostatitis really do not have a microbial infection of the prostate. Their low back pain, mild early morning discharge, irritative urinary symptoms, and testicular ache are not caused by an infectious agent but rather by congestion. Sexual stimulation brings about an increased blood supply to the prostate and other adjacent involved organs. In addition there is an increase in the production of prostatic fluid. When sexual stimulation is not followed by orgasmic relief, congestion occurs. This is noticed by men after prolonged petting sessions. "It appears," wrote one physician, "that the seminal vesicle, reacting to the stimulus of anticipated sexual activity and ready to perform its function according to nature's plan, but having no brains and no morals, accepts disappointment with poor grace."[60]

Despite anatomical differences, women may also experience the same problem for the same basic reason. Repeated petting sessions unrelieved by orgasm may result in pelvic pain not caused by disease. Occasionally vaginal discharge may occur. In addition, for women who have borne children the importance of orgasmic relief, once the

[59]Anne Bro-Jørgensen and Tage Jensen, "Gonococcal Tonsillar Infections," *British Medical Journal,* Vol. 4, No. 5788 (December 11, 1971), p. 661.
[60]Hans Lehfeldt, "Pelvic Pain After Petting," *Medical Aspects of Human Sexuality,* Vol. 3, No. 9 (September 1969), p. 47.

considerable pelvic congestion of sexual stimulation is present, should not be underestimated. A competent medical authority considers that "chronic pelvic congestion furthered by inadequate or absent orgasmic release fosters a pelvic condition conducive to many disorders interfering with impregnation, pregnancies and general health."[61] This is especially true with formerly pregnant women who have intercourse often. Pregnancy may result in some varicosities and chronic congestion of the pelvic veins. For such women added chronic venous congestion may be considered harmful.

[61] E. S. Taylor, *Essentials of Gynecology* (Philadelphia, 1962), p. 472, cited in Mary Jane Sherfey, "The Evolution and Nature of Female Sexuality in Relation to Psychoanalytic Theory," *Journal of the American Psychoanalytic Association,* Vol. 14, No. 1 (January 1966), p. 73.

the sexual life **3**

the biological logic of mutuality

THE PRIMORDIAL FEMALE

"In the beginning, we were all created females; and if this were not so, we would not be here at all." [1] This remarkable statement is the culmination of years of biological research. In their first stage of development, the sex organs of the mammalian embryo (including the human) consist of two elevations of tissue. These are the *genital ridges*. Each ridge contains the cells necessary for the development of either an ovary or a testis. Since it can develop in either direction—female ovary or male testis—each genital ridge must be considered an undifferentiated primitive gonad. (A gonad [Greek *gone, seed*] is a gland producing spermatozoa or ova.) The outer rind of each undifferentiated gonad is capable of becoming an ovary; the inner core is capable of becoming a testis. However, although genetic sex is established at conception, the sex genes do not exert their influence until the fifth or sixth week of life. At that time, if the genetic instruction is to produce a male, the inner cores of the embryonic gonadal ridges develop into testes. For this to occur, it appears that some active secretory process is necessary. (Should this process fail to happen, the tendency of the embryo's genital ridges is to develop ovaries.) Once the primitive testes have been formed, they secrete both the male hormone androgen, and a second substance. This latter, second substance inhibits the development and causes the regression of those embryonic tissues that could become the organs of the female internal reproductive system (tubes, uterus, and vagina). The androgen produces the development of the male internal and external reproductive system. The male substances thus overcome the female pattern.

However, if the genetic instruction is to produce a female, the

[1] Mary Jane Sherfey, "The Evolution and Nature of Female Sexuality in Relation to Psychoanalytic Theory," *Journal of the American Psychoanalytic Association*, Vol. 14, No. 1 (January 1966), p. 43.

processes by which testes, androgen, and female-inhibiting substance are produced do not take place, nor do the subsequent events. The outer rinds of the genital ridges—the female cellular potentials—proliferate into ovaries. In the absence of androgen and the female-inhibiting substance, a female results from the already existing, and thus primordial, tissue.

Scientists have conclusively proven that in the absence of embryonic androgen the female potential develops regardless of the genetic sex. They have removed the undifferentiated gonads of a male rabbit embryo within the uterus by means of exquisitely delicate surgical techniques. In the absence of testes (and, therefore, androgen), the genetic male was born with completely female external genitalia. When the undifferentiated gonads of a female embryo in the uterus were removed, the genetic female rabbit was, of course, born without ovaries, but with completely female genitalia. The ovarian hormone estrogen is not needed for differentiation into a female; however, androgen is essential for differentiation into a male. Clearly, then, the external female sex organs are not rudimentary, imperfect, inadequate versions of the male sex organs. "Nature's prime disposition is to produce females; maleness only results from something added—androgens."[2] In other words, "only the male embryo is required to undergo a differentiating transformation of the sexual anatomy; and only one hormone, androgen, is necessary for the masculinization of the originally female genital tract."[3] The female genital tract develops independently, without cellular transformation by a hormone. Thus, it is the female whose tissue is primordial; and the sex organs of the male are an outgrowth of her original tissue. The penis develops from the primordia of the clitoris; the scrotum, from the primordia of the labia; the male, from the female. Embryologically, man comes from woman.[4]

THE MALE BRAIN: AN ANDROGENIZED
FEMALE BRAIN

Recent research has revealed some startling additional information about androgen. The results of experiments with laboratory animals support the following concept:

It does appear that one of the principle actions of androgen during development is to organize the immature central nervous

[2] Warren J. Gadpaille, "Research Into the Physiology of Maleness and Femaleness," *Archives of General Psychiatry,* Vol. 26, No. 3 (March 1972), p. 195.
[3] Mary Jane Sherfey, "The Evolution and Nature of Female Sexuality in Relation to Psychoanalytic Theory," p. 45.
[4] These findings lend themselves to speculation. Is woman "superior," since she was embryologically first? Is man "superior," since he is "furthest along the evolutionary line"? Doubtless it is most sensible to put aside the notion of "superiority" and, instead, to use this new information for a more mature, realistic, and therefore enjoyable appreciation of the opposite sex.

system into that of the male . . . we are talking about an active process; that is, the presence of androgen during development acts upon the brain to program, in effect, patterns of maleness. The absence of androgen permits the ongoing process of femaleness to pursue its natural course. The evidence to support this theory is now abundant.[5]

Thus "the brain makes do with one type of anatomic system . . . The male brain is an androgenized female brain."[6]

What do some of these findings suggest? As has been pointed out, modern biological knowledge mitigates against the sexual subordination of woman. In addition, these studies suggest an explanation for the greater prevalence of divergent sexual behavior among males. Most behavioral scientists agree that homosexual behavior (see pages 297–316) is more prevalent among men than women. This difference is even more marked when other forms of divergent sexual behavior are considered, such as bestiality, sadism, masochism, and pedophilia (see pages 325–29). Indeed, some forms of bizarre sexual behavior, such as necrophilia (see page 325) seem to be limited to men.

Elsewhere in this book, reference is made to the fragility of the male as compared to the female (see pages 159–61). It has been suggested that his comparative weakness is not limited to the more physical aspects of life. The male's "reproductive function and psychosocial development is much more easily tipped off-balance or derailed than that of the female."[7] It is the male embryo that is subject to the added chances for error caused by formidable androgenic changes. It is the male whose embryonic brain patterns must be radically altered. The female embryo is the original one; it develops autonomously. Furthermore, the changes necessary for the production of a male take place at a critical period in the development of the embryo.

The power of the critical period is so great that a single pulse of hormone in the laboratory may set for life the gender behavior

[5] Seymour Levine, "Sexual Differentiation: The Development of Maleness and Femaleness," *California Medicine*, Vol. 114, No. 1 (January 1971), p. 13. Other research has indicated a relationship between a high IQ and an overproduction of fetal androgen or hormones with an androgenlike side effect. Included in the study were fifty-three female hermaphrodites and seventeen males who, it was determined, had also experienced an overproduction of fetal androgen. Sixty percent displayed an IQ of over 110; in the general population the expected percentage of such an IQ is 25 percent. An astonishing 13 percent had an IQ of over 130; this level is reached by only 2.2 percent of the general population. Corrective hormone therapy after birth apparently does not change the disproportionate ratio of high IQ's. The significance of this discovery is being studied. In the general population, there are no marked differences between the sexes in IQ. (John W. Money, "Pre-natal Hormones and Intelligence: A Possible Relationship," *Impact of Science on Society*, Vol. 21, No. 4 [1971], pp. 285–90.)

[6] Robert J. Stoller, "The 'Bedrock' of Masculinity and Femininity: Bisexuality," *Archives of General Psychiatry*, Vol. 26, No. 3 (March 1972), p. 209.

[7] Warren J. Gadpaille, "Research Into the Physiology of Maleness and Femaleness," p. 203.

as masculine or feminine (without there being any anatomic change in the body, for by this time the development of the reproductive anatomy is complete).[8]

the roots of sexual behavior

The presence or absence of androgen does more than determine physical reproductive function. By its organizing effect on the hypothalamus and nearby nervous tissue, it produces a change that predictably affects masculine or feminine sexual behavior. "Only if the fetal brain (hypothalamus) is organized by androgen does masculine behavior result. And, if normally occurring androgens are blocked in the male, then . . . femininity appears."[9] This has now been established beyond question by both clinical observation and laboratory experimentation with animals.

THE ROLE OF LEARNING IN GENDER IDENTITY

There are, however, more pervasive factors influencing the child's gender identity than the hormonal influences. These are the culturally learned patterns of behavior and thought that are inculcated in the child from birth by the parents and by society as a whole. What the child is taught by the culture concerning gender identity transcends the effects of chromosomes, hormones, and other physiological factors.

> *It is . . . clear that gender of assignment and rearing predictably take precedence over and override all contradictory determinants: chromosomes, hormones, gonads, internal and external sexual morphology [structure] and secondary pubertal changes . . . the critical period for core formation of gender identity may be between 12 and 18 months . . . after about 2 to 2½ years of age, shift of core identity cannot take place, even when all sexual determinants are those of the other sex. Thus far in the literature there are no reported cases of successful shift after that age; there are, on the other hand, numerous case reports of psychological havoc and tragedy brought about by efforts to effect or enforce such a shift after the critical period."*[10]

[8] Robert J. Stoller, "The 'Bedrock' of Masculinity and Femininity: Bisexuality," p. 210.
[9] Ibid., p. 209. See also Warren J. Gadpaille, "Research Into the Physiology of Maleness and Femaleness," p. 194. Significantly, moreover, it is the male hormone testosterone (see page 35) that most strongly influences sexual desire in both sexes. Females secrete most of their male hormones in the adrenal glands. Women who have had their adrenal glands surgically removed lose their sexual desire. Women who have had their ovaries removed, with subsequent loss of estrogens, rarely lose their sexual desire.
[10] Warren J. Gadpaille, "Research Into the Physiology of Maleness and Femaleness," p. 200.

The higher a creature is placed on the evolutionary scale the greater is the importance of learning in sexual behavior. Among all animals, it is most important in man. The learning experience of peer group juvenile sex play seems to be of greater significance for the achievement of competent adult sexual function than even mothering.[11]

The overwhelming influence of learning on the child's sense of gender identity can be most clearly seen in the case of hermaphrodites. There are various kinds of hermaphrodites; a *true* hermaphrodite, however, has both ovarian and testicular tissue either separate or in the same gonad.[12] The individual is physically a member of both sexes and the appearance of the external genitalia is inconclusive. If the parents are continuously uncertain about the sex to which their hermaphroditic child should be assigned, the child will go through life believing that he or she is of neither sex or of both sexes. However, if the parents are certain of the child's gender (whether male or female), the child will also be certain. This is true even when the genitalia are ambiguous. "There is no genetic or innate mechanism to preordain the masculinity or femininity of psychosexual differentiation . . . The analogy is with language. Genetics and innate determinants ordain only that language can develop . . . but not whether the language will be Arabic, English or any other."[13]

Different interpretations of maleness and femaleness have been made not only in various cultures but also during various periods of history. Is it the male who is always sexually aggressive? Not among the Muria in India. They expect the woman to be as aggressive as the man. "The Andaman Islanders like to have a man sit on his wife's lap in fond greetings, and friends and relatives, of the same or opposite sex, greet one another in the same manner after absences, crying in the affected manner of the mid-Victorian woman."[14] In many European countries embracing men are unnoticed. In the United States such behavior in everyday encounters would be noticed with amused (and hopefully tolerant) doubts about gender identity, although embracing among women is acceptable. However, men may publicly embrace with impunity in this country under specific circumstances. Upon scoring a touchdown, football players not only embrace vigorously, but have been known to weep and to add an affectionate pat on the bottom to their expressions of affection. (The father who pats the mother's bottom in front of the children is

[11] Ibid., p. 202.
[12] John W. Money, *Sex Errors of the Body* (Baltimore, 1968), pp. 42–43. (This wise and authoritative little book is highly recommended to anyone interested in this field.)
[13] Judd Marmor, "'Normal' and 'Deviant' Sexual Behavior," *Journal of the American Medical Association,* Vol. 217, No. 2, citing John Money, "Developmental Differentiation of Femininity and Masculinity Compared," in S. M. Farber and R. H. L. Wilson, eds., *Man and Civilization* (New York, 1963), pp. 56–57.
[14] Judd Marmor, "'Normal' and 'Deviant' Sexual Behavior," citing M. K. Opler, "Anthropological and Cross-Cultural Aspects of Homosexuality," in Judd Marmor, ed., *Sexual Inversion: The Multiple Roots of Homosexuality* (New York, 1965), pp. 108–23.

considered a good educator of the advantages of sexuality.[15]) In the case of the football players, the sudden release from the tensions of violence seems to initiate an acceptable blur of the learned, culturally imposed differences between the sexes.

Nor do clothes make the man—or woman. The colorful beads and shirts worn by many young men in this country today were worn by many young men in this country years before them—the Navajo Indians. Nor were the bejeweled, berouged, perfumed, powdered, curly-wigged, girdled, mini-skirted, panty-hosed, high-heeled males of former days particularly noted for their indifference to women. Indeed, it was not until relatively recent times that women's legs replaced those of men as objects of sexual admiration, and "unmentionables" were anything else but male garments.[16]

on the physiology of the human sexual response

William H. Masters and Virginia E. Johnson, of the Reproductive Biology Research Foundation at St. Louis, have written the most authoritative recent account of the physiology of the human sexual response.[17] Most of the discussion in this section is based on their work.

In their discussion Masters and Johnson divide the sexual responses of both sexes into four phases: the *excitement phase,* varying from a few minutes to hours; the intense, shorter (thirty seconds to three minutes) *plateau phase;* the three- to ten-second *orgasmic phase* (sometimes longer in women); and the *resolution phase,* lasting ten to fifteen minutes with an orgasm, and, without orgasm, lasting as long as twelve to twenty-four hours.

It should be emphasized that sex is more than a total body experience. It is an experience of the whole personality. One distinguished psychiatrist considers the female orgasm to be "the manifestation of that all-pervading instinct for survival of the child that is the primary organizer of the woman's sexual drive and by this also of her personality." [18] Other people totally reject this notion; they believe it to be still another outmoded and restrictive idea about woman's sexual expression. Whatever the opinion, it is well to remember that since there is no human equation, some individual variations are common and should be expected.

---

[15] "The greatest form of sex education is Pop walking past Mom in the kitchen and patting her on the fanny and Mom obviously liking it. The kids take a good look at this action and think, 'Boy that's for me.'" William H. Masters quoted in Mary Harryington Hall, "A Conversation with Masters and Johnson," *Psychology Today,* Vol. 3, No. 2 (July 1969), p. 57.

[16] Una Stannard, "Clothing and Sexuality," *Sexual Behavior,* Vol. 1, No. 2 (May 1971), p. 30.

[17] William H. Masters and Virginia E. Johnson, *Human Sexual Response* (Boston, 1966).

[18] From "Female Sexuality," a panel meeting of the American Psychoanalytic Association held in Detroit, Michigan, May 6, 1967, and reported by Warren J. Barker, *Journal of the American Psychoanalytic Association,* Vol. 16, No. 1 (January 1968), p. 126.

IN THE FEMALE

Even the early feminine responses to adequate sexual stimulation (during the excitement phase) are not limited to the pelvis. They are widely distributed. From contracting great muscles of the thighs, abdomen, and back, to the tiny muscle fibers often erecting the nipples, the woman's sexual attention is total. The distention of the breast veins as they become engorged with blood and the marked increase in breast size is called *tumescence*—swelling. (Tumescence occurs in all distensible parts of the body and is the major feature of the sexual response in both sexes. It results from the enormous increase of blood in the surface circulation. In these areas blood is forced in through the arteries faster than it can leave via the capillaries and veins. The presence of a special erectile tissue in some areas—the walls of the inner nose, the nipples, vaginal entrance, clitoris, and penis—makes them particularly susceptible to the swelling tensions of tumescence.) During the late excitement phase, or early in the plateau phase, in perhaps three-fourths of women and one-fourth of men, there begins the *sex flush*. Much more noticeable in fair-skinned people, this temporary, measleslike rash first appears on the skin of the abdomen. As sexual excitement intensifies, the rash spreads but it will disappear immediately after coitus. Often it does not occur. The clitoris also undergoes tumescence, and the vagina had begun early to secrete a lubricating fluid by a process not unlike sweating. This fluid aids penetration of the penis, thereby facilitating coitus. As sexual excitement continues, a sudden contraction of muscles encircling the vagina may cause some of this accumulated fluid to spurt out. This has led to the completely mistaken notion that women ejaculate as do men. In this first phase, the inner two-thirds of the vagina increases in size and the uterus contracts rapidly and irregularly. The reaction of labia depends on whether the woman has had children. If she has not, the labia majora will thin and flatten; if she has had children, they will enlarge. In both instances the labia minora increase in size. Bartholin's glands may, in this stage or the next, and during prolonged coital activity, produce a slight secretion to ease the entrance of the penis. The heart rate quickens, and, as is to be expected with sexual excitement, the blood pressure rises.

In the second phase, the plateau phase, tumescence and the sex flush reach their peak. From head to toe, muscle tension reflects the physical and emotional absorption with the impending climax. Evidence of this is in the facial grimace, the flaring nostrils, rigid neck, arched back, and tensed thighs and buttocks. Now respiration increases and the heart rate and blood pressure remain high. It is in the plateau phase that the clitoris withdraws from its normally overhanging position, pulling back deeply beneath its hood. Contraction of the encircling muscles of the vagina causes it to tighten about the penile shaft. Within these vaginal muscles, the veins become engorged with blood. Added to this venous congestion is that occurring in the veins of the irregularly contracting uterus as well as the other pelvic organs. And it is when the woman reaches the plateau phase of her sexual tension that her labia minora change color in a remarkable way. The color change of the labia minora with the woman who has never borne a child varies from a pink to a bright red. The labia minora of the woman who has borne children varies from a bright red to a deep wine. So specific are these color changes of the labia minora, that they have been termed the "sex skin." In the premenopausal woman, the sex skin is absolutely indicative of the impending orgasm. The *pelvic congestion* is relieved by the third level of the woman's sexual cycle, the orgasmic phase.

The orgasm is the pleasurable peak of the sexual experience. This explosive release of body-wide purposively developed, neuromuscular tension lasts from three to ten seconds. Hearing, vision, taste—all the senses are diminished or lost. It was during the excitement phase that this loss of sensory awareness had begun. It has been said that only a sneeze is as physiologically all-absorbing as an orgasm. But a sneeze is mostly a local experience and an orgasm is not. Although the sensation of orgasm is centered in the pelvis, the whole body responds to it. Of all the widespread muscle responses, the muscle contractions in the floor of the pelvis that surround the lower third of the vagina cause the most unique phenomenon. These muscles contract against the engorged veins that surround that part of the vagina and force the blood out of them. This creates the orgasm. These contractions, in turn, cause the lower third of the vagina and the nearby upper labia minora to contract between three to fifteen times. The strength and number of these orgasmic contractions vary greatly and normally, as does the whole sexual experience.

The resolution phase of the woman's sexual response is marked by prompt disappearance of the sex flush, the fading of the sex skin color, the decline of muscle tension and tumescence (detumescence), and her general return to the prestimulated condition.

IN THE MALE

Masters and Johnson have emphasized the physiological similarities of the sexes in their sexual responses. All the phases and the general changes, such as muscle contractions and tumescence, also occur in the male. In the excitement phase, blood that is delivered to the penis enters the spaces of its spongy erectile tissue. The structure within the penis efficiently prevents return of most of the blood from that organ into the general venous circulation. Penile enlargement and stiffening result. (There is no relationship whatsoever between the size of the penis and either virility or fertility.) During the male's plateau phase, the tumescent testes are elevated and become so congested with blood that they increase in size from 50 to 100 percent.

Orgasm and *ejaculation* occur simultaneously. The contractions of the epididymis, vas deferens, seminal vesicles, and prostate produce the sensation of imminent ejaculation. The force of perineal muscle contractions causes the seminal fluid to squirt out from the penis. This ejaculation accompanying the male orgasm is the most singular physiological difference in sexual response between the sexes.

General detumescence of the male is rapid (resolution phase). Penile detumescence usually occurs in two stages. After ejaculation the penis quickly returns to be about 50 percent larger than its prestimulated flaccid state. Although complete erection increases the actual size of the penis considerably, it often seems that the initial stage of penile detumescence has not actually caused much diminution of the erection. Depending largely on the kind and duration of the stimuli of the excitement and plateau stages, final detumescence requires a longer time. After orgasm, the male experiences a *refractory period*—a temporary resistance to sexual stimulation. During this period, the sexual stimulation that excited him earlier is no longer effective. It may be distasteful. But restimulation of the woman after her orgasm may result in one or more orgasms. Nothing will help more in understanding this complex human difference than honest communication. The man, for example, may learn to delay his orgasm until his wife has been satisfied. Consistent premature ejaculation with loss of erection is a frequent problem that can be effectively helped (see pages 294-96).

In 1970 Masters and Johnson published the results of their studies of the major problems of sexual expression in their book *Human Sexual Inadequacy*. A summary of some of their concepts and treatments of these problems is presented in Chapter 9.

sexual intercourse

POSITIONS

Much has been written about the "best" position for sexual intercourse. The only wrong positions are those that are nonstimulating. Any position that is exciting and comfortable and agreeable to both partners is the best. A couple may also try a variety of positions during a single sexual encounter. No major religious group in this country forbids any sexual position between man and wife. Variety in coital positions was recommended both by Mohammed and in the Talmud. Nor are all societies devoted to the male-superior posi-

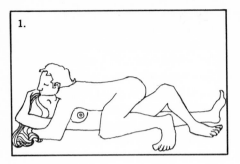

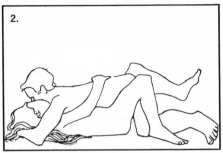

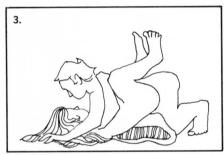

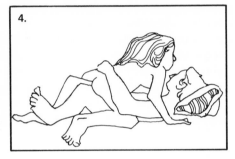

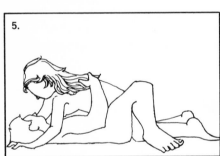

3-1 some coital positions

1. Man above, his thighs outside
2. Man above, her thighs outside
3. Man above, pillow raises hips
4. Woman above, her thighs outside
5. Woman above, his thighs outside

6. Sitting

7. Both on side

8. Entry from the rear

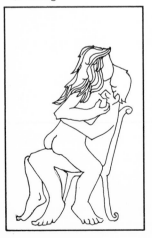

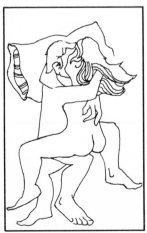

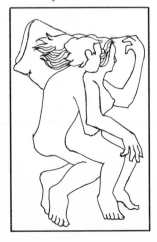

tion. Amused South Sea Islanders refer to it as "the missionary position." Indeed, there are times when variety in coital positions is recommended for medical reasons. Masters and Johnson advise certain variances for some of their patients who are being treated for sexual inadequacies (see Chapter 9). Moreover, the female-superior position may help relieve a husband with a heart condition of the need for overly vigorous coital thrusting and pushing. During the last three or four months of pregnancy, a face-to-face position can be most useful in relieving pressure on the woman's abdomen (see page 201). The same is true when one of the partners is obese. Direct penile contact with the clitoris is easy only in the female-superior and face-to-face positions.

The woman who desires added friction in her clitoral area may respond better with a small pillow under her hips to elevate the pelvis. She may, in addition, flex her thighs toward her abdomen in order to insure her husband's deeper penetration. For some, entry of the penis from the rear has its advantages as a coital position. Many men and women find such rear entry sexually stimulating, particularly if it is part of a variety of positions. Moreover, the man's hand is comfortably free to stimulate the clitoral body or mons. This enables him to delay his orgasm while he brings his wife closer to orgasm with his hand. Upon her signal, he can then resume his thrusting. If desired, simultaneous or near simultaneous orgasm might be achieved in this manner.

ORAL-GENITAL SEXUAL EXPRESSION

In this culture oral-genital contact is extremely common. As is the case with varying coital positions, no major religious group in this country interdicts the practice when it is a prelude to coitus between married partners. It is of interest to note that "mouth-genital contact in complete privacy between husband and wife, each consenting to and desirous of the act, is under the laws of most states a sex offense. The maximum penalty can be years of imprisonment." [19] In one state the minimum punishment is life imprisonment at hard labor. In that same state, a proven sexual connection with a cow is punishable by a sentence of five years.

Some individuals are reluctant to practice *fellatio* (oral stimulation of the penis) or *cunnilinction* (oral stimulation of the vulva) for aesthetic reasons. They are repelled by the association with urine or feces or by the nearby anus. To this the answer is simple enough: scrupulous cleanliness. Certainly, communicable disease is no more likely to be spread through oral-genital contact than through genital

[19]Paul H. Gebhard, John H. Gagnon, Wardell B. Pomeroy, and Cornelia V. Christenson, *Sex Offenders* (New York, 1965), p. 3.

contact[20] (see pages 76-77). Men may enjoy and accept cunnilinction more readily than women enjoy and accept fellatio.[21] Communication between the man and woman can do much to remove psychological impedimenta. Among the more educated, oral-genital contact increases in frequency.[22] Oral-genital contact may be rightly regarded as another way by which a great number of people give intense sexual pleasure to someone they love. When adult oral-genital contact is the only source of sexual expression, the practice is considered by some students of sexuality to be a sign of immature sexual development.

When oral-genital contact is refused by one of the partners, the other may attempt to induce it with patient tenderness. Many women not only learn fellatio but also enjoy it. The same is true of men in regard to cunnilinction. As with all sexual practices, oral-genital contact must be agreeable to both partners. Under no circumstances should it be physically enforced or be gained by exploitive exhortations. When one partner persistently refuses oral-genital contact, alternative methods of stimulation may be tried.

The great seventeenth-century philosopher Spinoza (1632-77) wrote: "Pleasure in itself is not bad but good, pain in itself is bad."[23] Sexual intercourse should be a pleasurable, not a painful, experience.

sexual similarities

Some essential similarities between the male and female sexual response may be noted from the above sections. The sexual response of each may be divided into four phases. Both sexes respond to touch, and a variety of stimuli may serve to arouse either sex. Nor is it true that the female responds much more slowly to sexual stimuli than does the male. Her history of a tardy response is due to cultural repression. When the female is able to time her own responses, when she herself regulates the rhythm and intensity of her stimuli (as occurs with masturbation), the time she requires to reach an orgasm approximates that of the male. In addition, both the male and female share the phenomenon of tumescence. And, despite the male ejaculation, the physiology of orgasm is similar in both sexes.

[20] In answer to the question as to whether "there are any harmful effects associated with swallowing semen," one clinician writes, "We have never heard one mention any harmful effects: granted that this is not conclusive proof that reactions may not occur. However, none such have been brought to our attention, even though approximately 50% state that they swallow the semen." (Harry Pariser, "Semen Ingestion," *Medical Aspects of Human Sexuality,* Vol. 6, No. 5 [May 1972], p. 185.)

[21] Alfred C. Kinsey, Wardell B. Pomeroy, Clyde E. Martin, and Paul H. Gebhard, *Sexual Behavior in the Human Female* (Philadelphia, 1953), pp. 257-58.

[22] Alfred C. Kinsey, Wardell B. Pomeroy, and Clyde E. Martin, *Sexual Behavior in the Human Male,* (Philadelphia, 1948), p. 371.

[23] Benedict de Spinoza, *Ethics,* translated into English by R. H. M. Elwes (Washington, D.C., 1901), p. 211.

sexual differences

DIFFERENCES IN ADOLESCENT SEXUALITY

Nevertheless, there are some basic differences in the sexual responses of the male and female. These differences begin to be noticeable at puberty. True puberty is marked by change in the ovaries and testes and changes in their secretions. With the first ejaculation, or soon after, most boys produce viable spermatozoa. In the female, however, puberty does not necessarily include the ability to become pregnant. And if pregnancy should occur, it does not follow that the child can be carried to term. Ancient physicians were aware of this distinction. Puberty (Latin *pubes,* hair) indicated the time that certain body parts became covered with hair. Nubility (Latin *nubis,* veil) meant the time that a girl was able to wear the nuptial veil and be married. A girl may experience a period of *adolescent sterility.* Although this is ordinary, there are exceptions. And the length of time that the adolescent female remains sterile varies greatly. Many adolescent menstrual cycles do not include ovulation. This developmental difference between the adolescent boy and girl may account for the subtle yet profound differences in sexual arousal and response (see pages 92-94). In addition, the dissimilar development of the sexual cells may explain why a physically mature adolescent girl generally is not strongly impelled to seek physical expressions of her sexuality, while a boy is.

When ova do begin to mature completely, they do so singly and are discharged without accumulating. Unlike the female, the male adolescent is vexed by accumulated and trapped sexual fluids, which must escape by ejaculation. In the young girl, sexual stimulation results in a rather diffuse reaction that is dominated by the cerebral cortex. Her increased adolescent sexuality is socially oriented toward marriage. In the adolescent male, a similar amount of sexual stimulation results in the increased production of spermatozoa and the flow of secretions from the accessory sex glands. With this pressure the ejaculatory reflex is excited. His tensions can be relieved only by ejaculation. In the male this is not a diffuse but a local reaction. It is not as cerebral as it is genital. His increased adolescent sexuality is genitally orientated. Although he is capable of great tenderness at this age, only later does his sexuality become social. "This contrast points to a basic distinction between the developmental processes for males and females: males move from privatized personal sexuality to sociosexuality; females do the reverse and at a later stage in the life cycle." [24] Combine this with the ordinarily greater sexual imagery of the young male and the reasons for his earlier interest in sexual

[24] William Simon and John Gagnon, "Psychosexual Development," *Trans-action,* Vol. 6, No. 5 (March 5, 1969), p. 13.

relief becomes clear. However, despite his sexual urgencies, the young adolescent boy finds that girls his own age are quite indifferent to him. Indeed, they may be contemptuous of his clumsy shyness. The early sociosexual orientation of the young adolescent girl explains her interest in dating older boys. It is not sexual expression that she seeks; it is social expression. The awkward boys of her age lack the social sophistication that is necessary to gratify her needs.

DIFFERENCES IN ATTITUDE TOWARD SEXUALITY

The average man can more frequently achieve sexual gratification independent of love than can the average woman. For many women, sexual expression, particularly coitus, is inseparable from love. Married men rate sexual intercourse with the woman for whom they feel affection as the most important feature of their marriage. Most married women tend to rank sexual intercourse lower than security. For them a home and children are the most important elements of marriage. This difference the husband will do well to heed. For the male to bring casualness to the marital bed is to invite rejection, or worse, resentful submission. The wise husband will "seduce his wife romantically rather than erotically, to put her in the right frame of mind by romantic words and settings that appeal to her."[25] The greater emphasis on security rather than sexuality by most women may well be associated with their greater ability to endure sexual deprivation. For a great number of wives whose soldier-husbands are overseas, sexual abstinence is no myth. Although such matters are individual, the adulterous wife of the overseas soldier is not as ordinary as some writers seem to believe.

PSYCHOLOGICAL DIFFERENCES
IN SEXUAL AROUSAL

The sexes are not equally aroused by the same stimuli. It is believed that fewer women than men are sexually stimulated by nudity, erotic movies, or sexual stories. The fact that upper-class men seem to be more susceptible to stimulation by these than men of lower socioeconomic levels indicates that the response may be learned. Women seem to be more easily aroused by such stimuli as romantic movies and stories, although, again, cultural conditioning doubtless plays a part in their response. Moreover, sexual fantasies are much more common among men than women. During both masturbation and sexual intercourse, many more men than women are inclined to make use of sexual fantasies. Frequently the fantasy in which the man engages during these sexual expressions varies considerably from the

[25] Robert O. Blood, *Marriage* (New York, 1969), p. 360.

actual expression. This is not usually the case with women. Thirty years ago, the Kinsey group concluded that only about 10 percent of the total female population in this country experienced orgasmic sexual dreams in any single year.[26] During a like period, the occurrence of dreams with nocturnal emission was far more frequent among males. The Kinsey group also noted that by the age of twenty, only 33 percent of the females in the sample had masturbated to the point of orgasm, as compared with 92 percent of the males.[27] Of course, these differences may have been due to pressures on women to marry. It is likely that the Kinsey data is no longer descriptive of people today.

DIFFERENCES IN DEGREE OF SEXUAL RESPONSE

Among women, the variations in the degree of sexual response are much greater than among men. Some women, perhaps 10 percent, never reach an orgasm. Others do not have an orgasm until they are thirty or forty years of age. Among men, this is exceedingly rare. At the other end of the scale, however, women far exceed men in number of orgasms they can achieve in a given time period. Among a group of college students, for example, a few young women reported an average of twenty-five or more orgasms every week throughout their entire four-year college careers.[28]

The sexes also vary in regard to the age at which they reach their peaks of sexual activity. When all kinds of sexual activity are considered, the average male of this culture reaches his peak before he is twenty years old. Typically, the average female starts engaging in sexual activity at an older age and increases her responses and

[26] Alfred C. Kinsey et al., *Sexual Behavior in the Human Female,* p. 173.

[27] Ibid, p. 197. A newly developed method of determining human sexual preferences involves the use of the electroencephalogram (EEG). This instrument provides traces of the electrical activity of the brain. It has been useful in the diagnosis of a variety of conditions such as brain tumors and epilepsy. One of the brain waves that can be recorded is related to anticipation. For this reason it is called the *expectancy wave,* or *E-wave.*

Twelve single male and twelve single female students between the ages of eighteen and twenty-two were selected for a study. They were not screened for sexual experience or preference. They were shown a series of photographs of male and female nudes, and their electroencephalographic tracings were recorded. Although the pictures were not erotic, the genitalia were fully visible. Also included among the photographs was the shadowy outline of a fully clothed woman; her gender could not be readily determined. The results: the electroencephalographic tracings of the male students showed a markedly elevated E-wave response to the photographs of female nudes; the E-wave response of the female students clearly showed their preference for the male nudes. As the experiment continued, the male E-waves increased as they viewed the clothed, shadowy figure of the woman; her gender had become revealed to them.

A whole new area of investigation into thought processes is opened by this experiment. What are the expectancy waves of a patient on viewing a mother and father? How is the therapy of a drug-dependent person progressing? What will the expectancy waves reveal when the patient is shown a picture of a needle and syringe or of a liquor bottle? (Ronald M. Costell, Donald T. Lunde, Bert S. Koppel, and William K. Wittner, "Contingent Negative Variation as an Indicator of Sexual Object Preference," *Science,* Vol. 177, No. 4050 [August 25, 1972], pp. 718–20.)

[28] *Sexuality and Man,* compiled and edited by the Sex Information and Education Council of the United States (New York, 1970), p. 28, citing Alfred C. Kinsey et al., *Sexual Behavior in the Human Female,* pp. 537–43.

activity more slowly to a peak at about age thirty. Until she is about fifty, and in many cases beyond that age, the average woman's sexual drive and activity remains at a relatively even plateau. There are, of course, individual variations.

THE PERIODIC (CYCLIC) INCREASE IN THE WOMAN'S SEXUAL DESIRE

Still another difference between the sexes may be partly attributable to female physiology. Many women report increased sexual desire before the onset of menstruation. A lesser number experience this heightened sexual interest following menstruation or at the time of ovulation, which occurs at the midpoint of the menstrual cycle. "Since those women who use rhythm [method of birth control] are deprived of sexual relations until the 21st to 23rd days of the cycle, it is clear that they are deprived of relations during two peaks of desire, the postmenstrual and ovulatory. This is a cause of frustration in many of these women."[29] Women whose sexual desire is greatest before the onset of menstrual bleeding may be stimulated by the pelvic congestion that is consequent to the increased amount of blood in that area.

This periodicity (or cyclicity) can be related to the activity of the hypothalamus of the female brain. It will be remembered that in the human embryo androgen acts on the brain to program maleness; the absence of androgen permits the ongoing pattern of femaleness to develop (see pages 79–80). It has also been shown that brain (hypothalamic) chemicals are responsible for the release of luteinizing and follicle-stimulating hormones from the anterior lobe of the pituitary gland (see page 31). On the average, the human female ovulates every twenty-eight days. As has been pointed out, this phenomenon depends on the periodic (or cyclic) release of (1) follicle-stimulating hormone (FSH) to promote the growth of the Graafian follicle, which produces estrogen and also houses the ova to be released at ovulation (see page 42) and (2) luteinizing hormone (LH), which induces the formation of corpora lutea and triggers ovulation (see page 43). Only pregnancy (see pages 190–208) interferes with this normal cycle in the female.

Male reproductive function shows no such cyclicity. Androgen organizes the hypothalamus of the brain of the male embryo to behave differently. Like the female, his hypothalamic brain patterns are organized to also provide chemicals to stimulate the release of both luteinizing hormone (LH) and follicle-stimulating hormone (FSH) from his anterior pituitary. In the male, however, the LH causes the development of those cells in the testes that are largely

---

[29] John R. Cavanagh, "Rhythm of Sexual Desire in Women," *Medical Aspects of Human Sexuality,* Vol. 3, No. 2 (February 1969), p. 39.

responsible for testosterone production (see page 35, footnote 3), and the FSH initiates spermatogenesis. But the LH from the anterior pituitary is not cyclically but continuously produced. And the release of FSH is timed to meet the demands of spermatogenesis, not oögenesis (the development of ova). That the pituitary gland itself is not sexually differentiated has been proven by transplantation experiments. A female pituitary transplanted into a male will not interfere with normal male functions; a male pituitary transplanted into a female will not interfere with completely female functions.[30] Thus, the cyclicity of the female's reproductive system and the acyclicity of the male's both appear to originate in the hypothalamus of the brain.

DIFFERENCES IN DESIRED FREQUENCY OF SEXUAL INTERCOURSE

How often do married couples have sexual intercourse? The answer depends on a wide variety of factors, such as how old they were when they got married and their individual needs. There are no rules, just differences. As is to be expected, sexual intercourse occurs more frequently early in the marriage. Kinsey reported that on the average married men had intercourse 2.8 times a week and women 2.6 times a week by the time they were twenty years old. By age thirty the frequency of intercourse had diminished to 2.2 times a week and by forty this had decreased to a median of 1.5 times a week. At age sixty the rate was 0.6 times a week.[31] As married people get older they become more preoccupied and fatigued by problems inherent in maintaining a family. This is one reason why both the quality and the quantity of the couple's sexual life suffers. This need not be (see pages 272-76).

There is some evidence to indicate that the average male desires sexual intercourse more frequently than the average female. The word *average* is here stressed. Some women prefer sexual intercourse more often than their husbands, although the majority of women report that they prefer it less often. It is noteworthy that husbands and wives often may give significantly different estimates of the actual number of times they have sexual intercourse with one another. This may be revealing of both their attitudes toward sexuality and their satisfaction with the marriage. For example, a woman who desires less intercourse may overestimate the number of times she has it, or a husband who wants to have sexual intercourse more frequently might estimate the actual frequency to be closer to what

[30] Seymour Levine, "Sexual Differentiation: The Development of Maleness and Femaleness," p. 14, citing A. Jost, "Embryonic Sexual Differentiation," in H. W. Jones and W. W. Scott, eds., *Hermaphroditism, Genital Anomalies and Related Endocrine Disorders* (Baltimore, 1958), pp. 15-45.
[31] Alfred C. Kinsey et al., *Sexual Behavior in the Human Female,* pp. 348-49.

he wants it to be, rather than to what it actually is. He may also report a greater frequency to emphasize his masculinity.[32]

The frequency of sexual intercourse is not as significant as is the frequency of rejection—and how the rejection is handled.

DIFFERENCES IN SEXUAL POTENCY

One of the most significant differences between the sexes lies in their relative potency. The fate of the comparatively frail male has already been considered on page 81 and will be further examined later (see pages 159-61). Compared to woman, man becomes ill much more often, and he dies at a younger age. In addition, his psychosexual structure appears to be comparatively fragile. But there is yet another area in which the male is relatively feeble. Man is not as sexually potent as woman.

Aside from ejaculation, there are two major areas of physiological difference between male and female orgasmic expression. First, the female is capable of rapid return to orgasm immediately following an orgasmic experience if restimulated before tensions have dropped below plateau-phase response levels. Second, the female is capable of maintaining an orgasmic experience for a relatively long period of time.[33]

Not only, then, are women able to be multiorgasmic, but they are also able to experience longer orgasms than men. Moreover, they need not undergo profound nervous system coordinations to prepare themselves anatomically for sexual intercourse as men do. For the man an erection is a prerequisite to intercourse. He cannot submit; he must always perform. For countless people, the stress of constant submission or performance is not conducive to sexual competence. Already mentioned (see page 87) is the striking difference between the sexes in their postorgasmic needs. During his refractory period, the man rejects further sexual stimulation; the woman may desire further stimulation in order to enjoy more orgasms.[34] The man and woman who are experienced with one another

---

[32] George Levinger, "Husbands' and Wives' Estimates of Coital Frequency," *Medical Aspects of Human Sexuality,* Vol. 4, No. 9 (September 1970), pp. 42-43, 47-48, 53, 57.

[33] William H. Masters and Virginia E. Johnson, *Human Sexual Response* (Boston, 1966), p. 131.

[34] Recent research suggests that the male rat already has a way of notifying the female of his sexual disinterest during his refractory period. After ejaculation he sings an ultrasonic song. The song corresponds to the period during which he cannot spontaneously initiate copulation. His song signals the female, who then refrains from sexually provocative behavior such as ear-wiggling and darting about. The measured frequency of the ultrasonic sounds of the male rat's "I'm out of action" song is exactly that of males who have been beaten in a fight, or of females who resist overattentive males. Thus "in general they appear to be desist-contact signals." (Ronald J. Barfield and Lynette A. Geyer, "Sexual Behavior: Ultrasonic Postejaculatory Song of the Male Rat," *Science,* Vol. 176, No. 4041 [June 23, 1971], p. 1349.) Demonstrating that the truly scientific mind is never idle, nor ever at a loss to turn pure science into some practical application, one journal published this reflection: "It should now surely be interesting to know what would happen if a rat colony was played continuous recordings of these antisocial signals. Could one devise an ultrasonic rat contraceptive?" ("A Song for the Male Who Has Had Enough," *New Scientist,* Vol. 55, No. 803 [July 6, 1972], p. 7.)

are usually able to resolve this. He, for example, can learn to defer his orgasm until she has had one or more. On the other hand, the female ability to be multiorgasmic should not lead one to assume that more than one orgasm is desired by all women. There is as much variability in orgasmic wants as in any other complex human function. Moreover, many young men are able to have several orgasms and ejaculations closely following the first; however, this capacity is generally lost by most males by the age of thirty.

PROBLEMS ARISING FROM DIFFERENCES
IN SEXUALITY

The differences in sexual expression between the sexes must be appreciated by both members of the marital couple. Otherwise lack of harmony may result. For example, the husband may misinterpret his wife's lesser interest in sexual intercourse. Convinced that she is indifferent to him, he may look elsewhere for a seemingly more agreeable sexual partner. Better communication may help the husband to find that his wife is more receptive than he had imagined.

The wife may attempt to meet her husband's sexual demands by submitting to intercourse and pretending orgasm. This is essentially insignificant if it happens only occasionally. When it persists, a deep-seated emotional disturbance may be suspected. (This is no less true about the husband who recognizes the pretense and accepts it.) Indeed, in these instances, differences in sexual desire may not be the basic problem. One woman fears the abandonment of orgasm. Another may be concerned that its very abandon makes her appear less attractive. By her pretense, a wife may express her hostility toward her husband. Subconsciously, she dares her husband to notice the fraud. When the husband fails to do so, the wife may then point to his deficiencies. A woman, who has gone through a period of pretending orgasm, may eventually begin to have and enjoy them. Then she may fear that her husband will notice the difference in her response. He may not. He might merely believe that "things are getting better and better." [35]

A woman has a profound responsibility in maintaining an active marital relationship . . . A wife sometimes finds that her husband's spontaneous desire for intercourse occurs more often than she is able actively to respond, no matter how much she would like to . . . If she enjoys it most of the time, she should certainly participate whenever he needs her.[36]

[35] Salo Rosenbaum, "Pretended Orgasm," *Medical Aspects of Human Sexuality,* Vol. 4, No. 4 (April 1970), p. 84.
[36] Maxine Davis, *The Sexual Responsibility of Women,* quoted in Robert O. Blood, *Marriage,* p. 374.

Not uncommonly, marital-sexual dissension arises not from the wife's lesser interest in sexual intercourse but from her greater desire. This, coupled with her potential for more and longer orgasms and her later development of peak sexuality, may make her husband feel threatened. Fearing a loss of masculinity, he may begin to reject sexuality. He may even become impotent (see pages 292–94). What he should realize is that "the female's orgasm most plausibly represents nature's gift to femininity and not woman's bonus to masculinity." [37] If he can learn to accept this, he may also come to enjoy it.

on woman's release from sexual slavery

> *Ah Love! could you and I with Him conspire*
> *To grasp this sorry Scheme of Things entire,*
> *   Would not we shatter it to bits—and then*
> *Remold it nearer to the Heart's desire!*[38]

The modern interest in the orgasm should surprise nobody. In this technological age, it is the technique rather than the art of love that sells marriage manuals. Yet, apparently technique alone does not suffice. Some college girls, who consider themselves sophisticated about sex, are often reduced to frustrated failure in achieving an orgasm. One psychiatrist writes:

> *An emphasis on orgasm pervades all age groups of our society . . . Among university students the search for the ultimate orgasm has become almost a competitive matter . . . the ultimate confession . . . I have seen girls who admitted cheating, stealing . . . and promiscuity with little shame but who wept violently when they confessed that they could not have orgasms.*[39]

It has been repeatedly observed that until recently in this culture the female half of the human species had much less experience with orgasm than the male. Not more than a hundred years ago, the opinion was held in Western cultures that only evil women ever admitted, even to themselves, that they enjoyed the sexual act. Sexual anesthesia was the price most women paid for the protection and support of their home and children. Society supported the male as ruler of the roost, and the double standard extended to the double bed. The male's sexual needs were gratified according to his, not his wife's, wishes. He chose the time. He felt no need to give. Once satiated, he rarely gave his docile mate a second sexual thought.

---

[37] Salo Rosenbaum, "Pretended Orgasm," p. 84.
[38] *Rubáiyát of Omar Khayyám,* translated into English by Edward FitzGerald.
[39] Seymour L. Halleck, "Sex and Mental Health on the Campus," *Journal of the American Medical Association,* Vol. 200, No. 8 (May 22, 1967), p. 687.

Moreover, he had deeply founded memories of another woman who, presumably, had also been a wife. She had provided for other hungers. With affection he remembered his mother. For such various reasons, then, did the male accept his monogamous arrangement. (And this one-sided relationship doubtless led to feminine feelings like those expressed in the lines from the *Rubáiyát* that introduce this section.)

The long overdue liberation of women changed all that. Enfranchised, and finding new employment and enjoyment opportunities open to them, women also, at last, expected equality in the marital bed. Many of their husbands then imposed upon themselves an unaccustomed husbandly duty—the sexual satisfaction of their wives. Many, but not all. College-matriculated men are apparently more concerned with wifely sexual gratification than are those with less education. In one study only 7 out of 51 men without college matriculation "expressed the slightest concern with responsibility for coital-partner satisfaction . . . Out of a total of 261 . . . subjects with college matriculation, 214 men expressed concern with coital-partner satisfaction." [40]

This concern of some men with the sexual satisfaction of their wives is to their credit; perhaps college is a civilizing influence, after all.[41]

VARIATIONS IN ORGASMIC QUALITY

"There is good evidence that the capacity for orgasm or sexual climax is a natural birthright of almost every healthy adult human being." [42] The quality of a human orgasm is to a great extent a matter of individual interpretation. Although an orgasm involves the same nervous pathways and the same total body responses in all humans, the degree of involvement varies with individuals and situations. This may be a factor causing subjective differences in the quality of different orgasms. On one occasion, for example, a woman may have sexual intercourse while she is depressed and tired. If her partner is matter-of-fact and pays no heed to her mood, she may have no orgasm or perhaps only a local clitoral sensation. But if her partner is sensitive to her mood, if he expresses his love and waits for her participation, she knows he cares. Then, even if her orgasmic experience is not intense (although it may very well be), the totality of her sexual experience will more likely be satisfying.

---

[40] William H. Masters and Virginia E. Johnson, *Human Sexual Response,* p. 202.
[41] Increased knowledge about female sexuality doubtless plays some part in the college male's interest in his sexual partner's satisfaction. The cultural double standard has progressed from the notion that sexual behavior is something that the man does *to* the woman, to something that he does *for* her. Now men (and women) must act on the premise that it is something he does *with* her. ("MDs Held Lacking in Sex Function Training," *Internal Medicine News,* Vol. 5, No. 14 [July 15, 1972], p. 24, quoting Mrs. William H. Masters [Virginia E. Johnson].)
[42] *Sexuality and Man,* p. 25.

John Money has written:

Whatever the antecedents to an orgasm that is better than others, the final common pathway is the same. The two lovers are able to experience a feeling of unrestrained and untamed abandonment to one another. It is not necessary for them to pay attention either to what the self is doing or what the partner is doing. All the movements take care of themselves, as if by means of a spinal reflex. The sensations greedily absorbed via the vulva, externally and through deep interior pressure, tell the vaginal cavity how to selfishly pulsate, ripple, quiver and contract on the penis in order to release itself in orgasm. Reciprocally, the penis selfishly probes and presses, twists a little, withdraws and tantalizes at the portals, and sinks deeply again, greedily building up its own orgasmic pleasure. The two bodies writhe, unheedingly. The two minds drift into the oblivion of attending only to their own feeling, so perfectly synchronized that the ecstasy of the one is preordained to be the reciprocal ectasy of the other. Two minds, mindlessly lost in one another. This is the perfect orgasmic experience. This is how an orgasm is made better than any that have ever preceded it. This also is how no orgasm is made the best—for orgasms can keep getting better and better than ever. Did you know that this is one of the tremendous payoffs of getting older?[43]

some myths and misconceptions about human sexuality

"The little rift between the sexes," wrote Robert Louis Stevenson, "is astonishingly widened by simply teaching one set of catchwords to the girls and another to the boys." Only too often is that rift widened even more by teaching them misconceptions about one another's sexuality. This is not usually deliberate. Most of the modern open-minded discussion about sexual matters is of recent origin. Unfortunately, much of today's talk about sexuality is based on yesterday's misinformation. What are some of the more common of these misconceptions?

Misconception No. 1: To have a satisfactory marital experience, the wife and husband must have an orgasm with each intercourse.

This generally unrealized ideal has been a hazard to many a marriage. The difference in the degree of sexual interest between the sexes has already been mentioned. As a marriage matures and in-

[43] John W. Money, "Why Are Some Orgasms Better than Others?" *Medical Aspects of Human Sexuality,* Vol. 5, No. 3 (March 1971), p. 17.

timacy deepens, the frequency of the wife's orgasms may increase. However, the wife will accomplish orgasm, and more often sooner, when she realizes that "the husband's enjoyment of the act has to take precedence over his efforts to please his wife. Otherwise, sooner or later, neither of them will have any pleasure at all." [44]

Both the young husband the and young wife approach their new roles with some guilt and anxiety. They do not suddenly awaken to maturity after a long period of sexual somnolence. Nevertheless, instead of preparing adolescents for their future sexual function, society merely controls them. Many of these controls are necessary. (Today, almost the only adult pleasure usually forbidden the unmarried teen-ager is sexual intercourse.) But this sexual control is matched by a conspiracy of parental silence about the subject. The growing boy is not helped by the slick magazine, nor by the refusal of his parents to talk about sexuality, nor by the embarrassment of his teachers. Too often, his education is a compound of the sniggering anxieties of his contemporaries and furtive, short-lived, basically uncomfortable liaisons. He drifts alone on the murky waters of opinionated misinformation. Sexuality is associated with something evil.[45] It may then be loaded with guilt and anxiety.

His young wife may be similarly ill-equipped. Her secret anxiety may be matched by her dreamy determination to equal the seemingly satisfactory creatures her husband sees in some magazine gatefolds. She owes it to him, the man she loves, to be the responsive and adequate wife.

No matter what their previous experience has been, marriage has ceremoniously thrust them into a new, often threatening role. They must prove themselves. Right now. Every time.

Thus does marriage pose anxieties that require patience, enormous understanding, and a sense of humor about oneself and one's mate. It will relax the couple to know that orgasm with each intercourse is not necessary to a happy marriage. Terman's research indicates that a wife's capacity for orgasm is not highly related to the couple's happiness.[46] And more recent research by Masters and Johnson suggests that the intensity and duration of a woman's orgasm is not necessarily related to her sense of sexual gratification. An orgasm of relatively low intensity and short duration, during a sexual experience with a husband she loves, may indeed be evaluated by the wife as a complete and fulfilling sexual experience.[47] The consistent sexual competency of the wife is not as important to marital happiness as understanding and patient communication.

[44] Milton R. Sapirstein, *Paradoxes of Everyday Life* (New York, 1955), p. 28.
[45] This association may have begun long before adolescence—on the day the small child is punished for examining the genitalia.
[46] L. M. Terman, "Correlates of Orgasm Adequacy in a Group of 556 Wives," in M. F. De Martino, ed., *Sexual Behavior and Personality Characteristics* (New York, 1966).
[47] Warren R. Johnson, *Human Sexual Behavior and Sex Education* (Philadelphia, 1968), pp. 50-51.

Feeling safe and feeling a sense of trust are no less profoundly involved with marital happiness than the orgasm.

Misconception No. 2: Simultaneous orgasm is absolutely essential for ultimate and satisfactory sexual expression.

This nonsense, a favorite of some marriage manuals, is another anxiety producer. The woman must, after all, either begin to have, or have, an orgasm before the man. If the former is true, simultaneous orgasms are possible. These are delightful experiences. However, many couples never have them, nor do they miss them. To insist on a simultaneous orgasm is, again, a way of putting oneself on trial. The man who is on constant trial does not relax. He may become unable to have an erection. This failure may, in turn, make him fear that he has lost his sexual prowess. Shame torments him. Sometimes a man may become impotent[48] (lose the ability to have sexual intercourse) with a wife with whom he feels on trial. Instead he finds himself potent with "another woman." Or, with his wife, he may have premature ejaculations,[49] with attendant guilt feelings. As will be pointed out later: "Problems of premature ejaculation . . . disturbed the younger members of the study-subject population." This was particularly true of college-matriculated men: "with these men ejaculatory control sufficient to accomplish partner satisfaction was considered a coital technique that must be acquired before the personal security of coital effectiveness could be established."[50]

With premature ejaculation, there is anxiety. Again the male doubts his potency. It is worth repeating that male sexual activity is circumscribed by a basic requirement. He must feel certain of his active role. He cannot, like his mate, submit to sexual intercourse. Although constant submission may relieve her of some of the stress of performance, it will bring her, not the fulfillment of a satisfying sexual expression, but the bitterness of sexual repression. For her, too, coitus should neither be a test nor a contest.

Some marriage manuals make effective chaperones.

Misconception No. 3: Direct clitoral stimulation during sexual intercourse is essential.

There are some misguided writers who detail the crucial importance of direct clitoral stimulation to arouse sexual desire. Research disputes this advice. For a great number of women the difference between clitoral excitement and irritation is slight. To their surprise (and in contradiction to many marriage manuals) many husbands discover that their wives find manual clitoral stimulation distinctly disagreeable, if not painful. Many, instead, prefer manual stimulation

---

[48]For a further discussion of impotence, see pages 292-94.
[49]For a further discussion of premature ejaculation, see pages 294-96.
[50]William H. Masters and Virginia E. Johnson, *Human Sexual Response,* p. 202.

of the general mons area. There is only one best way to find out. Ask.

Effective manual general-mons stimulation results in a clitoral retraction reaction (see page 85). The clitoris normally retracts upward.

This physiological reaction to high levels of female sexual tension creates a problem for the sexually inexperienced male. The clitoral-body retraction reaction frequently causes even an experienced male to lose manual contact with the organ. Having lost contact, the male partner usually ceases active stimulation of the general mons area and attempts manually to relocate the clitoral body. During this "textbook" approach, marked sexual frustration may develop in a highly excited female partner . . . Once . . . clitoral retraction has been established, manipulation of the general mons area is all that is necessary for effective clitoral-body stimulation.[51]

Misconception No. 4: This is a double mistake: (1) that there is a vaginal orgasm distinct from the clitoral orgasm, and (2) that clitoral orgasm is immature; only vaginal orgasm is mature.

These false concepts go back to the outmoded idea that female sexual organs are but incomplete male organs, nothing more than a perpetual case of arrested genital development. Thus hopelessly sexually retarded, it was even thought impossible, if not indecent, for woman to enjoy, much less desire, sexual intercourse. Freud did not fall into this trap, but he did fall for the idea of the female as an incomplete, hence inferior, male. He considered woman biologically dependent on the male. Lacking a penis, she was thought to be passively envious. "Freud's theories buttressed all the prevailing prejudices and promoted the notion that the female was a deficient male and a second-class citizen." [52] Reflecting the patriarchal culture of his time, he attributed to biology what was, in reality, culturally prescribed. To this was added another error. Girls who masturbated usually did so by manual clitoral stimulation. This, it was decreed by many early writers, was immature. Hence, manual clitoral stimulation to orgasm by adults was immature. Although clitoral stimulation during intercourse was acceptable, only vaginal orgasm was the mark of the normal and sexually mature woman.

The trouble with all this is that it is wrong. What are the facts?

1. The sexually sensitive areas of the female genitalia are the clitoris, labia minora, and the lower third of the vagina (see pages 50–51 and Figure 2-4). (As a source of erotic arousal, the mons area

[51] Ibid., pp. 65–66.
[52] Leon Salzman, "Psychology of the Female," *Archives of General Psychiatry,* Vol. 17, No. 2 (August 1967), p. 195.

ranks with the clitoris and the labia minora; it is, however, not strictly a part of the genitalia. The labia minora are not as sensitive as the clitoral shaft and the mons area.)

2. The upper two-thirds of the vagina has a different embryological origin than the lower third; that is, it arises from a different group of cells. The lower third of the vagina and the labia minora have the same embryological origin; they arise from the same group of cells. Nor are the clitoris and the lower third of the vagina separable structures.

3. The upper two-thirds of the vagina plays no part in the orgasm. Nor does it play a part in the development of erotic feelings.

4. During sexual arousal, the lower third of the vagina and labia minora function as a unit. They are thought to be about equally sensitive to sexual stimulation. The clitoris is more sensitive than either.

5. With one exception, there are no nerve or muscle or blood vessel connections between the clitoris and the vagina. The exception is a network of veins from the clitoris that merges into a network of veins lying along the walls of the vagina. During sexual excitement, these veins are engorged with blood, causing tumescence. Within ten to thirty seconds after sexual excitement, a lubricating fluid appears on the vaginal walls. This fluid seeps onto the vaginal walls directly from the plexus of veins surrounding the vaginal barrel.

6. Like the penis, the clitoris is generously endowed with nerves and is capable of tumescence, spasmodic contraction, and detumescence.

7. During coitus, the penis rarely comes in direct contact with the clitoris. This is because of the above-mentioned retraction reaction. The traction of the penis on the sensitive labia minora stimulates the shortened, hidden clitoris. (By varying positions during sexual intercourse, more direct contact may be achieved, see pages 87–89.) The thrusting movements of the penis

create simultaneous stimulation of the lower third of the vagina, labia minora, and clitoral shaft and glans as an integrated, inseparable functioning unit with the glans being the most important and, in by far the majority of instances, the indispensable initiator of the orgasmic reaction . . . it is a physical impossibility to separate the clitoral from the vaginal orgasm.[53]

8. During the female orgasm, the male often feels contractions on the shaft of his penis. What are they? Does the vagina produce these contractions of orgasm? No. Then what does contract? It was

[53] Mary Jane Sherfey, "The Evolution and Nature of Female Sexuality in Relation to Psychoanalytic Theory," p. 78.

pointed out above that the orgasmic contractions are of the muscles located in the floor of the pelvis that surround the lower third of the vagina. With female orgasm, these muscles contract, not directly against the vaginal wall, but against the network of engorged chambers of veins and blood channels about that part of the vagina. In this way the venous passages are emptied of blood (detumescence). These muscle contractions about the vaginal veins cause the lower vaginal walls to be passively pushed in and out. Moreover, these muscle contractions cause the upper labia minora to contract. That is what the male feels. "Therefore there is no such thing as an orgasm of the vagina. What exists is an orgasm of the circumvaginal venous chambers." [54]

9. Thus, one cannot distinguish between vaginal orgasm and clitoral orgasm. Regardless of how it was stimulated, the nature of the orgasm is the same.

Present knowledge of the origin, anatomy, and function of the female genitalia should help to dispel many a female fear. Long depressed by the idea of the inferiority of the clitoral orgasm, many women blamed either themselves or their husbands for their failure to achieve "vaginal orgasm." The whole notion, however, of a vaginal orgasm separate from clitoral orgasm is biologically impossible and, therefore, utterly invalid. And to consider clitoral orgasm immature and vaginal orgasm mature is senseless. "The tendency to reduce clitoral eroticism to a level of psychopathology or immaturity because of its supposed masculine origin is a travesty of the facts and a misleading psychologic deduction." [55]

Misconception No. 5: The size of the genital organs (penis or vagina) is related to sexual prowess.

This error is based on myths that have been dispelled by considerable research, most recently by that of Masters and Johnson. [56]

First, the size of the penis is in no way related to the size of the man. In a group of 312 men ranging in age from twenty-one to eighty-nine years, it was found that the longest penis in the flaccid (soft) state belonged to a man five feet seven inches tall who weighed 152 pounds; the smallest penis was that of a man four inches taller and twenty-six pounds heavier.

Second, upon erection, a larger penis does not necessarily increase to a greater size than does a smaller penis. For example, one man's penile measurement in the flaccid state was 7.5 cm. (2.95 in.); in the erect state its length increased to more than double its flaccid state—it lengthened 9 cm. (3.5 in.) to equal 16.5 cm. (6.5 in.). Another man's flaccid penis was 11 cm. (4.3 in.) long; it increased only 5.5 cm. (2.2

[54] Ibid., p. 84.
[55] Leon Salzman, "Psychology of the Female," p. 196.
[56] William H. Masters and Virginia E. Johnson, *Human Sexual Response,* pp. 191-95.

in.) as a result of erection; erect, its length also totalled 16.5 cm.[57] The extent to which misinformation about penile length can concern some individuals is demonstrated by the young man who reportedly tied weights of increasing size to his penis every day in an attempt to lengthen the organ. He failed.[58]

Third, during the late excitement or early plateau phases, the vagina lengthens and also expands in its upper (deeper) area of the cervix. This creates a receptacle to receive the seminal pool that is about to be deposited. This overdistension of that upper part of the vagina makes some women feel that the penis is "lost in the vagina." This sensation has nothing to do with penile size. It is more apparent in the woman whose vagina has been traumatized during childbirth and then inadequately repaired. However under ordinary circumstances, it is most unusual for the vagina to be so large as to interfere with coital pleasure. A vagina is rarely so small that accommodation of the penis is difficult unless the woman is highly aroused. The same is occasionally true in the case of the woman who has passed the menopause or who has not had sexual intercourse for a long time. In summary, "penile size usually is a minor factor in sexual stimulation of the female partner. The normal or large vagina accommodates a penis of any size without difficulty. If the vagina is exceptionally small, or if a long period of continence or of involution [shriveling] intervenes, a penis of any size can distress rather than stimulate, if mounting is attempted before advanced stages of female sexual tension have been experienced."[59]

Misconception No. 6: Permanent or even temporary abstinence from sexual intercourse will invariably result in neurotic or psychotic behavior.

Sexual intercourse is a means of fulfillment for the human personality. It can be a way of providing basic human needs for intimacy, sharing, and commitment. True, as in the animal world, coitus is a biological act of procreation. But it can also be a profound expression of humanness.

However, to equate temporary or permanent abstinence from sexual intercourse with invariable emotional disorder is an error. Coitus is an expression of the whole personality, but it is not the personality per se. Neurotic and psychotic behavior are expressions

---

[57] Does the penis ever decrease in size from the flaccid (soft) state? Yes. Cold, severe exhaustion resulting from undue and prolonged physical strain, advanced age, surgical castration—these are among the reasons that the size of the penis diminishes from that of its usual flaccid state in an individual. Prolonged impotence (see pages 292-94) of over two years may also have this effect. It may also occur immediately after a man has attempted but failed to have sexual intercourse. This last cause fortifies the belief that lessening of penile size, like erection, is not only the result of a spinal reflex, but is also profoundly influenced by stimuli from the higher brain centers. (William H. Masters and Virginia E. Johnson, *Human Sexual Response*, pp. 180-81).

[58] Eugene Schoenfeld, *Dear Doctor Hip Pocrates* (New York, 1968), p. 19.

[59] William H. Masters and Virginia E. Johnson, *Human Sexual Response*, p. 195.

of a disorder of the whole personality. Sexual disorders may be part of disordered personality expressions, but they are usually the result, not the cause, of neurotic or psychotic behavior. It should, however, be stressed that people may suffer disturbances of sexual function without demonstrating severely neurotic or psychotic behavior.

Coitus is the only physiological function that a person can choose to keep unfulfilled. Some people choose to permanently refrain from sexual intercourse. In his "On the Good of Marriage," Saint Augustine wrote: "To many, total abstinence is easier than perfect moderation." (In his *Confessions,* however, he wrote: "Give me chastity and continence but not yet.") Many people have led long and purposeful lives without experiencing the meaningful pleasures that can be part of sexual intercourse.

Of course, such individuals are in the minority. However, at various times in their lives, many people defer sexual intercourse for considerable periods of time. There is no evidence whatsoever that this leads to emotional illness.

Misconception No. 7: The treatment of sexual inadequacy is always difficult, costly, and time-consuming.

By no means is this true. Sometimes seemingly severe sexual problems have simple causes and need relatively minor adjustment for their solution. To cite some examples: one man was delighted with the totality of his wife's sexual responses, yet they embarrassed and inhibited him, particularly when her uninhibited screaming and shouting during orgasm occurred while their children or guests were in the house. A second man lost penile sensation and also worried about the adequacy of the size of his penis because his wife was prone to use an excessive amount of spermicidal jelly "just to be on the safe side." Another man was married to a demure little woman whose pelvic movements during coitus were so vigorous that penis and vagina were too soon parted. Instead of an uncontrollable desire to have an orgasm, the husband had an uncontrollable desire to laugh. Fearing to hurt his wife's feelings he controlled his merriment, but his sexual life was adversely affected. To avoid soiling the bed sheet, still another couple were wont to rush to the bathroom immediately after the husband's ejaculation. Soon they found the price of this tidiness too high; their sexual life suffered. All such problems, if they are candidly discussed, can be corrected with obvious minor adjustments.[60] They require neither prolonged nor expensive attention.

[60]The cases cited above are from John L. Schimel, "Some Practical Considerations in Treating Male Sexual Inadequacy," *Medical Aspects of Human Sexuality,* Vol. 5, No. 3 (March 1971), pp. 24, 29–31.

controlling
human
reproduction

birth control

Birth control is not a modern development of a civilized society. Primitive societies limit population in various ways. Although less common than formerly, *infanticide* still occurs. Some African tribes practice *coitus interruptus* (coitus in which the penis is withdrawn from the vagina before ejaculation). The primitive Achinese of Sumatra use a vaginal suppository containing tannic acid. This primitive group has hit upon a valid scientific principle; tannic acid is an effective spermicide.[1]

Ancient writings are replete with instructions on birth control. In the Petri papyrus (1850 B.C.), crocodile dung is recommended. Twenty-seven hundred years later, the Arabian physician Qusta ibn Tuqa substituted elephant dung for that of the crocodile. Few if any prescriptions, contraceptive or otherwise, persisted for as many years as did dung.[2]

Coitus interruptus is described in the Bible (Genesis 38:9). It was practiced by the ancient Hebrews. Infanticide is also mentioned in the Bible.[3] It was condemned by Jew and Christian alike.[4] Nevertheless, in eighteenth- and nineteenth-century Europe infanticide was practiced. "It was not an uncommon spectacle to see the corpses of infants lying in the streets or on the dung hills of London and other large cities."[5]

The views of Saint Thomas Aquinas have been vastly influential.

[1] Norman E. Himes, *Medical History of Contraception* (Baltimore, 1936), p. 63.
[2] Ibid.
[3] See, for example, Leviticus 18:21; Deuteronomy 12:31; II Kings 3:27, 16:3; II Chronicles 28:3, 33:6; Psalms 106:38; Isaiah 57:5; Jeremiah 19:5; Ezekiel 16:21.
[4] In China's first official document against infanticide, in 1659, Choen Tche (1633-62) wrote: "I have heard that the sad cry uttered by these girl babies as they plunged into a vase of water and drowned is inexpressible. Alas! that the heart of a father or mother should be so cruel." (Fielding H. Garrison, "History of Pediatrics," in Arthur Frederick Abt and Fielding H. Garrison, *History of Pediatrics* [Philadelphia, 1965], p. 3.)
[5] William L. Langer, "Checks on Population Growth—1750 to 1850," *Scientific American,* Vol. 226, No. 2 (February 1972), p. 95.

In the *Summa Theologica,* he wrote: "In so far as the generation of offspring is impeded, it is a vice against nature which happens in every carnal act from which generation cannot follow."

An Englishman, Francis Place (1771–1854), was the first to attempt mass education concerning contraception. Place was followed by many disciples, but none is better known than Margaret Sanger. As a nurse among the poor of the lower East Side of New York, she had been moved by the poverty of large families. She became an ardent worker for contraception. Her first contraceptive advice station in Brooklyn, in 1916, and her constant brushes with the law[6] testify to her militance. When she died, some years ago, she was widely mourned.

BIRTH CONTROL FOR THE FEMALE

oral contraceptives and clots

Table 4-1 presents the most common birth control methods available today. Oral contraceptives merit special discussion. In this country all the currently marketed oral contraceptive pills are composed of synthetic estrogens and synthetic progesterone (progestin).[7] They are administered in one of two ways, either in combination or in a sequential fashion.

Each of the combination oral contraceptive pills is identical; each contains synthetic estrogens and progestins. There are different kinds of estrogens and progestins and the kind and the amount of estrogens and progestins in an oral contraceptive pill varies with the brand. Most combination pills are taken for twenty-one days, then discontinued for a week before beginning a new cycle. However, some brands add seven "sugar pills" to be taken at the end of the cycle so that a pill is taken every day of the month. The sequential oral contraceptive pills are not identical. The first fifteen or sixteen pills in a cycle contain only synthetic estrogens; the last five pills contain estrogens and progestins. Like the combination type, the amount and kind of the synthetic hormones and the dosage taken in a monthly series varies with the brand. Oral contraceptives should never be used without the advice of a physician, and he will prescribe the brand he thinks is most advisable for the individual patient. In most cases he will prescribe one of the brands of pills that has the lowest dosage of estrogen (not more than .05 milligrams of estrogen in each pill). Why? This entails some understanding of thromboembolic disease.

A *thrombus* is a clot in a blood vessel (or in the heart) that is formed by the coagulation of blood. It remains at the site of its formation. An *embolus* is a clot that has left the site of its formation.

[6] In 1915, she was jailed in New York for trying to distribute her pamphlet *Family Limitation.*
[7] For a discussion of estrogen and progesterone, see pages 31-32.

TABLE 4-1 a summary of birth control methods

METHOD	WHAT IT IS AND HOW IT WORKS	EFFECTIVENESS AND ACCEPTABILITY
Oral contraceptives (the pill) (see pages 109, 113–17)	It is generally accepted that the synthetic hormones contained in oral contraceptives (estrogens and progestins) inhibit ovulation. There are two contraceptive pill methods. The most commonly used method is often referred to as the "combination" or "balanced progestin-estrogen" method. This method is by far the one most commonly prescribed (more than 90 percent). Each pill contains a combination of both synthetic estrogen and progestin to assure inhibition of ovulation. When no egg is released from an ovary, a woman cannot become pregnant. In the other one, called the "sequential" method, two different pills are used each month. When this method is used, a pill containing synthetic estrogen is taken daily for the first 14, 15, or 16 days of the cycle. This pill inhibits ovulation. The second pill, containing a mixture of synthetic estrogen and progestin, is then taken for 4, 5, or 6 days to assure orderly bleeding within 3 to 5 days after the last pill is taken in each cycle. The pills are usually taken for 21 or 28 consecutive days in each menstrual cycle.	Except for total abstinence or surgical sterilization, the combination pill is the most effective contraceptive known to man. Failures, even when occasional pills are omitted are extremely rare, numbering less than 1 per 100 women per year. The sequential pill method, when used correctly, is only slightly less effective, with failures of about 1.4 per 100 women per year. No woman should take the pill until she has had a physical examination by a physician who knows her medical history and has approved its use. Reexaminations are usually performed at 6- to 12-month intervals. Initial and refill prescriptions must be authorized to obtain the pills from a pharmacy or clinic. There are definite contraindications, important warnings, and precautions to both the user and the prescriber, as well as a number of side reactions reported to be associated with the use of the pill. The pill is by far the most acceptable method in terms of numbers because it is reliably effective and its nonmessy convenient use is unrelated to the timing of sexual play and coitus. It does not interfere with the spontaneity and passion of love-making.
Intrauterine devices (IUD)	Objects of different shapes made of plastic or stainless steel are inserted into the uterus by a physician. They may be left in place indefinitely. How the devices prevent pregnancy is not completely understood. They do not prevent the ovary from releasing eggs. At the moment the evidence suggests they probably speed descent of the egg or the egg may reach the uterus at a time when it cannot nest there.	The protection afforded by the IUD is superseded only by the pill. Protection with the IUD is greater than with such "traditional" methods as the diaphragm or condom, even when these methods are used without any deviation in their regular use. Failures are about 2.7 per 100 women per year. Some women cannot satisfactorily use the devices because of expulsion, bleeding, or discomfort. Contraindications to insertion include pregnancy or suspected pregnancy, abnormalities that distort the uterine cavity, infection or inflammation of the uterus or adnexa, a history of postpartum endometritis, or of infection with abortion within the past three months, and endometrial disease (hyperplasia, carcinoma, polyps, or suspected malignancy). Serious problems reported to be associated with the IUD are pelvic inflammatory disease and perforation of the uterus. Pregnancy can occur

Table 4-1   Continued

METHOD	WHAT IT IS AND HOW IT WORKS	EFFECTIVENESS AND ACCEPTABILITY
		with the device in place. Insertion in nulliparous women is restricted because of their narrow cervical canals. Expulsions limit immediate postpartum insertions. IUDs are now inserted in about 7 percent of an obstetrician's contraceptive users. Few general practitioners use them. IUDs are very acceptable when sustained motivation is lacking, when the user is fearful of using the pill, or when other methods cannot be used successfully.
Diaphragms	Flexible hemispherical rubber domes used in combination with cream or jelly which women insert into the vagina to cover the cervix, provide a barrier to spermatozoa. They must be left in place at least 6 hours after intercourse and may be left in place as long as 24 hours. They must be fitted by a physician; refitted every 2 years and after each pregnancy.	Offers a high level of protection although occasional method failures may be expected because of improper insertion or displacement of the diaphragm during sexual intercourse. A rate of 2 to 3 pregnancies per 100 women per year would seem to be a generous estimate for meticulously consistent users. If motivation or self-control is weak, much higher pregnancy rates must be expected. On the average, therefore, failures are about 17.5 per 100 women per year. Many women use the diaphragm successfully. Others have difficulty inserting it correctly, or dislike the procedure required.
Rhythm (see pages 117–18)	This depends on abstinence from intercourse during the time of month when a woman is fertile. Due to menstrual irregularity in many women and the inability to accurately determine the time of ovulation, success with this method may require abstinence for as long as half of every month. While some couples have successfully worked out this system for themselves, most couples will require assistance from a doctor or rhythm clinic.	Self-taught "rhythm," haphazardly practiced, is one of the least effective methods of family planning. For most couples the practice of rhythm is a guessing game. Failures are to be expected in at least 24 per 100 women per year. However, the effectiveness of the rhythm method may approach that of the diaphragm and condom when it is correctly taught, understood, and religiously practiced. Rhythm is generally an unacceptable method, not only because it is unreliable but also because success requires that the woman have regular menstrual cycles (few have) and that both partners accept long periods of abstinence each month.
Surgery: Vasectomy (see pages 119–22)	A vasectomy involves a relatively simple operation to prevent the spermatozoa from entering the ejaculate through the tubes (vas deferens) leading from the testes to the urethra in	Once the spermatozoa have been prevented from entering the ejaculate after a vasectomy, the male is considered sterile and his sperm can no longer fertilize the female egg. Many

Table 4-1 Continued

METHOD	WHAT IT IS AND HOW IT WORKS	EFFECTIVENESS AND ACCEPTABILITY
	the male. Cutting and tying or ligating of the vas deferens can be done under local anesthesia and performance usually in less than 30 minutes in the doctor's office or hospital. Ligation of the vas deferens should be considered a permanent procedure since there is no guarantee that fertility will be regained with the tubes reopened.	men find this method highly acceptable since it decreases neither the desire or the ability for sexual intercourse nor the amount of ejaculate. Some men, however, experience psychologic effects from a feeling of guilt or fear of lost manhood after this surgical procedure.
Tubal ligation (see pages 118–19)	Tubal ligation involves blocking the Fallopian tubes through which the fertilized egg travels from the ovary to the uterus. This procedure, which involves cutting, separating, and tying the tubes, can be done primarily through the abdominal wall or sometimes vaginally and is often performed just after childbirth. Reuniting the tubes is a major surgical procedure, and success may be defined by the fact that the tubes are reopened, but this does not necessarily mean that fertility is restored.	A tubal ligation is virtually 100 percent effective but failures with this method have been reported. While a tubal ligation is more involved than a vasectomy and must be performed in a hospital, it has become more acceptable to more women who desire permanent sterilization.
Condom	This is a thin, strong sheath or cover, made of rubber or similar material, worn by the man to prevent spermatozoa from entering the vagina. (The woman may also use a vaginal foam, cream, or jelly to provide added protection and lubrication.)	A high degree of protection is offered if the man will use it correctly and consistently. Some couples find the use of condoms objectionable. Failures are due to tearing of the sheath or its slipping off after climax. The condom rates in effectiveness with the diaphragm. There are approximately 16 failures per 100 women per year. The condom is universally accepted as one of the best preventives against venereal disease. A distinct advantage is that it can be purchased without a prescription.
Chemical methods:	These products are inserted into the vagina. Their purpose is to coat vaginal surfaces and cervical opening, and to destroy sperm cells; these products may act as mechanical barriers as well. They provide protection for about 1 hour.	The effectiveness of these vaginal chemical contraceptives used alone is lower than if they are used in combination with a diaphragm or a condom. Nevertheless, significant reductions in pregnancy rates may be obtained by the use of these simple methods. Among these contraceptives the vaginal foams are the most effective, followed by the jellies and creams. Foaming tablets and suppositories are the least effective. Failures with the foam, the best of these methods, are about 28 per 100 women per year. Drainage of the chemical materials from the vagina is objectionable to

Table 4-1   Continued

METHOD	WHAT IT IS AND HOW IT WORKS	EFFECTIVENESS AND ACCEPTABILITY
		some couples. Foaming tablets may cause a temporary burning sensation. The foam is acceptable to many women primarily because it is available to them without a prescription.
Vaginal foams	The foam is packed under pressure (like foaming shaving cream); it is inserted with an applicator.	
Vaginal jellies and creams	These are inserted into the vagina with an applicator.	
Vaginal suppositories	These small cone-shaped objects melt in the vagina. They must be inserted in sufficient time to melt before sexual intercourse.	
Vaginal tablets	The tablets are moistened slightly and inserted into the vagina; foam is produced. They must be inserted in sufficient time for tablet to disintegrate before sexual intercourse.	

Source: Adapted from "Contraceptive Methods Requiring Consultation with Physician," Searle & Co., San Juan, Puerto Rico.

It is carried by the blood stream from a vessel and forced into a smaller one, where it obstructs circulation and may cut off the blood supply to a part of the body. Thromboembolic disease has always been a serious medical concern. That concern has increased with the widespread use of oral contraceptives. In one major study, death from pulmonary embolism[8] occurred in fifteen women who took oral contraceptives. This was four times the expected number for women of their age.[9] Other investigators reported that "in the absence of other predisposing causes the risk of developing deep vein thrombosis, pulmonary embolism, or cerebral thrombosis is increased about eight times by the use of oral contraceptives, while the risk of developing coronary thrombosis[10] is apparently unchanged."[11]

By 1970, the Food and Drug Administration of the U.S. Department of Health, Education, and Welfare had published the results of

[8]Pulmonary embolism refers to a clot obstructing the pulmonary artery (or one of its branches), which brings blood to the lungs.

[9]W. H. N. Inman and M. P. Vessey, "Investigation of Deaths from Pulmonary, Coronary, and Cerebral Thrombosis and Embolism in Women of Child-bearing Age," *British Medical Journal,* Vol. 2, No. 5599 (April 27, 1968), p. 193.

[10]Coronary thrombosis refers to the formation of a clot in a coronary artery which supplies blood to the heart. With blood supply to the heart blocked, the heart suffers a lack of oxygen and is thus damaged.

[11]R. Doll, cited in the *Second Report of the Advisory Committee on Obstetrics and Gynecology,* Food and Drug Administration (August 1969), Chairman's Summary, Louis M. Hellman, M.D.

a survey of the available data concerning the connection between oral contraceptives and thromboembolic disorders.[12]

The association between thromboembolism and the use of oral contraceptives was confirmed, and the sequential type of oral contraceptives seemed to be associated with more risk than the combination type. Since contraceptives containing relatively higher doses of estrogen seemed to be connected with a greater risk of thromboembolic disease, "good therapeutics would indicate the use of the lowest effective dose of estrogen."[13] On January 12, 1970 these findings were made available in the form of a newsletter to almost all the physicians in the United States. Considering the widespread use of oral contraceptives, it must be pointed out that the risks are of a low order of magnitude. Indeed, the possible risk of death from the use of oral contraceptives is even lower than the extremely low (and decreasing) risk of death from pregnancy. The recognized adverse effects of the pill certainly do not warrant its removal from the market at this time.[14] The best insurance is for the woman to

[12] John J. Schrogie, "Oral Contraceptives: A Status Report," *FDA Papers,* Vol. 4, No. 4 (May 1970), pp. 23-25.
[13] "Oral Contraceptives and Thromboembolic Disorders," *FDA Current Drug Information* (April 24, 1970).
[14] Philip E. Sartwell, "Oral Contraceptives and Thromboembolic Disease," *Journal of the American Medical Association,* Vol. 220, No. 3 (April 17, 1972), p. 416. This remains true despite several additional reports pointing to problems associated with the use of birth control pills. An ophthalmologist (eye specialist) writes that "dry eyes from oral contraceptives are a . . . fairly frequent finding in refitting contact lenses in our office. If the patient decides to discontinue the medication, it is our clinical impression that adequate tears for wearing contact lenses may not return for a year. Some patients taking the pill develop symptoms of burning and photophobia" (abnormal intolerance to light). This intolerance to light may occur with patients taking the pill even when they do not wear contact lenses. Relief is obtained by the installation of artificial tears or other eye drops. ("'The Pill' Can Dry Up Contacts," *California Medicine,* Vol. 115, No. 1 [July 1971], p. 33, citing Paul R. Honan, extracted from *Audio-Digest Ophthalmology,* Vol. 7, No. 24, in the Audio-Digest Foundation's Subscription Series of tape-recorded programs.)
A second report indicates that women using birth control pills experience bodily depletion of vitamin C. Previous animal experiments had shown that estrogens (a major component of the contraceptive pill) increase the breakdown of vitamin C. Studied were eighty-eight women: thirty-one were controls; eighteen were pregnant; and thirty-nine were taking oral contraceptives. In each group were European, Asian, and African women. The findings showed that when compared with the controls and the pregnant women, the women who were taking the contraceptive pill had significantly lower vitamin C levels. Apparently, the pill partially inhibits the breakdown of vitamin C for body use. The investigators suggest that the induced deficiency of vitamin C due to the pill may account for some of the reported side effects attributed to oral contraceptive medication. Consequently, they recommend that consideration be given to the use of supplementary vitamins for women taking oral contraceptives. Interestingly, the injected contraceptive that was studied did not appear to influence vitamin C levels. (Michael Briggs and Maxine Briggs, "Vitamin C Requirements and Oral Contraceptives," *Nature,* Vol. 238, No. 5362 [August 4, 1972], p. 277.) It is not known whether women taking oral contraceptives suffer more episodes of upper respiratory infections than women who do not. Despite the opinion of one of the world's most eminent scientists, adequate proof that a lack of vitamin C is related to an increased susceptibility to the "common cold" does not exist. Nevertheless, this area does merit further investigation.
The contraceptive pill has been noted to have other effects pertaining to nutrition. Exclusive of the fetus, membranes, and amniotic fluid, the weight gain of a woman during pregnancy is about ten pounds; most women gain about six pounds when they begin to take oral contraceptives. In both instances the weight gain may be due to fluid retention, breast enlargement, and some impairment of carbohydrate metabolism. Moreover, there may be an increased need for one of the components of the vitamin B complex called *pyridoxine.* "Clinical investigators have already reported that women who have annoying headaches or depression as a result of the pill often obtain marked or complete relief when they take supplements of pyridoxine. Some have experienced relief from nausea and vomiting, but it is important to note that [controlled]

follow the advice of her physician—advice that is tailored to her individual requirements. A woman who has any of the conditions listed below may be denied oral contraceptives by her physician, since they may be unsafe in her particular case:

Heart disease and any abnormality associated with the circulation, including very high blood pressure

Liver disease, such as hepatitis

Kidney disease

Diabetes

Cystic fibrosis

Epilepsy

Migraine headaches

Tumors and cancer of the breasts, ovaries, or uterus

Severe emotional disturbance, particularly after the birth of a baby

Asthma

If a woman is taking oral contraceptives, she should have regular physical exams, including a Papanicolaou test, and should inform her physician of any of the following symptoms, which may indicate an improper reaction to the brand of pill being taken, or to pills in general:

Severe depression

Frequent, severe headaches

Very heavy menstrual periods, and heavy or persistent bleeding between periods

---

studies must be performed for firm conclusions." (Robert E. Hodges, "Nutrition and the Pill," *Journal of the American Dietetic Association,* Vol. 59, No. 3 [September 1971], pp. 215-16, citing M. Baumblatt and F. Winston, "Pyridoxine and the Pill," Letters to the Editor, *Lancet,* Vol. 1, No. 7651 [April 18, 1970], p. 832; D. P. Rose and I. P. Braidman, "Oral Contraceptives, Depression, and Amino-Acid Metabolism," Letters to the Editor, *Lancet,* Vol. 1, No. 7656 [May 23, 1970], p. 1117; and A. L. Luhby, P. Davis, M. Murphy, and M. Gordon, "Pyridoxine and Oral Contraceptives," Letters to the Editor, *Lancet,* Vol. 2, No. 7682 [November 21, 1970], p. 1083.) It is of interest to note that pyridoxine is sometimes used in the treatment of nausea and vomiting during pregnancy. Reports about its benefits vary.

Still another observation concerning the contraceptive pill has been reported by a Baylor College of Medicine gynecologist. "The most frequent cause today for copious vaginal discharge unrelated to vaginal pathogens [any disease producing microbe or material causing vaginal disease] is the taking of birth control pills." The chief source of this type of functional secretion is the cervix. He believes that the sequential type of contraceptive pill causes more secretion than the low estrogen dosage combined type. This is due to its relatively high dosage of estrogen. However, a profuse vaginal discharge may be due to a variety of causes. The diagnosis includes laboratory analysis of both normal and possibly abnormal vaginal microbes. (Herman L. Gardner, "Unexplained Leukorrhea," *Medical Aspects of Human Sexuality,* Vol. 6, No. 5 [May 1972], p. 181.)

More than two missed menstrual periods (if the pills have been taken properly, there is almost no chance of pregnancy; the hormone levels may be too high and are probably suppressing the menstrual period)

A high degree of water retention, as may be manifested by swollen legs, feet, or hands, a large weight gain

Jaundice (yellowing) of the skin or eyes

Any change in vision, especially double vision or loss of vision

Overly tender breasts and the secretion of milk or fluid from the breasts

Weakness in the arms or legs and sudden pain in the chest followed by coughing

The woman who has started taking the pill may experience some mild side effects that are usually not serious. For the first few months, she may experience nausea, similar to the morning sickness of pregnancy. Her menstrual period may not be as heavy and may not last as long. Between periods she may suffer some slight bleeding. If this continues after the first three months on the pill, a physician should be consulted.

The pills should be taken at the same time every day. If a pill is forgotten, it should be taken as soon as this is realized, and the next pill should be taken at the regular time. If two pills are missed, two pills should be taken each day for the next two days. If two or more pills are missed, another contraceptive method must also be used throughout that cycle as the pills alone are not then completely effective.

FIGURE 4-1

THIS LABEL
IS REQUIRED
BY THE FOOD AND DRUG
ADMINISTRATION

————•◦•————

ORAL CONTRACEPTIVES

•[Birth Control Pills]•

DO NOT TAKE THIS DRUG
WITHOUT YOUR DOCTOR'S
CONTINUED SUPERVISION.

The oral contraceptives are powerful and effective drugs which can cause side effects in some users and should not be used at all by some women. The most serious known side effect is abnormal blood clotting which can be fatal.

Safe use of this drug requires a careful discussion with your doctor. To assist him in providing you with the necessary information, a booklet has been prepared that is written in a style understandable to you as the drug user. This provides information on the effectiveness and known hazards of the drug including warnings, side effects and who should not use it. Your doctor will give you this booklet if you ask for it and he can answer any questions you may have about the use of this drug.

Notify your doctor if you notice any unusual physical disturbance or discomfort.

The FDA has ordered the enclosure of an informative brochure with each prescription of oral contraceptives. It is reproduced on page 116.

the rhythm method and recent research to improve on it

The rhythm method is approved by the Roman Catholic church. It may be practiced in two ways: by the computation of the safe, or nonfertile, period, and by the temperature method.

The computation of the safe, or nonfertile, period   This period is the interval during which a mature ovum is not available for fertilization (see Figure 2-5, page 41). The rationale on which this method is based is discussed on pages 43–44.

Because most women do not menstruate as regularly as they think, an accurate record of the length of each menstrual cycle must be kept for no less than one year. This is essential for any degree of success. The shortest and longest cycle is noted. By subtracting nineteen from the number of days in the shortest cycle the number of safe days during the first half of the cycle is obtained. By subtracting eleven from the number of days in the longest cycle the number of safe days during the second half of the cycle is found. For example, if the shortest cycle is twenty-four days, five days counting from the first day of the menstrual flow are safe. If the longest cycle is twenty-eight days, the seventeenth day of the cycle to the beginning of the next menstrual period is safe. Between the fifth and the seventeenth day of the menstrual cycle fertilization of the ovum (conception) is possible.

It will be noted that the unsafe period of fertility, in Figure 2-5 on page 41, is from the ninth to the eighteenth day of the menstrual cycle. This is because the calculations for that illustration are based on one regular twenty-eight-day cycle. Few women menstruate regularly every twenty-eight days.

The temperature method   This method is based on the fact that the temperature of most women is relatively low during their menstrual period and for the eight days that follow it. When they ovulate, there is first a decline in temperature and then a sharp increase of between 0.5 to 0.7 of a degree. This is the unsafe period. This rise in temperature continues until about two days before the next menstrual period. The woman who wishes to use the temperature method must first practice by taking her temperature upon awakening for six months to a year. In this way she learns to predict her safe period. This method is complicated by inaccuracies in reading a thermometer and by ordinary variations in human temperature. In addition, the correlation between the temperature rise and ovulation is not dependable. It can vary by as much as four days. Moreover, the average woman who relies on this method cannot spare the time in the morning to remain in bed and take her temperature.

Possible improvements on the rhythm method   Several promising new methods of predicting the safe period are presently being investigated that are of particular interest to those who wish to use the rhythm method. It has recently been discovered that the amount of an enzyme in the saliva, called alkaline phosphatase, increases just before ovulation. Every day the woman places in her mouth a paper strip containing a chemical that reacts to a high level of alkaline phosphatase. When the paper strip turns blue, the woman is ovulating. The woman can then avoid intercourse accordingly.

Another method of determining the safe period depends on the changing quality of the mucus in the vagina during the menstrual cycle.[15] Studies have indicated that following menstrual bleeding there is a variable number of days in which there is no vaginal discharge. Then an increasing amount of a cloudy, sticky secretion becomes noticeable. The duration of this, too, is variable. Before ovulation, the consistency of the mucus changes. It becomes clear and slippery, has the characteristics of raw egg white, and produces a feeling of lubrication. This lasts from one to two days; the last day of its occurrence is called the "peak mucus symptom" and is closely correlated with the day of ovulation. After ovulation, the mucus becomes thick and opaque for a variable number of days. It has been suggested that conception may be avoided by abstaining from intercourse during the peak of mucus symptom and for four days afterward. One advantage of the method is that under a physician's supervision it can be easily learned. Women are advised not to have intercourse during the menstrual cycle in which they are learning the method. Disadvantages of the method include the irregularity of ovulation in some women and the confusion of the ordinary mucous discharge with one that requires treatment. The reliability of the method is being further studied by various physicians.

tubal ligation

Tubal ligation is an effective method of birth control.[16] By a surgical procedure, the Fallopian tubes are tied and cut or cauterized, so as to avoid another time-consuming and expensive hospitalization, the operation is best performed immediately after the woman has had

[15] E. L. Billings, J. J. Billings, J. B. Brown, and H. G. Burger, "Symptoms and Hormonal Changes Accompanying Ovulation," *Lancet,* Vol. 1, No. 7745 (February 5, 1972), p. 282.
[16] Contraception allows intercourse between fertile partners while preventing conception. As a tubal ligation renders the female infertile it is not a contraceptive method although it is a method of birth control.

a child. If the ligation is done after vaginal delivery, an extra day may be required for recovery. If the child is born by Caesarean section, no extra time is required for recuperation. Although the structures may sometimes be rejoined later, tubal ligation is usually irreversible. A new method of tubal ligation that can be performed with local anesthesia is now being tried. Only one abdominal incision is necessary, and the operation can be an outpatient procedure. An instrument is inserted into an incision that is approximately the diameter of a finger. It has a light so that the Fallopian tubes can be located and cauterized. Also being developed is an instrument that will apply a clip around the tubes rather than cauterize them.

The majority of women who have had tubal ligations suffer no emotional problems as a result. Many, totally freed from the nagging fear of pregnancy, report enhanced coital enjoyment. As is the case with vasectomy in men, the incidence of emotional problems following tubal ligation varies with the individual and with circumstances. The woman who previously has had a difficult pregnancy, or whose husband's earning power is threatened, or who fears that her child might have a hereditary defect, may find that the tubal ligation increases her sexual pleasure. However, the woman who considers the operation to violate her religious beliefs, or who feels that her feminine image depends on her fertility may regret the ligation and experience diminished sexual enjoyment.[17]

BIRTH CONTROL FOR THE MALE

There are fewer contraceptive methods available to the male than to the female. Aside from condoms (see Table 4-1) and coitus interruptus the only birth control method currently in use is vasectomy.[18] Vasectomy is the surgical removal of a portion of the vas deferens (see page 35). When the operation is complete, the spermatozoa that are formed in the testes no longer reach the ejaculatory ducts (which lie on each side of the prostatic urethra) via the seminal vesicles. Therefore newly formed spermatozoa cannot become part of the semen. However, after vasectomy, residual spermatozoa are left in that part of the vas deferens on each side that remains connected to the seminal vesicles. It requires several ejaculations for the residual spermatozoa to leave the body. During that time the man remains fertile. After five or six seminal emissions more than 90 percent of the semen is sperm free. Several postoperative microscopic examinations of the semen for spermatozoa are necessary to ascertain sterility.

[17] Eleanor B. Easley, "Sexual Effect of Female Sterilization," *Medical Aspects of Human Sexuality,* Vol. 6, No. 2 (February 1972), p. 58.
[18] Like a tubal ligation a vasectomy is not a contraceptive method although it is a method of birth control.

Vasectomy is legal in all fifty states, although in Utah it may be performed only if medically indicated. In 1972, the Utah statute was being challenged in the courts. Usually only local anesthesia is required. Two very small incisions are made in the scrotum. The vas deferens is then easily exposed and cut. A tiny section of each vas deferens is removed. The cut ends are then sutured. A few stitches close the skin incision. By the day after the operation, about two-thirds of all patients can move about normally. The rest require a day or two longer to recuperate. Approximately one man in four has moderate pain at the operative site or some swelling of the testicles. Neither is usually cause for concern, and they subside in a week or two. Failures are uncommon. The vas deferens may recanalize itself, and the patient again become fertile. This is rare. In some cases the operation can be reversed, however, this possibility cannot be predicted. The man who is considering a vasectomy at this time should count on the unlikelihood that he will ever again be fertile. For some men, this realization may have adverse psychological effects.

Antibodies to spermatozoa have been identified in the blood of some men who have had vasectomies. The blocked-up sperm may act as an antigen (antibody generator). The antibodies have remained in the blood stream for at least a year, and they may further diminish the chances of reversing the effects of the operation.[19] Even if the operation were successfully reversed, the man might be producing an immunity to his own spermatozoa that could prolong his infertility.[20]

The problem of the irreversible vasectomy is being investigated. Now under study is a mechanical device made of gold and stainless steel. It is permanently implanted in the vas deferens and has a tiny faucetlike valve that may be set on or off. A second operation is necessary to change the position of the valve. Other experimental instruments that may make vasectomies reversible employ clips, threads, chemicals, and catheters as blocking mechanisms.

Vasectomy does not affect erection, climax, ejaculation, or volume of ejaculation. Thus it usually does not affect the man's response during sexual intercourse. Moreover, the operation has no known effect on the production of spermatozoa or of the male sex hormone testosterone (see pages 33-35). Almost all patients report both no change in physical health and a significant increase in coital frequency following the operation. They claim to feel freer and more satisfied with sexual intercourse, and report little change in "duration of ejaculation, control of ejaculation," and ease and "strength of erec-

[19] "Antibodies to Sperm May Form after Vasectomy," *Journal of the American Medical Association*, Vol. 217, No. 10 (September 6, 1971), p. 1310.
[20] Harold Lear, "Vasectomy—A Note of Concern," *Journal of the American Medical Association*, Vol. 219, No. 9 (February 28, 1972), p. 1207, citing A. M. Phadke and K. Padukone, "Presence and Significance of Autoantibodies Against Spermatozoa in the Blood of Men with Obstructed Vas Deferens," *J. Reprod. Fertil.*, Vol. 7 (1964), pp. 163-70.

tion." In the opinion of most husbands, "wives seem less restrained in intercourse and . . . over half of them obtain climax more easily."[21] It is emphasized that these are patient opinions.

> *Interestingly, careful psychological study does not entirely support the opinions of the patients . . . Although the effects were not dramatic . . . adverse changes in psychological functioning following vasectomy were confirmed . . . The data suggest that the operation is responded to as though it had [a] demasculinizing potential, with a result that the behavior of the man after vasectomy is more likely to be scrutinized by himself and others for evidence of unmasculine features.*[22]

Sometimes the operation led to self-scrutiny that was actually beneficial. Some men were able to improve their formerly immature and indecisive behavior pattern. In others, however, the operation was followed by an increased level of anxiety that interfered with marital harmony. This observation has been confirmed by other studies that suggest that "vasectomized men, their friends, their relatives, and their physicians equate vasectomy with castration and masculine inferiority"[23] and that "other couples denigrated those who chose vasectomy as a method of birth control."[24]

How frequent are postvasectomy psychological problems? "The most optimistic surveys indicate a potential three percent casualty rate, and others report a much higher incidence of psychological implications."[25] Such difficulties occur much more frequently in men who have experienced sexual dysfunctions or emotional problems before vasectomy, who have not sought and obtained wholehearted agreement from their wives, and who have not rationally considered all the implications of the operation, including its probable permanence. If a man divorces and remarries, he meets with a new marital situation that may cause him to bitterly regret his vasectomy. The same may be true should he become a widower. Vasectomy should never be considered casually.

The wife may also be troubled about her husband's vasectomy, and she should be included in the decision about the operation. The

[21] Andrew Ferber and William L. Ferber, "Vasectomy," *Medical Aspects of Human Sexuality,* Vol. 2, No. 6 (June 1968), p. 34.
[22] F. J. Ziegler, D. A. Rogers, and S. A. Kriegsman, "Effect of Vasectomy on Psychological Functioning," *Psychosomatic Medicine,* Vol. 28 (1966), p. 50.
[23] A. S. Ferber, C. Tietze, and S. Lewit, "Men with Vasectomies: A Study of Medical, Sexual, and Psychosocial Changes, *Psychosomatic Medicine,* Vol. 29, No. 4 (July-August 1967), p. 354.
[24] D. A. Rogers, T. J. Ziegler, and N. Levy, "Prevailing Cultural Attitudes about Vasectomy: Possible Explanation of Postoperative Psychological Response," *Psychosomatic Medicine,* Vol. 29 (1967), p. 367.
[25] Harold Lear, "Vasectomy—A Note of Concern," p. 1207, citing *Vasectomy: Follow-up of 1,000 Cases, Simon Population Trust Sterilization Project* (Cambridge, England, 1969); and H. Wolfers, "Psychological Aspects of Vasectomy," *British Medical Journal,* Vol. 4, No. 5730 (October 31, 1970), pp. 297, 300.

decision is best made in a conference between the physician and both marital partners.[26] One obstetrician-gynecologist writes that "the rising number of male vasectomies in the United States has produced, in some cases, a source of functional gynecological complaints."[27] Although the frequency of sexual intercourse may increase in these cases, interest in it diminishes. Some wives feel that the ligation makes their husbands more attractive to other women, and they become jealous.

The frequency of vasectomy often increases among groups of men, such as firemen, whose work brings them together.[28] In 1971, over three-quarters of a million men in this country elected to have the operation.[29] Perhaps, as vasectomy is more thoroughly explained and accepted, adverse reactions will diminish. Certainly, serious reactions are in the minority, and vasectomy is an excellent method of birth control in selected cases.

In India vasectomy is widely accepted. Throughout July 1971 a sterilization festival was held in one Indian district. About sixty-three thousand men were sterilized at the vasectomy fair. Vasectomy fairs are now being planned for each of India's 320 districts.[30]

semen banks: fertility insurance?

The relative permanence of present vasectomies has stimulated the development of frozen semen banks. There is little evidence that, with present techniques, such banks will be able to preserve spermatozoa for as long as five or ten years. By 1972, the longest well-documented time in which thawed spermatozoa had been successfully used for insemination was sixteen months after freezing.[31] Approximately 400 children in the world had been born as a result of impregnation with thawed spermatozoa, of whom the oldest was sixteen. To date, no undue increase of genetic problems has been noted; however, longer term studies are necessary.

RESEARCH FOR CONTRACEPTIVES

Extensive research on contraceptives is being conducted both in this country and abroad. By mid-1971, no less than fifteen experimental methods were being tested on consenting men and women.

[26] Pauline Jackson, Betson Phillips, Elizabeth Prosser, H. O. Jones, V. R. Tindall, D. L. Crosby, I. D. Cooke, J. M. McGarry, and R. R. Rees, "A Male Sterilization Clinic," *British Medical Journal,* Vol. 4, No. 5730 (October 31, 1970), pp. 295–97.
[27] James A. FitzGerald, "The Female Response to Male Vas Ligation," *Medical Insight,* Vol. 4, No. 1 (January 1972), p. 26.
[28] E. S. Livingstone, "Vasectomy: A Review of 3200 Operations," *Canadian Medical Association Journal,* Vol. 105, No. 10 (November 20, 1971), p. 1065.
[29] "Vasectomy Patients Multiply, but Doubts Linger," *American Medical News,* Vol. 15, No. 6 (April 24, 1972), p. 8.
[30] "Vasectomy in India," *Population Profile* (Washington, D.C., 1972), p. 2.
[31] "Vasectomy Patients Multiply, but Doubts Linger," pp. 8–9.

The list includes: daily, weekly, and monthly pills for use by women; semi-permanent under-skin capsules for men or women; intermittently-used vaginal inserts or chronically used intra-uterine inserts which act as carriers of . . . infertility agents; pills taken intermittently by women on the basis of coital exposure—before or after; intravenous infusion to terminate an early pregnancy . . . a remarkable foreign body placed in the vas deferens to impair male fertility; vaginal tablets to induce menstrual flow—whether or not a fertilization has occurred, or to cause abortion at a later stage.[32]

One of these, requiring the oral ingestion of small, daily doses of progestin (the synthetic form of the hormone released by the corpus luteum, see page 46), appears to be so safe and effective that it may be marketed in the United States in 1972. It has been suggested that progestin chronically changes the consistency of the cervical mucus, thus preventing adequate passage of spermatozoa.[33]

Another promising method also involves the use of progestin. The synthetic hormone is stored in a small Silastic container that is inserted under the skin. Minute doses of progestin are released into the blood stream. Studies of this contraceptive method are being conducted in the United States, India, Chile, Brazil, and Italy. With its use, the risk of forgetting to take the daily pill is averted. Still another product containing a synthetic progesterone can be injected intramuscularly and remain in place as a depot. From this focal point, measured amounts of the hormone are released into the blood. By midsummer 1968 "a long-acting contraceptive administered to women by injection once every three months . . . proved effective during three years of clinical trial."[34]

A nine-year study of 907 Mexican women between nineteen and forty-five years old of proven fertility provides encouraging data about the acceptability of contraceptive injections despite their sometimes disagreeable side effects. The study population comprised one group of 839 low-income women in Mexico City and a second group of 68 women who lived in a remote rural area. The rural women received only injectable contraceptives. The city women had a choice between injectable and oral contraceptives. One-half of the city women chose the injections. One of the reasons for this was the women's belief that injections were more effective than oral medication. Three injectable contraceptives were used. Side effects included irregular periods of bleeding, headache, dizziness, and nervousness.

[32] Sheldon J. Segal, "Beyond the Laboratory: Recent Research Advances in Fertility Regulation," *Family Planning Perspectives,* Vol. 3, No. 3 (July 1971), pp. 17–21.
[33] Ibid., p. 18, citing H. W. Rudel, J. Martinez-Manautou, and M. Maques-Topete, "Role of Progesterones in Hormonal Control of Fertility," *Fertility and Sterility,* Vol. 16 (1965), p. 158.
[34] "The Long-Acting Contraceptives: Quarterly Injections Pass Three-Year Trials," *Journal of the American Medical Association,* Vol. 204, No. 11 (June 10, 1968), p. 35.

Only a very small percentage of the women discontinued the injections for these reasons. The majority of the women were pleased to be relieved of the need to take a daily pill and were grateful for the long-acting (up to eighty-four days) injectable contraceptives. The most serious of the complications was occasional severe bleeding, which could be a problem with women suffering malnutritional anemia.[35] The ability of Silastic to store and gradually release birth control drugs is being used in still another way. Progestin is being incorporated into Silastic vaginal rings. When placed in the vagina, the rings release a small amount of progestin that is absorbed by the blood via the vaginal mucous membrane.

Morning-after pills are also under investigation. A recent study demonstrated their effectiveness. "One thousand women of childbearing age were given, within 72 hours of sexual exposure, 25 mg (milligrams) of diethylstilbesterol twice daily for five days. No pregnancies resulted and there were no serious adverse reactions."[36] Diethylstilbesterol is one of the synthetic estrogens. The hormone apparently acts on the uterine lining, making implantation unlikely. It may also increase the speed of the descent of the ovum. Since the probability of conception from a single unprotected coitus is between 1 in 50 and 1 in 25, these results are indeed promising.[37] The effects of their long-term or frequent use have yet to be intensively studied, nor has the significance of their disagreeable aftereffects in some persons been ascertained.

In much smaller doses, diethylstilbesterol has been used for many years to treat the symptoms of menopause, certain types of uterine bleeding, and a variety of other conditions. Recent studies suggest an association (not necessarily a cause and effect relationship) between a woman's ingestion of stilbesterol during pregnancy and the development, years later, of cancer of the vagina in her offspring.[38] In November 1971, the U.S. Food and Drug Administration warned physicians of this statistically significant association.[39] On the basis of data obtained from animal experiments, diethylstilbesterol is now thought to be a carcinogen; it should not be added to chicken feeds or be present in beef for human consumption.[40] It is not used during

[35] "Contraceptive 'Shots' Prove to be Effective," *Journal of the American Medical Association,* Vol. 220, No. 8 (May 22, 1972), pp. 1061-65.
[36] Lucile Kirtland Kuchera, "Postcoital Contraception with Diethylstilbesterol," *Journal of the American Medical Association,* Vol. 218, No. 4 (October 25, 1971), p. 562.
[37] Ibid., citing C. Tietze, "Problems of Pregnancy Resulting from a Single Unprotected Coitus," *Fertility and Sterility,* Vol. 11 (September–October 1960), pp. 485-88.
[38] A. L. Herbst, H. Ulfelder, and D. C. Poskanzer, "Adenocarcinoma of the Vagina: Association of Maternal Stilbesterol Therapy with Tumor Appearance in Young Women," *New England Journal of Medicine,* Vol. 284, No. 16 (April 22, 1971), pp. 878-81. P. Greenwald, J. J. Barlow, P. C. Nasca et al., "Vaginal Cancer After Maternal Treatment with Synthetic Estrogens," *New England Journal of Medicine,* Vol. 285, No. 7 (August 12, 1971), pp. 390-92.
[39] "Diethylstilbesterol Contraindicated in Pregnancy: Drugs Used Linked to Adenocarcinoma in the Offspring," *FDA Bulletin* (November 1971).
[40] Frederick B. Hodges, "Diethylstilbesterol: Problems of Unusual Drug Dosage and Administration," Public Health Reports, *California Medicine,* Vol. 116, No. 2 (February 1972), p. 84.

pregnancy. In the above-mentioned research on the "morning-after pill," it was emphasized to the subjects that the administration of diethylstilbesterol was strictly an emergency measure. It was not to be considered as a method of continuous contraception. Its use as a contraceptive should be carefully controlled.

A family of body chemicals that may be used to control fertility are the *prostaglandins*. These hormonelike substances are found in many tissues and fluids of the body. Prostaglandins are an important component of human seminal fluid and are also found in menstrual fluid. Despite their name, they are formed in the seminal vesicles (see page 35), and not the prostate.[41] The effect of the prostaglandins on the body is astonishingly versatile. For example, they are involved in the regulation of blood pressure and the stimulation and relaxation of smooth muscle. The extent of their action is just beginning to be understood. Since the prostaglandins stimulate contractions of the uterus, they have been found effective in inducing labor and terminating unwanted pregnancies. They are also being tried as an "after-the-fact" method of birth control. The contracting uterus brings on menstruation; the ovum is expelled, whether or not it has been fertilized. The mechanism by which menstruation is induced is not yet known.[42] In addition, the prostaglandins have been suggested as a possibly effective means of inducing menstruation in cases of menstrual failure. Although much research remains to be done, the use of prostaglandins is considered by some researchers to be the most important advance in fertility control since the introduction of oral contraceptives.

Since surgical abortions after the first trimester are not as safe as those performed earlier, the prostaglandins eventually may be used to induce abortions at a later stage of pregnancy.[43] At present, they do not seem to be always effective. Several prostaglandins have already been synthesized in the laboratory. It should be emphasized that prostaglandins act on almost all body systems. Much needs to be learned not only about their side effects, but also about how they are metabolized in the body. Present prospects for an effective oral form of prostaglandins (that might be used as a method of birth

---

Nevertheless, it was not until late summer of 1972 that the Food and Drug Administration reversed its previous defense of synthetic diethylstibesterol (DES). The ban on its use was not to become effective until the beginning of 1973; until then, the use of this cancer-causing substance with meat animals was to be permitted in the form of a pellet implanted in the animal's ear. This caused considerable concern among scientists, who considered the FDA's change of position belated. "On the day following its ban, the Senate health subcommittee passed a bill proposing a complete and immediate ban on DES. Maybe the FDA decided to act against the carcinogen [cancer-causing substance] before Congress did it for them." (Nicholas Wade, "FDA Invents More Tales About DES," *Science*, Vol. 177, No. 4048 [August 11, 1972], p. 503.)

[41] John E. Pike, "Prostaglandins," *Scientific American*, Vol. 225, No. 5 (November 1971), p. 84.

[42] "Birth Control Method Tried 'After-the-Fact,'" *HSMHA Health Reports*, Vol. 87, No. 1 (January 1972), p. 84.

[43] Carl Djerassi, "Fertility Control Through Abortion: An Assessment of the Period 1950–1980," *Science and Public Affairs: Bulletin of the Atomic Scientists*, Vol. 28, No. 1 (January 1972), p. 43.

control) are dim because of the very rapid destruction of natural prostaglandins in the body. The development of a synthetic prostaglandin analogue "could not be expected before the next decade at the earliest."[44]

why no male pill?

"1984 appears to be an exceedingly optimistic target date for development of a male contraceptive pill ready for use by the public."[45] Why? First, the basic knowledge of male reproductive biology is even less advanced than that of female. To improve on that knowledge would require extensive research with exceedingly expensive and still relatively unavailable infrahuman primates, such as chimpanzees.[46] This obstacle will take years to overcome. Second, as will be seen in the discussion that follows, the presently known variety of chemical agents that affect the fertility of male animals such as the rat are either toxic or potentially poisonous to man.[47] Third, evolutionary changes necessary to insure human survival have occurred much more frequently with the female.[48] One example of such a change is the limited production of ova by the human female that are capable of being fertilized—about 400 in a lifetime. The human male still produces millions of spermatozoa. However, the human female usually releases but one egg at a time, and each egg is nourished singly to come to maturity in its own elaborately ripened follicular abode. Fourth, the male has fewer steps in his reproductive cycle that are vulnerable to controlled interference. The maturation of the ovum, ovulation, the pick-up and beginning transport of the ovum down the Fallopian tube, its fertilization, the continued transport down the tube of the beginning life in the resulting zygote, and the eventual implantation in the prepared uterine endometrium—these are some episodes in the woman's reproductive history that are possibly amenable to scientific interference. Added to these are conditions that influence the possibilities of fertilization, such as the penetrability of the cervical mucus to spermatozoa, and the changing state of the endometrium. In contrast, the male reproductive cycle is vulnerable at only its three basic steps: the production of spermatozoa in the testes, the storage and maturation of spermatozoa in the epididymis, and the transportation of spermatozoa via the vas deferens. Along

---

[44] Ibid., p. 44. For a discussion of the potential of LH-RH as a contraceptive see page 32, footnote 2.

[45] Carl Djerassi, "Birth Control After 1984," *Science*, Vol. 169, No. 3949 (September 1970), p. 946.

[46] Carl Djerassi, "Fertility Control Through Abortion: An Assessment of the Period 1950-1980," p. 41. This article is also essential to learn more about the female's reproductive process.

[47] Carl Djerassi, "Birth Control After 1984," p. 947, citing "Developments in Fertility Control," *World Health Organization Tech. Rep. Ser.*, No. 424 (1969).

[48] Most of the discussion in the following section is from Sheldon J. Siegel, "Contraceptive Research: A Male Chauvinist Plot?" *Family Planning Perspectives*, Vol. 4, No. 3 (July 1972), pp. 21-25.

with these areas of interference, scientists have thought of the possibility of changing the chemical composition of the seminal fluid. Research is presently being directed into all these possibilities.

Research to impede the production of spermatozoa   It has been pointed out that the gonads of both sexes—testes and ovaries—are stimulated by the same hormones of the anterior lobe of the pituitary gland (see page 30). These pituitary sex hormones (called *gonadotropins*) are the follicle-stimulating hormone (FSH) and the luteinizing hormone (LH) (see pages 31-32). It has also been demonstrated that the production and release of both FSH and LH by the anterior pituitary are controlled by a hypothalamic chemical factor, the luteinizing hormone-releasing hormone (LH-RH). (That FSH has its own hypothalamic factor has yet to be shown, see page 31.) This remarkable hypothalamic substance is the same for male and female. Thus the sexes share the same brain factors and anterior pituitary sex hormones. In the female, the contraceptive pill is based on the secondary suppression of the ovary (ovulation) by stopping the anterior pituitary's production of gonadotropins. Cannot, then, progestin, for example (a component of the female contraceptive pill), also stop the production of male gonadotropins and thus, secondarily, inhibit spermatogenesis in the testes? Yes. However, the doses required to accomplish this also inhibit libido and potency. But, since estrogens (also part of the female contraceptive pill) suppress gonadotropins and ovulation in the woman, cannot testosterone (an androgen) stop gonadotropin production and spermatogenesis in the male? Again, the answer is in the affirmative. However, present dosages and methods of administration have seriously adverse effects on the prostate and blood chemistry. It is feared that prostatic tumors may be initiated and, moreover, elevated androgen levels are associated with fatal heart attacks and the shorter male life span. "Male combination" methods, such as mixtures of progesteronelike compounds and possibly harmless androgen dosages, are now under study, particularly by the Population Council's International Committee for Contraceptive Research.

In recent years a variety of nonhormonal substances have been proved to be effective in stopping spermatogenesis. They have also been proved to be excessively toxic. Also studied has been the effect of heat on spermatogenesis. In one experiment, volunteer medical students submerged their scrota in hot water for a half hour each day. An elevation of scrotal temperature by just a few degrees did result in diminished spermatogenesis. In a variation of this, the codeveloper of the contraceptive pill, Dr. John Rock, had his volunteer medical students wear an insulated scrotal supporter. However, both hot water and the "Rock Strap" (as it was inevitably called) produced results that were too variable for practical use. The immunization of human males with animal testicular extract to produce sterility has been tried. It was hoped that the extract would act as an antigen and produce antibodies against spermatozoa. This has not been successful. The whole concept of interfering with sperm production poses special problems. First, only a small number of viable spermatozoa may cause pregnancy; therefore, all sperm production must be stopped. Second, any possibility whatsoever of genetically damaged spermatozoa surviving must be eliminated.

Research to impede the maturation and fertilizing capacity of spermatozoa   Spermatozoa probably begin to mature in the hundreds of seminiferous tubules of the testes and in the ducts that connect them to the epididymis (see page 35). However, they are hardly ever studied at that stage because of their inaccessibility. It is during their storage in the epididymis that spermatozoa continue to mature, and it is there that they first become motile. Progestin has been found to interfere with the completion of the maturation of spermatozoa. As has been stated above, however, the substance presents dosage problems for the male. Another approach is based on the knowledge that spermatozoa must develop complex enzymes in order to penetrate the membrane of the ovum. Inhibitors of these enzymes are being studied.

Research to impede the transportation of sperm   The condom, as well as jellies, creams, and foams that are lethal to spermatozoa have long been used. Recent research has improved methods of vasectomy; other recently devised ways of blocking the path of the vas deferens have already been mentioned on page 120.

Research to adversely affect the chemistry of the seminal fluid   Experimental work suggests that adding a deleterious substance to the seminal fluid, rather than removing something already present, may someday provide a method of bringing about male sterility. The problem is the toxicity of the potential substances. Still to be discovered is a nontoxic, ingestable or injectable sperm-killer that can reach the seminal fluid.

Aside from functional anatomy, other problems beset the researcher for a male contraceptive pill. The male cycle takes about twelve weeks. Adequate testing of a contraceptive, if one were available, would require at least six months. "Women can easily be assembled for clinical studies through their association with Planned Parenthood clinics and individual obstetricians or gynecologists; there exists no simple mechanism for assembling similar groups of males for clinical experimentation.The prisons and the armed forces are the only convenient sources."[49] Even if these groups were used, the results of the studies would depend on spermatozoa obtained by masturbation, and not to fertility in a population.

There is no doubt that a relatively safe male oral contraceptive would be an important addition to family planning. A major objection to the presently available oral contraceptive for the female is its prolonged use. A male chemical contraceptive would make alternate use by the sexes possible.[50] However, the present unavailability of such a contraceptive is due not to male chauvinism but to male biology. "It is not surprising . . . that the number of approaches under study is fewer for male than for female methods. What is surprising . . . is not that we do not have more male methods, but that we came so far for so long with *only* male methods, and of the most primitive type."[51]

abortion

A viable fetus is one that has reached such a stage of development that it can live outside the uterus. The premature expulsion from the uterus of a nonviable fetus or an embryo is considered an *abortion*. Abortions are not just *criminal* or *therapeutic* (medically indicated). For a variety of reasons, many occur *spontaneously*. Lay people refer to a spontaneous abortion as a "miscarriage." Ten to 15 percent of pregnancies end in abortion or miscarriage. Recent state legislation in this country has certainly changed the legal interpretation of many thousands of abortions that were formerly considered criminal.

The causes of spontaneous abortions are numerous and sometimes unclear. Maternal illnesses, such as malnourishment, German measles, and possibly influenza, are often causative. Of the traumas that cause abortion, only one in a thousand is nondeliberate.

Traditional indications for abortions are diminishing. Heart disease was once a common reason for medical interruption of pregnancy. Heart surgery has changed this; that reason for the interruption of a pregnancy has become less frequent. Nevertheless, chronic hypertension and kidney disease, breast and uterine cancers are considered valid indications by many physicians. Most hospitals have a therapeutic abortion committee composed of distinguished medical staff specialists. They review each case. Their decision is final. Therapeutic abortions are not done in Catholic hospitals.

Only a generation ago, abortion, like contraception, was rarely

[49] Carl Djerassi, "Birth Control After 1984," p. 948.
[50] Ibid., pp. 947–48.
[51] Sheldon J. Siegal, "Contraceptive Research: A Male Chauvinist Plot?" p. 25.

discussed in public. There are ample reasons for this change. First, *the sheer number of abortions* makes the procedure a major concern. Throughout the world, every year, some twenty-five million legal and illegal abortions are performed. Illegal abortions remain a major cause of maternal deaths. In Latin America half of all pregnancies end in illegal abortions. The resultant cost of mothers' lives is a shocking tragedy. It is fully four times greater than in countries in which abortions are legal. Formerly, about one million abortions a year in this country killed more than ten thousand women. For many women, extensive infection, the most common complication of illegal abortions, resulted in death. Only too often, the criminal abortionist is an incompetent, operating in atrociously unsanitary conditions. Second, *medical knowledge now warns of possible abnormal babies.* Maternal infection with German measles (rubella) virus in the first trimester, for example, results in a high percentage (20 percent) of abnormal babies. Such information has stimulated interest in legal abortion. Third, *the failure of contraception in overpopulated countries* has brought about a reevaluation of abortion. Fourth, some think present *abortion laws* penalize the poor, are unenforceable, and are less applicable to married than to unmarried women[52]—these impressions have added to the widespread discussion. Moreover, limited objective studies so far indicate that "there was little new psychiatric illness that appeared after therapeutic abortion that could be related to the abortion."[53]

In 1962, a model law, proposed by the American Law Institute, allowed therapeutic abortion to save the life or health of the mother, prevent the birth of a deformed or mentally deficient child, or prevent the birth of a child conceived as a result of rape or incest. In June 1967, the American Medical Association Committee on Human Reproduction approved of these. However, they added two more prerequisites: two consulting doctors were to approve the abortion and, if agreed upon, the abortion was to be performed in an approved hospital.[54] A majority, although not all, of U.S. physicians agree. Based on the model law of the Law Institute, some liberalizing state legislation has been passed. Colorado was one of the states that passed such a law. During the first year of operation of the law there was an eightfold increase in the legal abortions in the state. Only 32 percent were from out-of-state. Of the 407 women who were aborted in the first year, only 138 were married; 12.7 percent were under sixteen; 33 percent were between sixteen and twenty-one. Seventy-two percent of the abortions were done for psychiatric reasons. Forty-six percent of the legal terminations of pregnancy

[52] *M.D., Medical Newsmagazine,* Vol. 12, No. 2 (February 1968), p. 105.
[53] R. Bruce Sloane, "The Unwanted Pregnancy," *New England Journal of Medicine,* Vol. 280, No. 22 (May 29, 1969), p. 1209.
[54] "AMA Policy on Therapeutic Abortion," *Journal of the American Medical Association,* Vol. 201, No. 7 (August 14, 1967), p. 544.

were performed on patients with a family income of less than $6,000 yearly.[55] New York has also passed a liberalized abortion law; its provisions and the response to it are discussed below.

Numerous ethical and theological problems arise when fallible men attempt to define indications for abortion. One of these is the scientific limitation in predicting abnormal births. Another lies in the variable interpretation of "health" of the mother. The family of a poor woman would suffer more, perhaps, with the addition of another child. Her health might thus be adversely affected. Should she be more eligible for abortion than the wealthy woman? Complicating the issue even more is the present gulf between some scientists and some theologians.

"Life is a continuum," the scientists say,

it has evolved and survived over billions of years by the provision of fantastic margins of safety in terms of excess sperms and ova; the particular conjunction of sperm and ovum that leads to conception is not a unique event but is rather a matter of chance, the development of the individual from conception to full humanity is an unbroken process—who is to say when "life" began?[56]

Opponents of abortion place a sacred and infinite value on each separate beginning, on each potential life. Many consider that this value must be protected even beyond the mother's life. Threats to this concept, such as selfishness, irresponsibility, and sexual promiscuity, are especially condemned.

Both theologians and scientists revere life. To the responsible, both concepts surely have much to offer. Abortion laws, meticulously respectful of every human being's conscience, are now being considered and adopted in increasing numbers.

THE NEW YORK EXPERIENCE WITH ABORTION

In April 1970, the New York State abortion law was amended from extremely conservative to extremely liberal. The new law became effective on July 1, 1970. Formerly abortions were permitted only if a physician judged that the pregnancy endangered a woman's health or life. The new law permitted abortions on request within a period of twenty-four weeks after conception. It made no stipulation as to the place of the abortion, nor were there any residency requirements. An Obstetric Advisory Committee helped the Health Department to

[55] William Droegemueller, Stewart E. Taylor, and Vera E. Drose, "The First Year of Experience in Colorado with the New Abortion Law," cited in "The First Year of the 'Modernized' Colorado Abortion Law," *Briefs: Footnotes on Maternity Care,* Vol. 33, No. 5 (May 1969), pp. 67-69.
[56] "Abortion and the Doctor," *Annals of Internal Medicine,* Vol. 67, No. 5 (November 1967), pp. 1111-13.

establish standards, which included a stipulation that pregnancies that had progressed beyond the twelfth week had to be terminated in a hospital. Those of twelve weeks or less could be done in an outpatient facility if conditions permitted. If the outpatient facility was outside the hospital building, it had to be supported by a hospital located within ten minutes travel time. This requirement could be waived if the outpatient facility had available all the equipment of a minihospital, such as operating rooms and X-ray equipment.

data on abortions in New York City

Within the first eighteen months after the new law took effect, 278,122 abortions were performed in New York City.[57] More than half (65 percent) were performed on women who were not residents of New York City. The most common method of abortion was by vacuum aspiration; 58.9 percent of the abortions were by this method. Dilation and curettage was used in 26.1 percent of abortions; saline injection, in 14.2 percent; and hysterotomy, in 0.8 percent. (See pages 133–34 for a description of these methods.)

Approximately 81,000 of these abortions were performed in private, profitmaking hospitals. Another 105,000 were performed in private clinics. About 54,000 occurred in voluntary hospitals, and 39,000 in municipal hospitals. Most New York City residents had abortions performed in voluntary or municipal hospitals; most nonresidents made use of the private, profitmaking facilities.

Among New York City residents the ethnic distribution was: white, 46.2 percent; nonwhite, 43.4 percent; and Puerto Rican, 10.4 percent. Among nonresidents the ethnic distribution was: white, 89.1 percent; nonwhite, 10.4 percent; and Puerto Rican, 0.5 percent.

The majority of abortions were performed for women between the ages of twenty and thirty-four. Among residents of New York City who had abortions, 16.6 percent were under twenty and 10.1 percent were over thirty-five. Among nonresidents, 30.2 percent were under twenty and 8.5 percent were over thirty-five. The youngest person to receive an abortion was ten years old; she had already given birth to one live infant.[58]

During the first eighteen months of the new abortion law the death rate from legal abortions in New York City was 4.3 per 100,000.

[57] Data in this section from a news bulletin of the Health Services Administration of the City of New York, February 20, 1972.

[58] Jean Pakter, David Harris, and Frieda Nelson, "Surveillance of Abortion Program in New York City," *Bulletin of the New York Academy of Medicine*, Vol. 47, No. 8 (August 1971), pp. 853–74. In an extensive study of 42,598 patients conducted between mid-1970 and mid-1971 by the Joint Program for the Study of Abortions, which involved sixty hospitals and four independent clinics in twelve states, it was found that the most common patient was a young, single, white woman pregnant for the first time. The most common procedure was the vacuum aspiration technique (69.5 percent) compared to the once standard dilation and curettage (5.4 percent). ("Who Gets Abortions, How, and When," *Medical World News*, Vol. 12, No. 45 [December 3, 1971], p. 52.)

This compares favorably with the experience in other countries. In Great Britain the death rate during the first year of legal abortions was 17 per 100,000, and in Scandinavia it was 40 per 100,000. Although the rate of deaths from illegal abortions is unknown, it is certainly probable that the availability of legal abortions has saved many lives.

THE MOST COMMON LEGAL METHODS OF INDUCING ABORTION

There are five ways by which most abortions are today legally performed by competent physicians. Like all strictly medical procedures, their safety depends on the presence of an experienced and knowledgeable physician.

dilation and curettage (D and C)

In this procedure, the opening in the cervix (see Figure 2-4) is slightly dilated. A hand-instrument called a curette, a metal loop on the end of a long, thin handle, is inserted into the uterus through the cervical opening. With hand manipulation of the curette the physician gently scrapes the pregnancy tissue from the surface wall of the uterus and then removes it. Most physicians prefer to limit dilation and curettage to about the ninth week of pregnancy. Beyond this time complications occur somewhat more frequently.

vacuum aspiration (or suction)

This method is similar to dilation and curettage, however, it employs suction rather than the hand-manipulated curette. It is somewhat more expeditious than the D and C, and it usually results in less blood loss. As with all surgical procedures, there is some risk associated with this technique. This is because "the powerful suction needed to accomplish the procedure does pose a serious hazard to neighboring viscera in the event of uterine or cervical perforation." [59] In the hands of an experienced operator, such risks are minimal, and they very rarely occur. The vacuum aspiration technique is preferred for the abortion of pregnancies of more than nine weeks duration.

saline injection into the amniotic sac

In this procedure, a hypodermic needle approximately six to eight inches long is inserted through the abdominal wall into the amniotic sac (see Figure 6-1, page 194), and some of the amniotic fluid is withdrawn. This fluid is then replaced by a strong saline solution. The

[59] D. P. Swartz and M. K. Paranjpe, "Abortion: Medical Aspects in a Municipal Hospital," *Bulletin of the New York Academy of Medicine,* Vol. 47, No. 8 (August 1971), p. 848.

saline solution upsets the delicate water and chemical balance within the sac, placenta, and fetus. Fetal death is almost immediate and is hastened by the placental damage, which results in sharply diminished oxygen and food supplies to the fetus. In addition, the hormonal balance, so necessary to maintaining the pregnancy, is disrupted. The hormone oxytocin is released from the pituitary gland; it stimulates contraction of uterine musculature. Prostaglandins (see page 125) may also be released. From six to twelve hours after receiving the saline injection, the uterus begins to contract. The placenta and fetus are expelled from twenty-four to thirty-six hours after the injection. Most operators prefer the technique of introducing the saline solution into the amnion for pregnancies that have already progressed from sixteen to twenty weeks because, before that time, the amniotic sac is small and difficult to locate.

hysterotomy

With a hysterotomy an incision is made in the abdomen and then through the uterus, and the fetus is removed. This is obviously a major surgical procedure requiring hospitalization. Hysterotomy does not impair the woman's reproductive system, unlike a hysterectomy, or removal of the uterus, with which it is often confused.

oxytocin stimulation

Oxytocin is one of the hormones produced in the hypothalamus. It is stored in the posterior lobe of the pituitary gland (see page 30), which is situated at the base of the brain. Upon being injected, oxytocin stimulates contraction of the muscles of the uterus. It is used to induce active labor or to cause contraction of the uterus after the afterbirth (placenta) has been delivered. In the expert hands of a physician it is safe. Its use to terminate pregnancy may require several administrations over several days.

TRENDS IN ABORTION TECHNIQUES

In 1966 there were an estimated 6,000 legal abortions performed in the United States; a conservative estimate for 1971 was 500,000. This increase has been accompanied by a rapid change in abortion procedures. The traditional method of dilation and curettage is being abandoned for the vacuum aspiration technique. Although vacuum aspiration is primarily used in the first trimester of pregnancy, it is also being employed as late as the sixteenth week from the last menstrual period. Earlier and outpatient abortions are seriously being considered by medical authorities.

During the Bangladesh civil war, mass rapings led to the opening of outpatient emergency abortion clinics. "Lady family planning visitors," rather than physicians, performed aspiration procedures under medical supervision. A U.S. physician in Bangladesh recently demonstrated a relatively simple abortion technique; it employs a length of polyethyline tubing adapted for the purpose and a suction device. It has been reported that with proper patient relaxation six- to ten-week pregnancies can be terminated in a few minutes with little pain or blood loss. The dilation and curettage procedure requires forty-three instruments; polyethyline tubing aspiration requires only two. In this country outpatient procedures are illegal in most states. They are, however, being supported by some leading medical authorities, as is the use of nonphysician paramedical personnel to do the actual abortion.

Still another trend is "menstrual induction" or "menses extraction." In this procedure the uterus is evacuated with a vacuum aspiration tube of small diameter. Also being studied is a "Supercoil" as a substitute for the presently practiced saline induction of a second trimester abortion. The "Supercoil" is formed by inserting a series of up to eight coiled intrauterine devices. When they are removed in sixteen to twenty-four hours, fetal and placental tissue may then be removed by suction or curette. Some of the simpler abortion techniques present the danger of inviting self-abortion or abortions done by untrained individuals. This can only result in an increase in infections and other serious complications.[60]

ABORTIONS: CAUTION!

There is little question that the changes in abortion laws in New York, Washington, Hawaii, and Alaska, as well as in other states, have been legislated as a result of public pressure. Nor are physicians averse to changing their minds in this respect. A 1967 study noted that only 23.5 percent of 5,289 members of the American Psychiatric Association favored laws allowing abortion on request. By 1969, 72 percent of 2,041 psychiatrists polled favored such action.[61] Moreover, it is not necessarily true that abortion-on-request laws are accompanied by a decline in the use of contraceptive methods. This occurred neither in Japan nor in various European countries. Indeed, in these countries an increased number of abortions has resulted in an increase in the use of contraceptives.[62]

Nevertheless, there are dangers to abortion-on-request laws. One danger is that many young women may regard an abortion too

[60] "Two-Minute Abortion Is Here—Are We Ready?" *Medical World News,* Vol. 13, No. 19 (May 12, 1972), pp. 15-17.
[61] E. Pfeiffer, "Psychiatric Indications or Psychiatric Justification of Therapeutic Abortion," *Archives of General Psychiatry,* Vol. 23 (1970), pp. 402-07, cited in "About Abortion," *Journal of the American Medical Association,* Vol. 215, No. 2 (January 11, 1971), p. 286.
[62] "About Abortion," *Briefs: Footnotes on Maternity Care,* Vol. 35, No. 6 (Summer 1971), p. 91.

casually. Another is that the availability of inexpensive abortions may reduce the individual use of contraceptives. "Why use a contraceptive this time?" a young wife may ask herself. "Abortions are quick and easy and cheap and no trouble." But abortions can be trouble. An induced abortion temporarily interferes with the body's hormonal system. Although return to normal is the rule, postabortion medical help may be needed. Moreover, even skillfully induced abortions may be unavoidably connected with future problems. There is reliable opinion that the physical trauma of repeated induced abortions may be associated with both a later inability to conceive or to carry a child to full term.[63] In Hungary, Rumania, and the Soviet Union the most recently available records show a higher number of induced abortions than live births.[64] In Hungary the rate of premature births is also rising, and that country now has the highest rate in Europe. "It is widely felt that this change is the result of the free recourse to abortion possible in Hungary and particularly to the termination of first pregnancies."[65] This opinion may be particularly applicable to a growing experience in this country. In both California and Delaware, the first pregnancies in single women are the ones most frequently terminated. During the first two years of California's revised abortion law, girls younger than twenty years of age constituted almost 33 percent of all abortion cases. Fifty-three percent of all abortions were performed on childless women. In Colorado, more than 50 percent of all abortions are performed on women who have yet to bear their first child.[66] Physicians are concerned about the one-child-sterility syndrome—couples are unable to have a second child. Although not proven, it has been theorized that this may be due to low-grade infection.[67] Such infections can occur following abortion.

Although most abortions are surely justifiable, they should never be regarded as a substitute for a reliable contraceptive.

---

[63] Melita C. Gesche and Donald G. Dickinson, "Abortion and the Young," *Health News,* Vol. 47, No. 8 (August 1970), p. 6.
[64] Carl Djerassi, "Fertility Control Through Abortion: An Assessment of the Period 1950–1980," p. 12.
[65] Melita C. Gesche and Donald G. Dickinson, "Abortion and the Young," p. 6.
[66] Ibid., p. 13.
[67] Ibid., p. 14.

the human 5
beginning

Before I was born out of my mother generations guided me[1]

"in the beginning . . ."

Many millennia ago there was no life in the world. In a certain right time and environment, however, chemicals combined and were sparked into living fragments. That is, they reproduced themselves exactly. Sometimes they failed to do this and reproduced themselves inexactly. This accident was then duplicated exactly.

In time the living fragments became cells. Cells became tissue. Tissues were formed into creatures. Countless trillions of different individuals were born into a million species, and died. Some, like the dinosaur, perished forever. Others, like man, endured and became more complex. But, although man has found a way to get out of this world and back again, he still has, as an embryo, "gills" like a fish. His genes send ancestral messages, but his needs have modified the message. His "gills" become glands and major blood vessels. Genetic instruction and evolution dictate this.

genetics: molding a new person

The reasons for interest in heredity are several. The chromosomes within the nucleus of the human cell give directions that help decide the characteristics of man. Change those directions and man can be changed. Many scientists are apprehensive that man will "tamper with heredity." To better understand and control its destiny, this generation must understand some genetics.

Atomic energy provides a second reason for concern with genetics. The fallout from atomic testing may produce an effect, most likely deleterious, on human genes. But more than bombs are

[1] Walt Whitman, "Song of Myself," line 1162.

involved. Future generations will see a greatly expanded industrial use of atomic energy. The effect of possible atomic radiation on the progeny of posterity is urgent health business, and only an informed public can influence government policymakers to safeguard health.

The involvement of genetics with illness is yet a third reason the subject requires study. More than 1,600 varieties of birth defects perplex man. Some, like flat feet, are minor. Others, like Mongolism, are more serious. In all such disorders, genes play a varying role. Sometimes it is the gene that is basically at fault. In other cases it is the environment that disturbs genetic processes. And there are conditions for which the primary cause is unclear. But one concept is clear: all genetic processes must be considered within their ecosystems. Every gene interacts with its environment and is inexorably influenced by it.

THE CELL, UNIT OF LIFE

The *cell* is the basic unit of life. The cellular *protoplasm* is the chemical life of the cell. Protoplasm is composed mainly of cellular proteins, fats, carbohydrates, and inorganic salts in a watery medium. It contains thousands of *enzymes* (see footnote 6). Many enzymes contain *vitamins.* Enzymes are eventually used up and must continuously be created anew by the cell from available nutrients. Their vitamin component must be made by the cell or taken in with food. Cells also contain special materials involved with their particular activity, such as the *glycogen* seen as granules in the liver cell.

The ministructures in the cell's protoplasm, the *organelles,* function in concert with their intracellular environment. The membrane-encircled *nucleus,* the largest of the cell's organelles, contains and is surrounded by protoplasm. Protoplasm outside the nucleus is called *cytoplasm.* Thus, the two major parts of most cells are the nucleus and the cytoplasm. The events that occur in the cytoplasm, such as digestion, respiration, secretion, and excretion, depend on the activity within the nucleus. The nucleus is also essential for the reproduction of the cell.

the nucleus

Within the nucleus are the *chromosomes.* The chromosomes contain the *genes.* A gene is the unit of heredity. But it is even more. Because each gene is composed of *DNA,* it governs the life of the cell. Because DNA can reproduce itself during cell division, its code is transmitted to subsequent cells. The *nucleolus,* or "little nucleus," is an organelle that is not visible in some stages of cell division. It has no membrane. It may be a storehouse of chemicals for the reproduction of DNA.

In the cell community, red blood cells are unique. During their maturation in the bone marrow they lose their nuclei. Bereft of DNA, these cells cannot synthesize protein. Red blood cells live only so long as their enzymes last—about 120 days. Every second some 2.5 million red blood cells must be released into the circulation.

the cytoplasm, its membranous wall, and the endoplasmic reticulum

Policing the kind and amount of material entering the cell is its enveloping, porous *plasma membrane*. The plasma membrane admits some molecules that seek to enter the cell; it rebuffs others. It also permits the escape of waste materials from the cell but fastidiously retains essential substances. At various places the plasma cell membrane folds inward to extend into the cytoplasm of the cell as the *endoplasmic reticulum*. Thus is created a membranous transportation system of canals along which needed materials move deep into the cell's cytoplasm. The endoplasmic reticulum communicates with the nuclear membrane. By this route nutrients for the nucleus are delivered. Wastes can be carried out via these canals too.

the organelles within the cytoplasm

On part of the endoplasmic reticulum granules are clustered; these are *ribosomes*—the sites of protein synthesis. Seemingly continuous with the nongranular endoplasmic reticulum is the *Golgi complex*. This may be a sort of enzyme storage bin; protein enzymes, completed at the ribosomes, penetrate the membrane of the endoplasmic reticulum and possibly migrate, via its channels, to the Golgi complexes, to be kept and released when needed by the cell. Also in the cytoplasm of most cells are the *mitochondria* and *lysosomes*. Mitochondria are the cell's energy sources. Like tiny fuel furnaces distributed throughout the cellular cytoplasm, they convert the chemical energy of cellular nutrients into a high-energy compound called *adenosine triphosphate (ATP)*. ATP is released as needed for the cell's work. Mitochondria are enclosed by a membrane. So are the lysosomes, the cell's digestive organelles. Each lysosome contains enzymes that break down complex nutrients into simpler substances. Another duty of the lysosome is to act as a minute garbage disposal, ridding the cell of bacteria or worn-out materials.

Consider the treasure of past and future generations contained within the cell: the nucleus, the power-packed mitochondria, the digesting lysosomes, the Golgi complex of storage facilities for completed protein enzymes, the membranous network of endoplasmic reticulum that provides a transportation system for cellular nutrients and wastes and a ribosomal site for protein synthesis—all these active islands surrounded by a small sea of protoplasm, which, in turn, is enveloped by the meticulously selective plasma membrane. They speak of the balanced organization within the cellular ecosystem. Two tools have made the cell more accessible to scientific scrutiny—the *electron microscope* and the *ultracentrifuge*. The first has afforded magnifications of over one hundred thousand. The ultracentrifuge can whirl treated cell suspensions at speeds of sixty thousand revolutions per minute. Trapped in such an intense separating force, the microlayers of the cells separate to provide materials for the study of organelles. A new science, *molecular biology,* reveals both the normal and the abnormal at this level. Scientists in this field may soon discover what, for example, causes cancer, a disease of the cell.

MEIOSIS AND MITOSIS

There are two basic kinds of cells in the human body: germ cells (*gametes*) and somatic cells (Greek *soma,* body). A germ cell is a cell of an organism the function of which is to reproduce the kind; these are the ova (eggs) and the spermatozoa.[2] All other body cells are somatic.

When a mature sperm fertilizes a mature ovum, the resultant fusion is a cell called the *zygote*. To achieve the maturity necessary to participate in zygote formation, the germ cells, starting from *primordial sex cells,* must go through a special process of cell division called *meiosis*. Primordial sex cells have forty-six chromosomes, but when meiosis of a primordial sex cell is complete, the mature gamete has only twenty-three chromosomes (see Figure 5-1). Twenty-two of these are single, nonsex chromosomes and are called *autosomes*. The remaining chromosome is either an X or a Y *sex chromosome*. At the end of meiosis, the mature ovum carries a single X-chromosome; the mature sperm either an X-chromosome or a Y-chromosome (see Figure 5-2). It is a basic (although not the only) function of the Y-chromosome to direct the production of the male sex glands (testes).

When fertilization of the mature ovum by the mature sperm occurs, each parent contributes twenty-three chromosomes to the resultant zygote—twenty-two autosomes and one sex chromosome. A normal ovum always contains an X-chromosome. If an ovum is fertilized by a normal sperm containing an X-chromosome, the result is XX (female):

$$X \text{ (ovum)} + X \text{ (sperm)} = XX \text{ (female)}$$

---

[2]Women are born with their total supply of primitive eggs, which nestle immature in the ovary until puberty. Beginning at puberty, men continually replenish their supply of sperm cells.

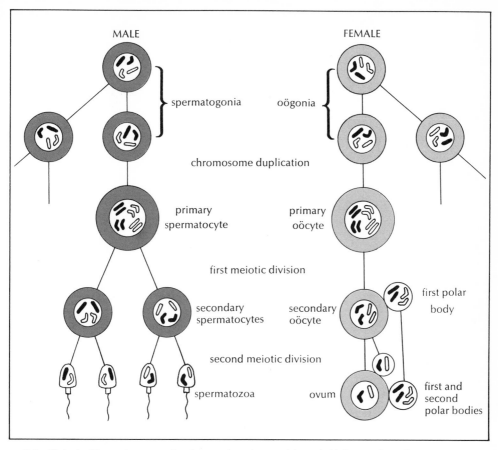

5-1 Meiosis. The mature gametes (spermatozoa or ova) have half the number of chromosomes that the primordial sex cells (spermatogonia or oögonia) had. During the maturation process, polar bodies simply degenerate. For simplicity, cells shown here have only four chromosomes.

If an ovum is fertilized by a sperm containing a Y-chromosome, the result is XY (male):

$$X \text{ (ovum)} + Y \text{ (sperm)} = XY \text{ (male)}$$

So the zygote and all subsequent body (somatic) cells normally contain twenty-three pairs of chromosomes (a total of forty-six chromosomes), of which twenty-two pairs are autosomes and one pair are sex chromosomes. Each autosomal pair is different in genetic content and usually in appearance from all other pairs.

As noted above, only the primordial sex cells multiply by meiosis. The zygote and all subsequent body (somatic) cells multiply by *mitosis*. In the process of mitosis, the threadlike chromosomes in the nucleus of a cell duplicate themselves; the duplicate sets are sepa-

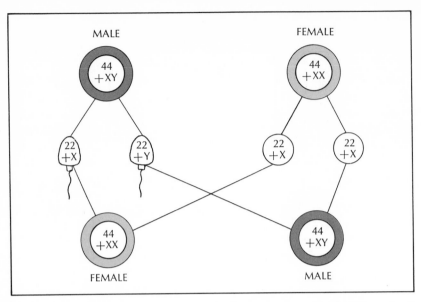

5-2 If a sperm carrying an X-chromosome fertilizes an ovum, a female (XX) results; if a sperm carrying a Y-chromosome fertilizes an ovum, a male (XY) results.

rated, with one set going to each of the two "daughter" cells produced by the division of the original cell. Thus in *mitosis* each of the two cells produced by the division of a single cell has a full set of chromosomes, whereas in *meiosis* each of the cells has *half* the number of chromosomes the original cell had. By mitosis the body replaces discarded cells and grows. In both meiosis and mitosis there are plenty of chances for errors. Should a cell, be it germ or somatic, fail to receive its proper share or composition of chromosomes, abnormality results.

CELLULAR ENGINEERING: GENETIC ORDER

By their union in the Fallopian tube (see page 46) the mature sperm and egg contribute their twenty-three single chromosomes to the fertilized egg to form a zygote with its full normal complement of forty-six. Mitosis begins. The zygote prepares to divide. Each of the forty-six chromosomes splits into two parts, which are exact replicas of one another. The cell divides. Now there are two body cells. Normally, each has its full share of forty-six chromosomes. Several hours later the two somatic or body cells cleave again. There are then four body cells. Normally, each still contains forty-six chromosomes. And so cell multiplication continues. Every day the somatic cell cluster continues to divide as it travels down the Fallopian tube toward the uterus. With each division these cells double in number. Normally, they never have fewer or more than forty-six chromosomes. At last, the tiny multiplying cellular mass[3] is implanted in the uterine endometrium. Membranes begin to form. Within two or three weeks after fertilization, the embryo is being fed via these membranes. In another week there is a heart. A week later the heart begins to beat. Now cell differentiation continues rapidly, and so does organ development. Differentiation began with the earliest division. For each cell must multiply in the limited space allotted to it and it is influenced by pressures from every other cell. And, as will be seen, each cell is instructed as to its future function. This is the nature of the cellular ecosystem.[4]

The cells of various organs are specific for those organs. In other words, the cells of the heart are different from those of the gut which, in turn, are different from those of the nerves, and so on. By birth, there have been about forty-four successive cell divisions resulting in trillions of marvelously organized cells. With normal cell division, every one of those trillions of cells contains the identical number of chromosomes as the original individual single zygote contained. How did this happen? How does one kind of cell end up as a part of a bladder muscle, another kind in the eye, still another in a toenail, and yet a fourth in a mole on the left cheek? How does each cell get the message telling it what to become?

The answer lies within the nucleus of the cell, in the chromosomes.

DNA, the master plan; RNA, the obedient worker

Chemically, a chromosome consists mostly of proteins combined with a substance called *deoxyribonucleic acid* (abbreviated as DNA). The chromosomal DNA is the material of the gene. Within it is stored the genetic information. Chromosomal DNA cannot itself leave the nucleus. It remains imprisoned within it, capable of duplicating itself with each cell division, and serving as a blueprint for the formation of *ribonucleic acid* (RNA) molecules. Thus, chromosomes also contain RNA. As will be seen, several kinds of RNA are made, and each plays a specific role in the building of cell proteins.

Outside the nucleus, as part of the cell's cytoplasm, there are still other proteins. Like all body proteins they are originally derived from food. Like all other proteins they are composed of amino acids. It is from this nutrient pool of cytoplasmic proteins that amino acids are taken and brought to the ribosomes.

---

[3]In the human, one week after fertilization, the developing organism is called an *embryo;* this term is applicable until the end of the second month; then the term *fetus* is used.
[4]*Embryology*, the science dealing with the development of the embryo, is discussed in Chapter 6, pages 191–96.

how the ribosomal factory is made

Peering through the electron microscope at an amphibian oöcyte,[5] biologists believe they have discovered how ribosomes originate. A gene is shaped like a carrot or spindle. Each gene is linked with every other gene like the beads of a necklace. Running from the broad base of the spindle to its tip is a thread. This thread is DNA—a tiny segment of a chromosome. The DNA of the gene directs the production of molecules of ribonucleic acid (RNA). These hairlike molecules, extending from the gene, spiral about the DNA thread and decrease in size from the base to the tip of the spindle. (The RNA is not an inherent part of DNA; the DNA merely governs the synthesis of RNA according to its present code.) The length of the RNA fiber and its structure are dictated by the DNA, which directs its synthesis from cytoplasmic amino acids. As it is synthesized, the RNA molecules appose themselves to part of the DNA pattern in such a way as to reflect specific chemical configurations. RNA is thus instructed by the DNA. According to DNA instructions, each RNA fiber breaks off and, when free in the nucleus, is broken up into segments, probably by an enzyme.[6] First one, and then a second part of the original RNA fiber leaves the nucleus, deserting the nuclear DNA, which cannot leave. Bearing the specific instructions of the DNA, these segments of the RNA fiber meet in the cellular cytoplasm to together form a single ribosome. John Lear has described this remarkable process:

> According to the biochemical evidence, the opening event in the sequence of the spindle's operation is the extrusion of the RNA fiber from the main thread of DNA. As the extrusion proceeds, the fiber is strung with a protein coat according to coded instructions from the DNA. This process goes on until each fiber reaches a predetermined length . . . , after which that particular RNA fiber separates from the DNA thread like a quill from a porcupine's back. The fibers depart individually after attaining individual maturity. En route they pass under an unidentified biological knife (presumably an enzyme) that chops each fiber into segments. The first segment to be severed is about one-sixth the length of the whole fiber. This segment moves into the cytoplasm very quickly and at once coils into a tiny sphere. The coiling apparently occurs in response to instructions the DNA thread imprinted on the RNA fiber before setting the fiber loose. That part of the fiber that remains in the nucleus is

---

[5] An *amphibian* is a vertebrate animal (a frog or a toad, for example) able to live both on land and in water; an *oöcyte* is a female gamete that has not reached full development; mature, it is an ovum.

[6] An enzyme is frequently a protein and has the power to initiate or accelerate certain chemical reactions in plant or animal metabolism.

subsequently chopped several times, until the surviving segment is about one-third as long as the original fiber had been. The final segment then moves out through the nuclear membrane into the cytoplasm, finds a tiny sphere formed by an earlier segment of fiber, and coils into a larger sphere alongside the tiny sphere. The two spheres together make a ribosome.[7]

how body protein is made

Consider what happens at a single ribosome.

An amino acid is brought and attached to it. Then a second amino acid is brought to it. With the assistance of an enzyme, the second amino acid is linked to the first. But only in a predetermined way. A third amino acid is brought to the ribosome. It is linked to the second—again in a manner previously decided, and helped by an enzyme. A fourth amino acid then reaches the assembly line at the ribosomal factory. It is linked to its predecessor. Still another follows it. Then another and another. To all the ribosomal depots, in all the body cells, whether in a developing embryo or in an aging man, amino acids, derived from the nutrient pool of cytoplasmic proteins, are brought and linked one to the other. At each ribosome, then, a series of linked amino acids, a chain, is formed. Bonds between these amino acid chains form complex proteins. The manner of arrangement of the amino acids determines protein structure. And protein structure decides body structure and, therefore, function. So the chemical arrangement of the amino acids at the ribosomes results in proteins that will become blue eyes or black eyes, liver or heart, a short or tall person. The variations in the arrangement of amino acids at the ribosomal workbench are no less endless than the variations of hereditary characteristics.

How do the amino acids get selected out of the cytoplasmic protein? How is their sequence determined? How are they brought to the ribosome? And, once at the ribosome, how does it happen that amino acids are so properly arranged? It is the nuclear DNA that governs all this. Only the DNA contains the genetic formula, so only the DNA can impart the genetic code, the hereditary instructions. But how can these DNA instructions reach the ribosome? It has been seen that the DNA cannot itself leave the nucleus to direct protein construction at the ribosome. It is imprisoned within the nucleus, irrevocably locked within the chromosomal pattern. It is fixed, a die, a stamp, a mold, a template of chemicals. Since the DNA is unable to carry its own message outside the nucleus, an intermediary is needed—a messenger.

That messenger must somehow obtain the exact complex message, the specific instructions, of the DNA. Like the ribosomal RNA

[7]John Lear, "Spinning the Thread of Life," *Saturday Review* (April 5, 1969), pp. 63-64.

before it, that messenger must, therefore, in turn become a template, a mold of the DNA code. And unlike DNA, that messenger must then be able to leave the nucleus. Obediently that messenger must wend its way to the waiting ribosome, bringing to it the DNA message of instructions. A special kind of RNA is that messenger. Somehow, *messenger RNA* (as it is called) must obtain the patterned message, established by the coded position of certain chemical elements in the DNA. (As will be seen, the message obtained by the messenger RNA is for a different purpose than that obtained by ribosomal RNA.)

Within the cell's nucleus, messenger RNA places itself in apposition to part of the DNA code. It arranges its chemical structure to exactly match that of the DNA. The RNA transcription of the DNA template is thus formed.[8] In this way the messenger RNA has itself become a template, a mold, a momentous master copy of the DNA basic chemical structure. Having incorporated within itself the instruction of the DNA, having acquired within its very structure the position of the coded chemical elements of the DNA, the messenger RNA deserts the DNA. It traverses the nuclear membrane. It enters into the midst of the cellular cytoplasm. There the DNA-code-carrying messenger RNA heads for a waiting ribosome. For, as has been stated, it is at the ribosomal workbench that protein is manufactured. And these synthesized proteins contribute to the specific characteristics of the creature-to-be.

Upon finding a ribosome, the messenger RNA is associated with it. Thus is established, at the ribosome, the copy of the DNA code of instructions. Now amino acids, taken from the surrounding cytoplasmic protein, must be brought to the ribosome. And, with the instructions awaiting their arrival, the amino acids must be properly arranged at the ribosome. This can only be done as instructed by the DNA. For although the DNA remains in the nucleus, it remains the master. The traveling messenger RNA, associated with a ribosome, remains but a copy, a slave. And now the readied ribosomal workbench (the synthesis of which was also specifically directed by the DNA) awaits amino acid delivery. To construct specific proteins, to create specific tissue as instructed, amino acid building blocks must be brought to the ribosomal factory from the nutrient cytoplasmic protein pool.

How is this accomplished?

While the ribosome was receiving its instructing messenger RNA, the DNA in the nucleus was not idle. It kept busy directing the production of still another, smaller type of RNA. This third RNA is called *transfer RNA*. Also instructed by the DNA, in a predetermined sequence, transfer RNA leaves the nucleus and enters the cytoplas-

---

[8] The rate at which messenger RNA is transcribed from the DNA is determined by the arrangement or sequence of the chemicals of the DNA. In some manner light affects this rate. It sets the biological clock.

mic protein pool of amino acids. For each separate amino acid there is a separate transfer RNA. On its way to the ribosome the transfer RNA picks up its selected amino acid from the protein pool. On reaching the ribosome, the amino acid leaves the transfer RNA and, helped by enzymes, attaches itself to the ribosome. One after another, in assembly line fashion, and as instructed by the messenger RNA, the amino acids are linked one to the other.

So transfer RNA keeps leaving the nucleus, picking up selected amino acids from the cytoplasmic protein pool, and delivering them to be linked to the growing amino acid chain at the ribosomal protein factory. But recent work suggests that this factory is not merely an inert organelle—that it is more than a passive building site. It is postulated that the ribosome moves. The message that is brought to the ribosome from the DNA by the messenger RNA is in the form of a string of chemicals arranged in a specific sequence. Along this messenger RNA these chemicals are arranged in groups of three, and each group is called a *codon*. Each codon specifies a particular amino acid. So the messenger RNA associated with a ribosome is like a string of beads; each bead is a codon, which is composed of an exact sequence of three chemicals. And each codon waits for transfer RNA to bring to it an allocated amino acid. It is the codon, then, that the transfer RNA must recognize to know at what point at the ribosome to bring its amino acid. Imagine such a string of messenger RNA beads or codons (see Figure 5-3) and, for the present purpose, give each codon a number from 1 through 10. (There are many more, and this is done for the sake of explanation.) Also for convenience, number each molecule of transfer RNA carrying its particular amino acid. Transfer RNA number 1 brings its specific amino acid, number 1, from the cytoplasmic pool to the ribosome, which is now located at codon number 1 of the messenger RNA. There, amino acid number 1 is attached to the ribosome. Transfer RNA number 1 is then released to seek another of its specific amino acids. Carrying its first amino acid, the ribosome moves on to codon number 2. There another transfer RNA (number 2) waits with its amino acid number 2. Amino acid number 2 is then bound to amino acid number 1. The ribosome moves on to the third bead (or codon) of the string of messenger RNA. The process is repeated and amino acid number 3 is bound to amino acid number 2. In this way one after another specific amino acids are bound to one another, as shown in Figure 5-3. In this sense the ribosome makes its own string of beads, and each bead is an amino acid. The completed amino acid chains are the components of complex proteins. Thus, the ribosome conducts the synthesis of proteins. Finally, and, as always, according to DNA instructions, the ribosome has had enough. There are no more codons for it to move along. The ribosome then rids itself of its linked chain of amino acids—of its protein component. What becomes of the complete

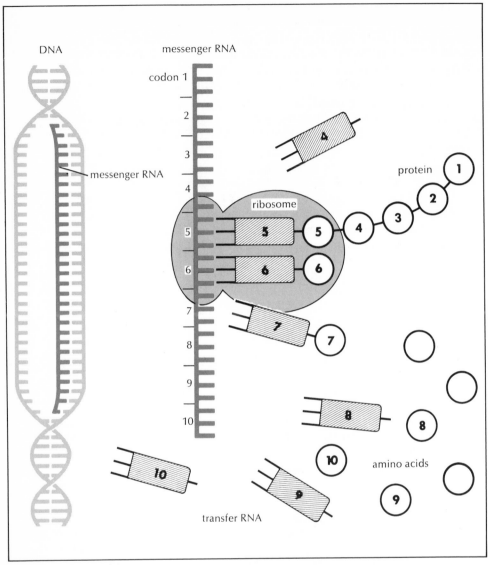

5-3 The synthesis of proteins. The diagram at the left represents the transcription of genetic information from DNA to messenger RNA. The rest of the illustration schematizes the process by which transfer RNA brings its specified amino acid to the ribosome, which is situated at the codon specifying that particular amino acid. Here amino acid number 6, specified by codon number 6, has just been bound to its site on the ribosome by the corresponding transfer RNA. Amino acid number 6 will bond to amino acid number 5, adding to the growing chain. Then the ribosome will move along the messenger RNA to codon number 7. In this example, the chain will be complete when amino acid number 10 has been bonded to it. (Most proteins, however, consist of two or more chains of amino acids.)

protein? It contributes to the body structure and function. It will contribute to the eye, or to the heart, or to an enzyme. Multiplied billions of times, this process accounts for the creation of a unique person.[9] The wonder is not that an occasional error or defect occurs. The wonder is that it occurs so rarely.

How extensive is all this activity?

If it were possible to assemble the DNA in a single human cell into one continuous thread, it would be about a yard long. This three-foot set of instructions for each individual cell is produced by the fusion of egg and sperm at conception and must be precisely replicated billions of times as the embryo develops.[10]

After birth too, and so long as the individual grows, develops, and ages, the genetic process by which cellular proteins are manufactured is repeated still more billions of times. As long as the person lives, it goes on.[11]

the new person: product of genetics? environment? or both?

DNA instructions are many and they are related one to the other. And the whole genetic process takes place in, and is affected by, an

[9] Here one can best comprehend the individuality of the single being. Within each new zygote formed by the union of sperm and ovum is a completely new organization of DNA, a new master plan, a new set of instructions. Never before had there been a zygote with exactly the same DNA code.

[10] Marshall W. Nirenberg, "The Genetic Code; II," *Scientific American,* Vol. 208, No. 3 (March 1963), p. 82.

[11] In 1970, the enzyme *reverse transcriptase* was discovered. It is found in cells that have been invaded by certain RNA viruses. The simultaneous announcement of the discovery of this enzyme by two young virologists, working in separate laboratories, ranks as a major scientific event of the beginning of the decade. Before its existence was proved, it had been believed that the genetic process was a one-way street. Helped by an enzyme, DNA was always thought to direct the production of RNA; RNA could only be transcribed under the direction of DNA. The formula DNA → RNA, then, was scientific dogma. But now it was learned that the newly discovered enzyme could reverse that transcription. Reverse transcriptase could initiate the transcription of DNA under the direction of RNA. Thus, an RNA virus, containing reverse transcriptase, could enter an animal cell, and, instead of acting as a messenger, it could (using the cell's organelles and energy) act as a template to direct the production of DNA. The classic formula DNA → RNA was reversed to RNA → DNA.

Reverse transcriptase is also called *RNA-dependent DNA-polymerase.* How did this enzyme get its formidable name? It will be remembered that an enzyme has the power to initiate or accelerate a chemical reaction. The word *polymerase* is simply a combination of *polymer* and the suffix *-ase.* A polymer is a compound of many molecules that have been formed by a combination of simpler molecules. The suffix *-ase* is used to designate an enzyme. The polymerase in question is involved in the production of DNA. And, as an enzyme, the DNA polymerase is indeed dependent on the existence of RNA.

Reverse transcriptase—or RNA-dependent DNA-polymerase—has been reported to be present in cells that are not thought to be actively infected with viruses. What is it doing there? On this there is, as yet, no agreement. One prominent theory holds that an infectious agent, called the C-type RNA virus, is possibly the underlying cause of all cancers, whether spontaneous or induced by chemical or physical agents. This virus, it is theorized, is actually incorporated into the mother's genes. Using the enzyme reverse transcriptase, the C-type RNA virus is transmitted from mother to child by genetic processes, as if it were a gene (or *oncogene*—a cancer causing gene). Such a dormant or covert or latent gene could be "switched on" or triggered, as it were, by some adequate stimulus, such as radiation, chemicals, or perhaps another virus.

all-encompassing environment. Each cell, each nucleus within the cell, each strand of DNA within the nucleus, each chemical component within the DNA, functions within the context of its environment. So there are genetic ecosystems.

If the whole genetic process operates in an environment, it is inexorably influenced by it. An individual is not merely the result of the *genotype*. "The genotype is the sum total of the heredity the individual has received, mainly . . . in the form of DNA in the chromosomes of the sex cells. The cytoplasm may also contain some heredity determinants; if so, they are likewise constituents of the genotype." [12] But with cell division and the resultant increase in the number of cells, with the growth of the organism, the constituents of the genotype must continuously reproduce themselves (replication). The material for this replication is taken from the environment. Consider just the change in size that occurs from man's beginning as a fertilized ovum to full adulthood.

> *A human egg cell weighs roughly one twenty-millionth of an ounce; a spermatozoon weighs much less; an adult person weighs, let us say, 160 pounds, or some fifty billion times more than an egg cell . . . The phenotype is, then, a result of interactions between the genotype and the sequence of the environments in which the individual lives . . . The "environments" include, of course, everything that can influence man in any way. They include the physical environment—climate, soil, nutrition—and, most important in human development, the cultural environment—all that a person learns, gains, or suffers in his relations with other people in the family, community, and society to which he belongs.* [13]

Thus, to say that an individual is genetically predetermined is more than an unjustified limitation on human potential. It is also scientifically invalid. And there is an element of absurdity to the "heredity versus environment" argument. For whatever happens in the genetic system is a happening in an environment. Genes are not fateful. By themselves, they decide little.

Nevertheless, practicality does require an answer to the question, "To what extent can genes predispose an individual to develop certain illnesses?" Some disorders are dependent on the presence of a particular genetic error (though not all individuals who carry such errors will necessarily manifest the disorders). Then what is the role of the surrounding environment? This varies. In some instances, such as

[12] Theodosius Grigorievich Dobzhansky, *Heredity and the Nature of Man* (New York, 1964), pp. 49-50.
[13] Ibid., pp. 50-51. The *phenotype* is the appearance of the trait; the *genotype* is the genetic basis of the trait.

hemophilia, the environmental influence, compared to the genetic, is surely small. With other conditions, the environment plays a more distinct role. Coronary artery disease, as an example, is greatly influenced by both genetic instruction and environment. Short stocky men with a history of heart attacks in their families are more prone to coronary heart disease than tall thin men without such a history. But diet (environment) plays an important role too. How long the condition remains latent and, when revealed, how severely it is manifested—these may be profoundly influenced by the environment. Another example: much has been written of the relationship between an XYY chromosomal pattern and aggressive behavior (see pages 155–56). The association may have some validity. Yet, most aggressive behavior is unrelated to the XYY chromosome. Moreover, a gentle, well-adjusted person may carry an XYY chromosomal aberration and harm nobody. Another with the same genetic disorder will be a violent, homicidal menace. The difference may be in the environment.

A few years ago, Charles J. Whitman, a twenty-five-year-old architectural engineering major, climbed to the observation deck of the University of Texas tower in Austin. He shot and killed fourteen persons who were on the campus below. Thirty-one others were injured. A few hours before, he had killed his wife and mother. Whitman's chromosomal pattern is unknown. This, however, is known: at autopsy, he revealed a highly malignant brain tumor. Could his brain tumor have contributed to his aggression? Perhaps. (He had presented no known neurological abnormality.) The chromosomal patterns of Lee Harvey Oswald and Jack Ruby are also unknown. But the terrible childhood of the former certainly helped lay the groundwork for the terrible act of his adulthood.[14] On the other hand, Ruby suffered from psychomotor epilepsy—a seizure disorder singularly resistant to treatment. During a seizure from this type of epilepsy, violence is not uncommon. Twice in his lifetime Ruby had been struck on the head by a pistol butt. Where did genetic influence begin? Where did the environment enter the behavioral picture? It is now impossible to tell. But neither factor can be ignored. What is needed is more alert study.

GENETIC DISORDER

Human genetic problems are related either to (1) an error in the physical or chemical *structure* of a chromosome or (2) an error in the *amount* of chromosomal material in the cell. This is generally expressed in terms of the *number* of chromosomes in the cell.

---

[14] David Abrahamsen, "A Study of Lee Harvey Oswald: Psychological Capability of Murder," *Bulletin of the New York Academy of Medicine,* Second Series, Vol. 43, No. 10 (October 1967), pp. 861–88.

disorders of chromosomal structure

Spontaneous mutations   Man was once a fish and within the uterus he still lives submerged in water like a fish. Slowly, over millions of years, he left the sea, and over still more millions of years he adapted to a new environment. All his adaptive changes were made possible by infinitely gradual gene changes or mutations (Latin *mutare,* to change). There are much more rapid changes due to environmental influence, as occurs when the German measles virus attacks the embryo. However, some genetic changes, although occurring in the environment, do not seem to be primarily caused by it. These are called *spontaneous.* A spontaneous change of some part of the chemical structure of the DNA takes place. If the change is not basically molded by the surrounding environment, how, then, may one account for the existence of a mutation in chromosomal structure? What causes a spontaneous change in DNA? The answer to this question remains unknown. Yet even one spontaneously mutant gene can result in profound developmental changes and hereditary health problems. Anatomical and, therefore, functional deviations from the normal ensue. There may be inborn errors of metabolism. Disorders of carbohydrate metabolism, such as diabetes mellitus, and of amino acid metabolism (phenylketonuria—PKU, see page 181) are examples. Or disease of the blood or blood-forming organs may result. Hemophilia is one of these. By no means are all mutations spontaneous, however. Some are plainly *induced* by an external environmental stimulus. An example is genetic disorder (see pages 166-67) caused by radiation.

Chromosomal translocation and deletion   This, too, may occur spontaneously, or there may be a direct external cause, such as radiation. Sometimes a chromosome breaks. DNA structure is disrupted. The chromosome may heal into a new and different structure. Or it may remain in fragments. Or it may be just partly repaired, leaving a piece out of its structure. Or two chromosomes may exchange pieces. *Translocation* occurs when a segment or a fragment of one chromosome shifts into another part of a noncorresponding chromosome. Sometimes, one of the products of such an exchange is so small it gets lost. This is called *deletion.* Whatever occurs the chromosome is adversely altered. Genetic instruction by the DNA of the affected chromosomes is awry. Usually a fertilized egg, containing a broken or wrongly formed chromosome, dies. Occasionally, the zygote lives. The individual develops to suffer various deficiencies.

disorders of chromosome number during meiosis or early mitosis

Sometimes it is not a changed chromosomal structure that results in disease. Rather it is an error in the total number of chromosomes that find their way into the cells. Normally, there are forty-six. With genetically related sickness, there may be too many or too few. How can this happen?

Errors during meiosis   Study again Figure 5-1 illustrating meiosis. This shows how the chromosomes, having duplicated themselves, separate. Consequently, after the first cell division, when two cells are formed, each cell normally has duplicates of only a single member of each original pair of chromosomes. Sometimes, though, something goes wrong. Nobody really knows why. During meiosis, the chromosomes of a pair do not separate. This is the basic error. One cell receives both chromosomes of the pair, while the other gamete receives none. This is called *meiotic nondisjunction.*

It will be further noted in Figure 5-1 that there are two meiotic divisions. Meiotic nondisjunction can also occur during the second meiotic division after a normal first division. Upon fertilization, should a gamete with a missing chromosome unite with a normal gamete, the zygote and all the cells consequent to its multiplication will have forty-five chromosomes instead of the normal forty-six. This condition is called *monosomy.* Should a gamete with an extra chromosome unite with a normal gamete, the zygote will have forty-seven chromosomes. This is *trisomy.* The trisomy and monosomy of meiotic nondisjunction can affect both the autosomal chromosomes and the sex chromosomes.

Trisomy 21. The most common trisomy affects the twenty-first autosome. *Trisomy 21* is one of the causes of *Mongolism* or *Down's syndrome.* In this illness nondisjunction occurs with chromosomes other than the X and Y. As a result of this autosomal aberration, the individual has forty-seven instead of forty-six chromosomes. Children with Down's syndrome[15] (named after a nineteenth-century English physician, John Down) are physically and mentally retarded. Muscle tone is poor. The tongue is large. The eyes are slanted, which accounts for the other name of the condition—Mongolism. Palm and footprints are abnormal. As the age of the mother increases, so do her chances of giving birth to a child with Mongolism.

Meiotic nondisjunction involving the X and Y sex chromosomes can result in gametes that may unite to produce zygotes that manifest some aberrant sex chromosome arrangements. How do these disorders occur?

[15] A *syndrome* refers to a set of signs and symptoms occurring together, as a group, in a disease state.

Turner's syndrome (Figures 5-4 and 5-5). Illness may result from nondisjunction of sex chromosomes during meiosis. Assume that during an error in meiotic division an ovum receives no X-chromosome. It is fertilized by a normal sperm containing an X-chromosome. The resultant individual acquires a chromosomal pattern as follows:

$$\text{No X (ovum)} + \text{X (sperm)} = \text{0X}$$

(0 refers to the missing X chromosome.)

An 0X zygote develops into an individual with a combination of characteristics called *Turner's syndrome (monosomy X)*. At birth the baby appears to be a female. But the child has tiny ovaries. Nor does the child develop secondary sexual characteristics. She is abnormally short and never menstruates. Turner's syndrome also results if a sperm with no X-chromosome fertilizes a normal ovum.

Klinefelter's syndrome (Figures 5-4 and 5-5). Sometimes, during meiosis, a single ovum receives both (XX) chromosomes. With fertilization by a sperm carrying the Y-chromosome, what happens? This:

$$\text{XX (ovum)} + \text{Y (sperm)} = \text{XXY}$$

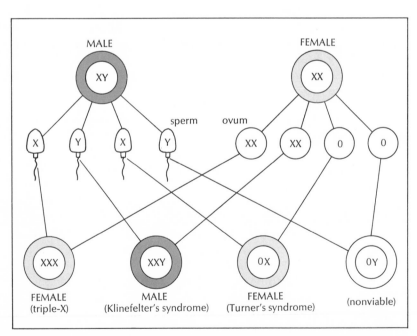

5-4 Nondisjunction in the mother, resulting in ova with either two X-chromosomes or none. When fertilized, these ova can give rise to the four chromosome combinations shown here. Three of them are abnormal; the fourth is nonviable—the complete absence of an X-chromosome is lethal to a zygote. (This diagram presents an abbreviated view of the development of spermatozoa and ova from the primordial sex cells. The process of meiosis is shown in greater detail in Figure 5-1.)

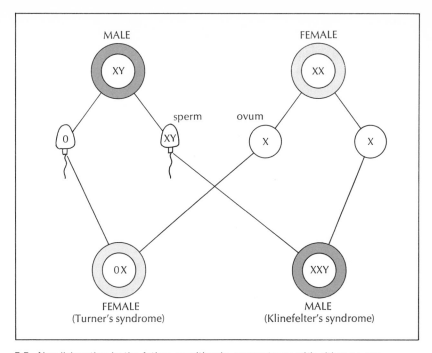

5-5 Nondisjunction in the father, resulting in spermatozoa with either no sex chromosomes or both an X- and a Y-chromosome. Ova fertilized by such spermatozoa can give rise to the two chromosome combinations shown here. Both of them are abnormal. (As in Figure 5-4, this diagram omits the step-by-step process of meiosis, which is shown in Figure 5-1.)

Here there is an excess X (female) chromosome (*intersex*[16]). The result: a *Klinefelter male,* as this individual is called. These people may appear normal, or be quite tall. They may have underdeveloped sexual structures. Ordinarily, they are sterile and are often mentally retarded.

Illness from nondisjunction of sex chromosomes during male meiosis can also result in the Klinefelter male.

Chromosomes and crime. Another abnormal arrangement of chromosomes that can result from nondisjunction of sex chromosomes in male meiosis involves an extra Y-chromosome. Figure 5-6 shows how a sperm carrying two Y-chromosomes is produced. When such a sperm fertilizes a normal ovum the *XYY syndrome* occurs. Recent research has brought considerable attention to individuals manifesting this syndrome. Tentative results indicate a startling association between the XYY disorder and criminal insanity.[17]

[16] Intersexuality should not be confused with homosexual behavior. The former is a genetic disorder. It refers to the abnormal intermingling, in varying degrees, of the characteristics of each sex in one individual. The incidence of homosexual behavior among intersexually abnormal patients is not higher than in the general population.

[17] Fathers and children of XYY are no more likely to have abnormal chromosomes than the average person in the population. The condition is innate, but not hereditary. Moreover, it should be

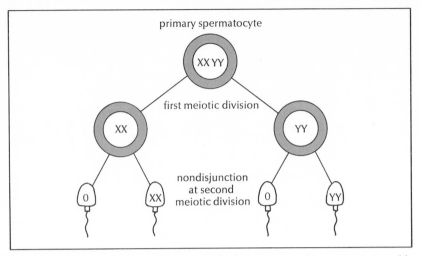

5-6 The XYY syndrome. Nondisjunction in the father may produce spermatozoa with two Y-chromosomes, as shown here. When such a sperm fertilizes a normal ovum (which has an X-chromosome), the result is the XYY male.

Richard Speck, the 1966 murderer of eight Chicago nurses, was found to have the XYY disorder. The XYY chromosomal error is by no means an absolute indicator of criminal behavior. Only a portion of XYY males develop criminal behavior. But it does appear much more commonly in prison populations. Its victims are unusually tall males,[18] often mentally retarded, with histories of aggressive violence. Should they be punished for their crimes? A French court has ruled affirmatively. An Australian court has said "no" and acquitted an XYY murderer. In this country, a final decision has yet to be made. Although society must be protected, many suggest that XYY aggressiveness should no more be punished than the genetic gentleness of the Mongoloid is rewarded. Everything possible should be done for the known XYY carrier. With such an individual, environmental conditions encouraging crime take on a special meaning.

Configurations with three, four, or no X-chromosomes. Rarely a person is born with an XXX configuration—the so-called "super-" or "hyper-" female. Males with two extra X-chromosomes (XXXY) have

---

reemphasized that present scientifically reported associations between human XYY chromosomal structure and criminal behavior are tentative. All that can be now indicated is this: possibly some people with an XYY chromosomal structure may be more susceptible to certain kinds of social stress than people without such a chromosomal structure. However, even this remains theoretical. Widespread and inaccurate news reports about a "proven" relationship between XYY chromosomes and criminality have created an unwarranted public stir. In this respect, it is appropriate to quote a distinguished newspaperman of another generation, Heywood Broun: "For truth", he wrote, "there is no deadline."

[18] Extraordinary height is not necessarily due to chromosomal abnormality.

also been found. Even more rarely, males and females with four X-chromosomes have been noted by investigators (XXXXY and XXXX). However, these prefixes refer only to the excess number and kind of chromosomes and not to "super-abilities"; such an individual is usually a nonfunctioning mental defective. The complete absence of an X-chromosome in a zygote is lethal.

Chromosomes and competition in athletics. Abnormal chromosome arrangements can become a matter for concern in international female athletic events. In former times, disputes arose when a performance was thought to be due to chromosomal maleness. Microscopic examination of cells usually settled the argument. Most experts disagreed with this superficial approach.[19]

Chromosomal analysis alone does not determine sex. Also to be considered is *nuclear sex*. In the cell nuclei of female mammals (including the human) is a structure not present in males (*Barr body,* see page 184). Yet, even these two—chromosomal sex and nuclear sex—are not adequate to definitely determine the appropriate sex of some people. Other important criteria include genital appearance, internal reproductive organs, structure of the gonads, influence of other endocrine glands, psychological sex, and social sex.[20] Thus, it was the opinion of some that it was unfair to disqualify the Polish track star Ewa Klobukowska from the 1967 Women's European Athletic Cup competition. In her case, apparently only nuclear and chromosomal sex indicators were used. (Incidentally, there have been instances of males who, disguised as females, won Olympic medals. "Claire," the bronze-medal winner in the 100-meter dash in the 1946 competition at Oslo, today answers to the name of Pierre, is a father, and lives on a farm near Metz, France.)

The differences between male and female performance in athletics is the reason for the concern over chromosomal sex. Three decades ago (1924), Johnny Weismuller won fame and a movie contract (as Tarzan) with his record swim of the 400-meter free style. But since 1924, no less than eleven women have surpassed Weismuller's record; among them was Sweden's Jane Cedergvist. "The fact that even Jane can now swim faster than Tarzan is certainly worthy of mention."[21] Today, the only two Olympic events in which men and women compete under the same rules are shooting and equestrian sports. For the other events, it is believed that anatomic differences place women at a disadvantage. Although, in these, the performance of some women equals or betters that of some men, individual records

---

[19] Some tests used in detecting abnormalities in chromosomes are mentioned in the section on genetic counseling on page 184.
[20] Sometimes sex is determined by surgical exploration, but only after all these and other factors have been carefully weighed.
[21] Warren Boroson, "Medicine and the Olympics," *Medical World News*, Vol. 13, No. 31 (August 18, 1972), p. 49.

do show a difference. Differences in track are between 10 and 18 percent, and in swimming events, 10 percent. Since the breast stroke, butterfly, and backstroke require more muscular effort, the difference in these events rises to 15 percent.

Prior to the competition in the 1972 Olympic Games in Munich, women athletes underwent careful screening. Tests were performed for X- and Y-chromosomes. If these were not decisive, a karyotope (chromosomal map) was constructed and examined. Sample cells were obtained from the mucous membrane of the inner cheek and the hair roots. When an irregularity was apparent, blood tests and gynecologic examinations were indicated. Cases of intersexuality (see page 155) or hermaphroditism (having sex organs of both sexes) were barred from competition. Results were kept in strict secrecy by the Medical Commission, and, since the examinations were conducted before the competition, would-be competitors could ostensibly be excluded without embarrassment. For each competing female, a "certificate of femininity" was prepared and signed by the President of the Medical Commission of the International Olympic Committee. Some people criticize the entire process as callous and discriminatory. However, it does not presently seem practical to "please everyone" by holding "several Olympic Games . . . to accommodate the different chromosomic groups."[22]

As the years go by, near-maximum performance will inevitably be reached in an increasing number of events. It will then be interesting to see how stable are the presently observed differences in male and female peak performances in some events. Moreover, one may speculate as to whether actual studies do prove that individuals with excluding chromosomal aberrations actually do have an advantage over women without them.

Errors during mitosis   Although most abnormalities from nondisjunction occur during meiosis, nondisjunction can also occur during mitosis. A normal sperm fertilizes a normal ovum. But during the early mitotic cellular multiplication following fertilization two chromosomes may fail to separate. In this way half the body cells of the affected individual have three rather than two of a particular chromosome (forty-seven total) and the other half of his body cells have one instead of the normal two (forty-five total). This is called *mosaicism*. Sometimes three types of cells may occur in one person's body, normal (forty-six chromosomes), trisomic (forty-seven), and monosomic (forty-five). Mosaicism can also result, not from failure of separation of chromosomes, but from the loss of a chromosome during the cell division of mitosis. In all these mitotic variables there is the potential of grave illness.

[22]Eduardo Hay, "Sex Determination in Putative Female Athletics," *Journal of the American Medical Association,* Vol. 221, No. 9 (August 28, 1972), p. 998. It is on this article that most of the material in the above section is based.

illness and the genes of sex and race

Illness patterns are profoundly influenced by such genetic factors as sex and race.

Sex   Fortunately, the union of the human sperm and egg results in about 140 males for every 100 females. Fortunately indeed. The male hold on life is relatively feeble. Even within the safety of the uterus, 50 percent more males than females perish. In all age groups up to the age of eighty, there is a consistent excess of male over female deaths (see Table 5-1). In 1968 over two-and-one-half times

TABLE 5-1 male deaths per 100 female deaths by age groups, United States, 1970*

AGE	MALE DEATHS PER 100 FEMALE DEATHS
Under 1	139.6
1–4	122.1
5–14	174.0
15–24	277.5
25–34	204.8
35–44	161.5
45–54	171.6
55–59	193.1
60–64	189.4
65–69	159.2
70–74	133.8
75–79	108.6
80–84	89.5
85 and over	64.5
Total all ages	128.2

*These data do not cover deaths of U.S. civilians or members of the armed forces that occurred outside the United States.
Source: National Center for Health Statistics, *Monthly Vital Statistics Report*, Provisional Statistics, Annual Summary for the United States, 1970.

as many males between fifteen and twenty-four died as did females in the same age group. Neither U.S. civilians nor members of the armed forces who died outside this country were included in these data. Moreover, the ratios were similar in 1960, a year in which the United States was not engaged in hostilities. For the fragile male, almost all disease categories are more lethal. Aside from the complications of childbirth, it is only in a relatively few disease categories that females die more frequently (see Table 5-2). Syphilis has been called "the chivalric disease." It surely shows special consideration for the female. For her, the disease is milder and is less likely to involve the heart and central nervous system. Syphilis kills less than half as many females as males. When suitable antibiotics are given to a male child with bacterial meningitis, his chances for survival are less than those of a female child of about the same age and in

TABLE 5-2 deaths in the United States due to selected causes, 1968 (according to sex)

CAUSE OF DEATH	TOTAL NUMBER	TOTAL RATE (per 100,000 population)	MALE NUMBER	MALE RATE (per 100,000 population)	FEMALE NUMBER	FEMALE RATE (per 100,000 population)
Tuberculosis, all forms	6,292	3.1	4,502	4.6	1,790	1.7
Syphilis and its sequelae	586	0.3	430	0.4	156	0.2
Meningococcal infections	741	0.4	424	0.4	317	0.3
Malignant neoplasms (cancers)	318,547	159.4	173,694	178.0	144,853	141.6
Benign neoplasms and neoplasms of unspecified nature	4,948	2.5	2,345	2.4	2,603	2.5
Asthma	2,688	1.3	1,234	1.3	3,751	3.7
Diabetes mellitus	38,352	19.2	15,781	16.2	22,571	22.1
Anemias	3,494	1.7	1,645	1.7	1,849	1.8
Major cardiovascular diseases	1,023,399	512.1	557,233	571.1	466,166	455.7
Influenza and pneumonia	73,492	36.8	40,562	41.6	32,930	32.2
Chronic and unqualified bronchitis	6,205	3.1	4,594	4.7	3,751	3.7
Peptic ulcer	9,460	4.7	6,438	6.6	3,022	3.0
Appendicitis	1,485	0.7	888	0.9	597	0.6
Hernia and intestinal obstruction	7,758	3.9	3,561	3.6	4,197	4.1
Cirrhosis of the liver	29,183	14.6	18,821	19.3	10,362	10.1
Cholelithiasis, cholecystitis, and cholongitis	4,385	2.2	1,897	1.9	2,488	2.4
Infections of kidney	9,395	4.7	4,347	4.5	5,048	4.9
Congenital anomalies	16,793	8.4	9,075	9.3	7,718	7.5
Certain causes of mortality in early infancy (birth injuries, difficult labor, etc.)	43,840	21.9	25,879	26.5	17,961	17.6
Symptoms and ill-defined conditions	23,656	11.8	14,183	14.5	9,473	9.3
Accidents	114,864	57.5	79,424	81.4	35,440	34.6
Suicide	21,372	10.7	15,379	15.8	5,993	5.9
Homicide	14,686	7.3	11,523	11.8	3,163	3.1
Total deaths due to all causes	1,930,082	965.7	1,087,220	1,114.3	842,862	824.0

Source: National Center for Health Statistics, *Monthly Vital Statistics Report, Advance Report, Final Mortality Statistics,* 1968.

the same circumstances. Adverse effects of atomic radiation are more frequent in boys than girls.

Why the disparity? There is a good theory. It has been stated that, of the forty-six chromosomes in the primordial sex cell of the ovum or sperm, two are sex chromosomes. The female has two X-chromosomes. These are equal. The male, however, has one X-chromosome and one puny Y-chromosome. Thus, the arrangement of the X- and Y-chromosomes is probably to the advantage of the female. If something goes wrong with one of her chromosomes, perhaps she can rely on the other. The male is denied such possible insurance. There is evidence, at present inconclusive, that this biological inequality may be gradually equalizing because of the inactivation of one of the female X-chromosomes. Nonetheless, the male is indeed the weaker sex.

About a queen's genes   A rare but deservedly famous disease involving sex chromosomes, in which blood clots slowly or not at all, is *hemophilia*. It is hereditary and sex-linked. Like color blindness, the gene for hemophilia is recessive and is carried on the X-chromosome. Since males have only one X-chromosome they are more likely to be bleeders than females, who must have two X-chromosomes carrying the hemophilia gene in order to be bleeders. Bleeder fathers transmit the defective gene not to their sons (since a male child does not receive an X-chromosome from his father) but to their daughters. Unless the daughter has also received an X-chromosome carrying the hemophilia gene from her mother, she will not be a bleeder, but she may transmit the disease to her children. (Female hemophiliacs do not live to maturity, since the onset of menstruation is fatal.)

The family tree of Queen Victoria was riddled with hemophilia. The son of the last tsar of Russia was a bleeder. This led to the reliance by the royal family on the corrupt quack Rasputin and hastened the decline of the Russian court. The last tsar of Russia shared this tragic situation with the last king of Spain, who also sired a bleeder. Both had married granddaughters of Victoria. "Thus two of the greatest dynasties of European history, the Spanish in the west and the Russian in the east, ended with uncrowned successors who were bleeders."[23]

Race   Sickle cell anemia is much more frequent among Negroes than Caucasians. In the United States, tooth decay is more common among Caucasians than Negroes. Among women in Japan, cancer of the breast is rare. One should, however, view with caution the varying frequency of diseases in races. True, heredity helps decide body reactions to disease. But socioeconomics rather than genes

[23] Fritz Kahn, *Man in Structure and Function*, Vol. I, translated and edited by George Rosen (New York, 1960), p. 215.

accounts for the comparatively greater frequency of such illnesses as tuberculosis and syphilis among Negroes in this country. Moreover, recent studies emphasize the association between the malnutrition of poverty and mental retardation.

Sickle cell disease   A major abnormality of the red blood cell's hemoglobin is *sickle cell disease*. It is inherited; the only way a person can have the disease is to be born with it. In this condition, there is a genetically transmitted abnormality in the chemical structure of the hemoglobin molecules within the red blood cells. As a result, the hemoglobin molecules can link together to distort the cell. Thus, the ordinarily doughnut-shaped red blood cell is forced into the shape of a sickle. The molecular change is minute; the human suffering caused by it is immense. In this country, sickle cell disease largely affects the Negro population. However, the disease can occur among Caucasians from the Mediterranean area and among the peoples of the Middle East and certain parts of India. More than 2 million U.S. Negroes carry the *sickle cell trait;* that is, they have the capacity to pass the disease on to their children. Over fifty thousand U.S. Negroes have the much more serious *sickle cell anemia.*

In some unusual circumstances, even those individuals with only the trait may become seriously ill. This is because some (although not all) of their red blood cells contain the abnormally structured hemoglobin molecule. In such people, sickling of the affected red blood cells can be brought on by extreme lack of oxygen. This can occur with a severe hemorrhage during a surgical operation, or with exposure to an atmosphere of reduced oxygen tension (as is the case in an unpressurized airplane or on a high mountain). Lack of oxygen during anaesthesia administration is also a matter of special concern with these individuals. However, in usual situations, people with the sickle cell trait do not have red blood cells that are shaped like sickles. They are, therefore, generally without symptoms.

For the person with sickle cell anemia the situation is much more dangerous. All his red blood cells contain the abnormally structured hemoglobin molecules; all his red blood cells are potential candidates for sickling. Sickle cell anemia is diagnosed during childhood, and a child with this disease can become desperately ill even without the occurrence of a special set of circumstances. Normally, the oxygen tension in the capillaries and small veins is low. In these tiny blood vessels, red blood cells containing abnormally structured hemoglobin will tend to sickle. Worse, the misshapen red blood cells clump together. In this way, they plug the small blood vessels and thus partly or wholly deprive needy tissues of blood and oxygen. Cells die, as do the tissues of which they are a part. Pain, loss of appetite, joint swellings, ulcers—these plague the afflicted child. (The pain is not dissimilar to the pain of coronary thrombosis [acute heart attack] and occurs for the same reason—lack of oxygen to the tissues.) Normally, red blood cells live more than one hundred days. Sickled, they are destroyed, mostly in the spleen, in ten to twenty-five days. The little patient is exhausted, wan, often desperately anemic. His belabored spleen cannot provide him with adequate immunity; he is at constant risk from infections such as pneumonia. Periodically, crises of intense sickness imperil his life.

Not long ago, it was expected that one-half of these patients would die before they were twenty; the other half would barely survive middle age. Now there is hope. It was first found that a chemical called urea unsickled the affected cells. This was followed by the discovery that it was not the urea, but a chemical, cyanate, in the urea solution, that accomplished the beneficial result. By midsummer 1972, intensive work was being done in this area. In addition, several valuable diagnostic tests have been developed, both for the sickle cell trait and sickle cell anemia. Those who suffer from the anemia can find hope in renewed research and recent treatments. Those who find that they carry the trait must make their own decision as to whether to risk passing on a tragic genetic legacy to future generations. However, early diagnosis remains essential. It makes possible not only early treatment[24] but also affords the time necessary to make thoughtful decisions about having children. Someday, genetic surgery may be of help. It may be possible to replace the gene responsible for the abnormal hemoglobin with a gene that codes for hemoglobin that is normal.

THE GENETIC ECOSYSTEM: THE FERTILIZED OVUM IN THE ENVIRONMENT

Within the nucleus of the cell, the basic genetic chemicals are arranged in relation to one another. And they are dependent on one another. So, inside the very nucleus there is environment with ecological balance or imbalance.

Within the no longer secret nucleus, the genes contain a pattern set to direct development. But no amount of healthy genetic instruction can bid cytoplasm, sickened by an abnormal environment, to be normal. Nor can a healthy cytoplasm expect beneficial patterns of instruction from a gene made deviant by environment. Normal

[24]Within the uterus, the hemoglobin produced by the normal fetus does not differ from that produced by a fetus with a potential sickle cell problem. Both produce fetal hemoglobin—labeled HbF. For this reason, parents cannot elect abortion to avoid the future problem in their child. Nor does a newborn baby give any indication of the disease. A newborn's hemoglobin is of the fetal variety. Within a few months the normal baby's HbF diminishes and he begins to produce adult hemoglobin—HbA. Babies with sickle cell anemia cannot produce HbA. Instead, they produce sickle cell hemoglobin (HbS). For this reason, the symptoms of HbS-producing children do not usually occur until between the sixth and twelfth month of life. The first manifestation of the disease may be disastrous. Death may occur from overwhelming infection or anemia. Thus, early diagnosis is of critical importance.

genetic action depends on a normal environment inside and outside the cell. The internal drama of the cell will be disarranged not only when the chromosomal players unaccountably neglect their proper parts but also when they are surrounded by destructive microorganisms, or hostile drugs, or searing radiation. That is why German measles (rubella) and thalidomide and atomic radiation kill and cripple the unborn. Consider now these and other influences.

nutrition

Pregnant women may need extra calories, proteins, minerals, and vitamins. However, such decisions, including vitamins and mineral therapy, should be made only by the physician. Deficient maternal diets mean more stillborn babies and more deaths among babies less than one month old. The child is affected by the mother's diet not only during his residence in the uterus but also long after birth. Babies born to poorly nourished mothers are more susceptible to infections in early life and have more birth defects. The child surviving the mother's poor nutrition may be smaller at birth and often will grow into a small adolescent and adult. There is a direct relationship between the economic status of the mother and the birth weight of her baby (see Table 5-3). Children born of poor mothers

TABLE 5-3 mean birth weights according to socioeconomic status

PLACE	POPULATION	SUBJECTS	MEAN BIRTH WEIGHTS (in grams)
Madras	Indian	Well-to-do	2,985
		"Mostly poor"	2,736
South India	Indian	Wealthy	3,182
		Poor	2,810
Bombay	Indian	Upper class	3,247
		Upper-middle class	2,945
		Lower-middle class	2,796
		Lower class	2,578
Calcutta	Indian	Paying patients	2,851
		Poor class	2,656
Congo	Bantu	"Very well nourished"	3,026
		"Well nourished"	2,965
		"Badly nourished"	2,850
Ghana (Accra)	African	Prosperous	3,188
		General population	2,879
Indonesia	Javanese	Well-to-do	3,022
		Poor	2,816

Source: World Health Organization, *Nutrition in Pregnancy and Lactation*, cited in Miriam E. Lowenberg et al., *Food and Man* (New York, 1968).

weigh less. And children with lower-than-normal birth weights have a greater tendency to physical defects in later life.

Should the mother fail to provide enough food for the child within her, will he suffer shortages? Or will he be able to avoid malnourishment by helping himself to whatever is available from his mother's reserve? The availability of the mother's reserve has been overestimated. Daily nourishment for the developing child comes from the daily nourishment of the mother. Even a temporarily inadequate diet, unnoticed by the mother, may wreak irreparable damage to an unborn child. With maternal malnutrition, the unborn infant suffers before, and more, than the mother.

A maternal diet that is poor in calcium may result in a child born with poor bone development and bad teeth. Inadequate iron results in anemia for both mother and child. Severe protein deficiency retards growth and development. Vitamin diseases, such as beriberi, rickets, and scurvy, are seen in the babies of mothers deprived of vitamins B, D, and C respectively. An iodine-deficient maternal diet may result in the birth of a child that will show the distressing signs of cretinism by the sixth to the eighth month of life. Marked by severe physical and mental retardation, cretinism is always a threat when the mother uses plain salt without added iodine. Animal experiments indicate that maternal diets deficient in zinc and manganese result in deformed babies. The effects of such shortages on human beings is unknown. A malnourished mother may not carry her child full term, and she is more inclined to develop complications of pregnancy.

Many pregnant women, understandably concerned about their figures, embark on a restrictive weight-watching program. To a limited extent this may be good sense; however, it can be seriously overdone. In 1970, the National Research Council Committee on Maternal Nutrition recommended an average weight gain during pregnancy of twenty-four pounds, with a range of between twenty and twenty-five pounds. "Weight reduction programs and severe caloric restrictions should not be undertaken during pregnancy, even for obese women, because of the possibility of adverse effects on the fetus' weight and neurological development."[25] For underweight women and pregnant teen-agers, weight restrictions may be particularly harmful. Moreover, women who smoke during pregnancy deliver babies of significantly lower weights; in their cases, weight restrictions are particularly risky for the child (see pages 173–75).

It used to be thought that weight reduction during pregnancy prevented *toxemia of pregnancy,* a serious and rare metabolic disorder marked by swelling of the body and increased blood pressure. Rarely, toxemia can lead to the more serious *eclampsia.* However,

[25] "Pregnant Weight Watchers Risk Harm to Babies," *Public Health Reports,* Vol. 85, No. 11 (November 1970), p. 964. The material in this section concerning the report of the National Research Council Committee in Maternal Nutrition is from this source.

there is no evidence that excessive weight gain, whether it be due to fat or water, causes eclampsia. Nor is there evidence that severe caloric restrictions diminish the chances that the toxemia of pregnancy will occur with a woman who gains too much weight, or that a woman who gains excessively is more prone to toxemia. There is, however, a marked association between low income and deaths due to the toxemia of pregnancy. Women in low-income groups die from this condition at a rate that is about three times that of women in high-income groups.

infection

Women who develop *German measles* (rubella) during the first three months of pregnancy are over five times (15 percent) more likely to give birth to a defective child than women who do not have the disease (2.8 percent). The heart, hearing, and vision (cataracts) are most commonly affected. *Regular measles* (rubeola) should not be confused with German measles (rubella). There is some medical opinion that a woman who contracts regular measles also has a greater chance of having a defective child. But many physicians think that this contention is unproved. There are now available effective vaccines to prevent both regular measles and German measles. There is limited evidence that *infectious hepatitis,* a third viral illness, can adversely affect chromosomes. Because *smallpox vaccine* is composed of a living virus, it may affect the unborn child. Consequently, pregnant women are not usually vaccinated against smallpox. *Syphilis* can also be transmitted from mother to unborn child. Adequate treatment of the mother can prevent tragedy for both.

An important infection that may be transmitted from the pregnant women to the fetus is *cytomegalic inclusion disease.* Its name is descriptive of some of its characteristics. *Kyto* (Greek, a hollow vessel) denotes relationship with a cell. *Megalic* is derived from the Greek *megalois* (magnificent) and refers to the unique large cells associated with the illness. The word *inclusion* describes the unusual inclusion bodies found within those cells. This illness, usually noted during the first month of life, is due to a viral infection. It is revealed by a wide variety and degree of malformations in the child. As with German measles, children with the disease may be contagious for months after delivery. They should, therefore, be isolated, particularly from pregnant women.

direct radiation

Excessive exposure of a pregnant woman to X-rays can result in either fetal death or a malformed child. Women should, therefore, always advise a doctor who plans to X-ray them of a possible, still unapparent, pregnancy.

There have been large-scale experiences with radiation. Seven out of eleven Hiroshima children were born retarded if, within the first twenty weeks of conception, their mothers stood within 1,200 meters of absolute center of the atomic bomb blast. Others, whose mothers were at a greater distance, had malformed hips, eyes, and hearts. Some, symptomless at birth, developed poorly.

In 1954 the United States made a test explosion of a nuclear device at Bikini. An unpredictable wind deposited significant amounts of radioactive material on the residents of four nearby islands as well as on twenty-three Japanese fishermen. Years later, children of the islands who were less than five years old at the time of exposure were found to be retarded in physical growth.

Why does radiation cause abnormal babies? The baby is a triumph of recent cellular multiplication. And radiation has a predilection for multiplying cells. It requires more radiation to kill a fly than a mouse. Why? As a maggot, the fly passes through all its phases of growth and development. As an adult, it has few dividing cells. Adult mice and men have many dividing cells. It is these that are sensitive to radiation.

Radiation reaching the testes or ovaries, and thereby the reproductive cells, can cause changes in the structure of the DNA (genes). Mutation rates are increased by radiation. Since over 99 percent of mutations are harmful and since they do accumulate in man, the threat to future generations is apparent. Depending on the amount, moreover, radiation may cause chromosomal breaks and translocations. So another danger of radiation, more recently recognized, is related to chromosomal aberrations. Thus, radiation may be one of the causes of a wide variety of genetic disorders, ranging from the mental retardation of phenylketonuria to the mental retardation of Mongolism.

chemical pollution

The placenta is no longer considered an effective barrier against environmental pollutants. Large molecules of polluting substances are now thought to merely cross the placenta more slowly than those that are small. Added to this are the constant risks that are taken by prolonged use of chemical pollutants without adequate knowledge of the effects they will have. The use of diethylstilbesterol in meat animals is but one example of this kind of error. Another example is the recent mercury pollution of water and fish that resulted in the poisoning of numerous Japanese; the women who ate the poisoned fish gave birth to blind and paralyzed children.[26] Still a third example

[26] Neville Grant, "Mercury in Man," *Environment,* Vol. 13, No. 4 (May 1971), p. 3. An excellent account of a recent and tragic outbreak of mercury poisoning in this country is given in Paul E. Pierce, Jon F. Thompson, William H. Likosky, Laurence N. Nickey, William F. Barthel, and Alan R. Hinman, "Alkyl Mercury Poisoning in Humans," *Journal of the American Medical Association,* Vol. 220, No. 11 (June 12, 1972), pp. 1439–41.

of the careless chemicalization of the environment is the use of PCB (polychlorinated biphenyls). Little is known of the effects of its prolonged use.[27] Since standard test systems for many chemical pollutants are extremely insensitive, it would seem reasonable to take as few chances as possible. Strict regulations should be imposed on chemicals that may possibly affect human beings in an adverse way.[28] And those regulations should be in effect, not after, but before human harm occurs.

noise

As a pollutant, noise has been attracting increasing attention. It has also been generating understandable irritation. A Canadian hygienist reported the story of a man who "was annoyed by a loud-playing portable radio on a bus. After reasoning with the owner to play the radio more quietly, the man banged her over the head with the radio. He was tried before a jury . . . but was not indicted. In an informal survey, 299 out of 300 persons applauded the act. The 300th person felt he should have waited until the woman got off the bus."[29] That undue noise can have a deleterious effect on animal reproduction is known.[30] What effect it has on the unborn or newborn human is being researched. One recent hospital study found that "under the plastic hood of the incubators the noise spectrum fell well above the recommended acceptance level and, due to the prolonged exposure time, very close to the danger area."[31]

One extraordinary observation has been made by Japanese scientists.[32] They noticed that the way babies reacted to aircraft noise depended on the length of the mother's stay in Itami City, which is near the Osaka International Airport. Three hundred and seven babies were chosen for a study. They were divided into four groups according to the length of time that they and their mothers had been exposed to the airplane noise of Itami City. The results showed that when a woman spent the last half of her pregnancy, or the period directly after the birth of the child, in noisy Itami, the child was much more likely to be disturbed by the aircraft noise. When the women

[27] "Chemical Pollution: Polychlorinated Biphenyls," *Science*, Vol. 175, No. 4018 (January 14, 1972), p. 156.

[28] Paul Sampson, "A Warning About Introducing New Teratogens," *Journal of the American Medical Association*, Vol. 221, No. 8 (August 21, 1972), p. 853, quoting Samuel S. Epstein, Professor of Pharmacology at Case Western Reserve University Medical School.

[29] L. K. Smith, "Noise in the News," *Canadian Journal of Public Health*, Vol. 60, No. 8 (August 1969), p. 306.

[30] Krishna B. Singh, "Effect of Noise on the Female Reproductive System," *Journal of Obstetrics and Gynecology*, Vol. 112, No. 7 (April 1, 1972), pp. 981-91.

[31] Frank L. Seleney and Michael Streczyn, "Noise Characteristics in the Baby Compartment of Incubators," *American Journal of Diseases of Children*, Vol. 117, No. 4 (April 1969), p. 450.

[32] "Stick Out the Noise Mums, and Your Kids Will Take It Better," *New Scientist*, Vol. 47, No. 713 (August 6, 1970), p. 270, citing Y. Ando and H. Hattori, "Effects of Intense Noise During Fetal Life upon Postnatal Adaptability," *Journal of the Acoustical Society of America*, Vol. 47 (April 1970), pp. 1128-30.

moved to Itami before conception, so that the babies spent their entire fetal life near the airport, 58 percent of the babies slept soundly during airplane noise, and only 6 percent awoke and cried. When women moved to the vicinity of the airport during the first five months of pregnancy, 47 percent of their babies slept soundly during airplane noise, and 13 percent awoke and cried. When women moved to Itami City during the last half of their pregnancies or after the birth of their babies, only 9 to 16 percent of the babies slept through airplane noise, and 45 to 50 percent awoke and cried.

During the early months of the baby's development within the uterus, the nervous system (and the hearing mechanism) is relatively undeveloped. It is possible that exposure to intense noise during the earlier months of pregnancy in some way may enable the child's nervous system to adapt to it. Other observers comment that "if Japanese researchers' results are borne out, it does give people living near airports or motorways the dubious satisfaction that, if only they can stick it out, their sons and daughters won't find it so bad."[33]

endocrine influences

The *pancreas,* lying in the abdomen behind the stomach, is a gland producing a juice that passes into the upper intestine through a duct. However, another of its products, *insulin,* is produced by specialized islands of cells (*islets of Langerhans*) and is released directly into the blood. Insulin regulates carbohydrate metabolism. Without enough insulin, diabetes develops.

Diabetes is a genetically transmitted disorder of metabolism. Diabetic mothers have malformed children ten times more frequently than the average. The reasons are undetermined. They may be genetic or endocrine or nutritional or, perhaps, all three.

the Rh factor

In 1969, in this country, about ten thousand babies died of *Rh blood disease.* The condition is also known as *erythroblastosis fetalis* (Greek *erythros,* red + *blastos,* germ + *osis,* increase). The increase in red germ cells refers to the numerous immature primitive red blood cells seen in the circulation of the affected child. Their development in the fetus accounts for the term *fetalis.* Why do they occur? To make up for the normal red cells that are destroyed. Why are the normal red blood cells destroyed? In this the Rh factor is involved. What is Rh?

Rh is a chemical substance. Its exact structure is unknown. It sits on the surface of the red blood cells of 85 percent of all people. They are then Rh positive. The 15 percent who do not carry it are

[33] Ibid.

Rh negative. Why is it called Rh? The *Rh*esus monkey also has the factor. Has Rh a known purpose? No. It just causes trouble. How?

One in eight marriages is between an Rh-negative woman and an Rh-positive man. If the child is Rh negative, like the mother, there is no problem. But the child may inherit the Rh-positive factor from the father. The Rh-negative mother thus carries an Rh-positive child. Erythroblastosis fetalis occurs when the Rh-positive blood of the child enters the mother's blood. The baby's Rh-positive factor is a foreigner to the mother. It is an *antigen*, an antibody generator. To neutralize her baby's Rh-positive antigens, the mother produces antibodies in her blood. When these antibodies enter the child, they destroy red blood cells. There are two ways in which the child's antibody-stimulating Rh-positive factor reaches the mother's circulation. One way is through the placenta during pregnancy. Usually only small amounts of baby antigen reach the mother in this fashion. During the time that she is carrying her first child, these minimal amounts are not thought to be enough to cause the mother to manufacture antibodies. The second way that the child's Rh antigen enters the mother occurs during delivery. Indeed, most of the child's Rh-positive blood reaches the mother during delivery, since, at that time, the afterbirth loosens and bleeds. Therefore, it is after delivery that she manufactures antibodies. Once she has manufactured such antibodies, she will be restimulated, in future pregnancies involving an Rh-positive fetus, to produce antibodies with only the small amount of antigen that enters through the placenta. That is why erythroblastosis fetalis usually affects the child of a later pregnancy more severely than an earlier one; a third child, for example, will be more adversely affected than a second; a fourth child, more than a third; and so on.

To repeat, then, in most cases the mother usually does not produce enough antibodies to harm the child during a first pregnancy. During the actual delivery of her first child, however, she receives enough Rh-positive blood to manufacture a high level of antibodies. These antibodies remain in the mother's blood. With the second child, harm is likely. As with the first child, the second may inherit the father's Rh-positive blood factor. The mother's antibodies, formed in response to the Rh-positive antigen of the first baby, now pass through the placenta of the second baby. The antibodies destroy the unborn second child's red blood cells. To recoup, the child hastily makes new cells. These are the primitive red blood cells of erythroblastosis fetalis. But, as immature cells, they do not make up for the destroyed mature red blood cells. Anemia results. Products from the child's red cell destruction seep into the skin. Jaundice occurs.

Well over 90 percent of babies with erythroblastosis are saved. Complete replacement of their blood is necessary. Of the most severely affected, only about 25 percent are saved. A relatively new technique has sometimes been helpful. Rh-negative blood is introduced directly into the unborn child. This may maintain life within the uterus long enough to result in a baby who, at delivery, is adequately mature for transfusion. To the baby with erythroblastosis fetalis, the new era of the surgery of unborn babies has brought renewed hope. It is now even possible to temporarily remove a child from the uterus, replace the child's blood, and then return that child to the womb to complete the intrauterine life. Although such spectacular fetal surgery is not generally needed in the treatment of erythroblastosis fetalis, the very fact that it has been accomplished successfully opens further the whole new field of the surgery of the unborn.

But in some cases erythroblastosis fetalis can now be prevented. Recently, a product containing antibodies against Rh-positive blood has proved successful. Within seventy-two hours of delivery of her first Rh-positive baby, the mother's blood is tested for antibodies. If she already has them in considerable amount, the product is useless. But if she does not have a significant level of antibodies, because not enough of the baby's Rh-positive antigen had passed through the placenta into her circulation, the mother is injected with the medicine containing antibodies against Rh-positive blood. These medicine-antibodies quickly combine with the baby's Rh-positive antigen that had reached the mother's blood during delivery. This happens before the mother has a chance to make her own Rh-positive antibodies. The Rh-positive antigen-antibody mixture is then washed out through the kidney. The mother does not have any antibody against Rh-positive blood to threaten her next baby.

the mother's age

As a rule, young mothers (under thirty) provide a relatively safer intrauterine environment for their children. Perhaps older women do not produce adequate endocrine secretions to guarantee proper development of ova. (In animals, both aged ova and sperm appear less likely to combine to produce healthy offspring than do fresh ones.) With increase in the mother's age, for example, the frequency of Mongolism, as well as some other rare abnormalities, increases (see Table 5-5, page 180).

It should not be concluded that the younger mother needs less medical attention than the older. Table 5-4 shows that child marriages and pregnancies in this country are but a small percentage of the total but they are by no means rare. The young-teen-aged mother presents a special problem. She is less likely to obtain early professional care and is more prone to be improperly nourished. Consequently, both her life and that of her baby are at greater risk.

TABLE 5-4 childbearing children in the United States, 1965

Number of Babies Born to Mothers Ten to Fourteen Years of Age

NUMBER OF CHILDREN BORN	WHITE	NONWHITE	TOTAL
One child	2,450	4,984	7,434
Two children	72	248	320
Three children	2	10	12
Four children	2	0	2
Total	2,526	5,242	7,768

Source: Lucille B. Hurley, "The Consequences of Fetal Impoverishment," *Nutrition Today*, Vol. 3, No. 4 (December 1968), p. 9.

the mother's emotions

Emotional stress, particularly early in pregnancy, may be related to cleft palates. Some emotions cause a hyperactivity of the outer part (*cortex*) of the adrenal glands. This hyperactivity causes the adrenals to produce the hormone hydrocortisone, which can pass through the placenta. If hydrocortisone is injected into mice while their upper palates are being formed, over 90 percent are born with cleft palates.

Many other factors such as abnormal fetal position or a faulty placenta may adversely affect the environment of the child developing in the uterus. A mother's high blood pressure and hyperactivity of the thyroid gland also detract from the safety of the embryonic and fetal ecosystem.

So, even within the environment of the uterus, there are numerous ways in which that delicate individual, the developing human, may be threatened. Heredity and environment interact. Both may be improved.

drugs and the beleagured baby

Knowledge about the effect of drugs on the unborn child is incomplete. Sensitivity to various drugs and their combinations may be inherited; an entirely new specialty devoted to studying this problem, called *pharmacogenetics,* has been acknowledged as an increasingly important field in medicine and pharmacy. Animal experiments may be inconclusive, as their results do not always apply to humans. The calamitous crippling of thousands of unborn children, in 1961 and 1962, by a German-made tranquilizer containing thalidomide, will long be a mournful reminder of the danger in the use of inadequately tested drugs. How complex such testing can be is illustrated by the facts that people are 60 times more sensitive to thalidomide than mice, 100 times more sensitive to it than rats, 200 times more than dogs, and 700 times more sensitive to the drug than hamsters. Thus, enormous doses, given to several species, might not indicate the danger to the human embryo and fetus.[34] (Nevertheless, despite its initial association with tragedy, thalidomide today shows promise in helping people with an ancient disease; it seems to prevent acute reactions of leprosy patients.) When one considers the real scientific problems that exist in establishing toxicity, the sheer foolhardiness of the abuse of illicit, unmeasured, untested, and grossly impure street-drugs becomes even more apparent.

Whether drugs will affect the unborn child depends on the stage of the child's development. During the first four weeks, the embryo cells undergo extremely rapid proliferation. Food supply and waste elimination are achieved by simple diffusion. Any drug that can diffuse quickly to the rapidly multiplying cells may cause changes that are significant enough to cause loss of the embryo. If this occurs between menstrual periods, the woman does not even know of her pregnancy. Drug action at a more advanced stage (the fifth to the eighth week) can cause abnormal tissue and organ differentiation. There are critical periods in the development of the human embryo in which various structures are being differentiated, and during which some drugs may have the most profoundly deleterious effects. Some of these are: the nervous system, days fifteen to twenty-five; eyes, days twenty-four to forty; heart, days twenty to forty; legs, days twenty-four to thirty-six.[35] By the eighth week of pregnancy, differentiation of these body parts is basically complete. After that, the hazard to the fetus diminishes greatly. It should, however, be understood that some drugs not responsible for immediately apparent effects, nevertheless, may retard growth and development.

Tobacco   Maternal smoking during pregnancy is apparently associated with an increased risk of spontaneous abortion[36] and still-birth.[37] How else does the child born to the woman who smokes during pregnancy compare with the child born to the woman who does not? The chances are greater that he will die during the first

[34] Paul Sampson, "A Warning About Introducing New Teratogens," p. 853.

[35] Bernard L. Mirkin, "Effects of Drugs on the Fetus and Neonate," *Postgraduate Medicine,* Vol. 47, No. 1 (January 1970), pp. 91–95.

[36] J. Frederick, E. D. Alberman, and H. Goldstein, "Possible Teratogenic Effect of Cigarette Smoking," *Nature,* Vol. 231, No. 5304 (June 25, 1971), p. 529, citing C. S. Russell, R. Taylor, and C. E. Law, *British Journal of Preventive Soc. Med.,* Vol. 22, No. 119 (1968). Alton Ochsner, "The Health Menace of Smoking," *American Scientist,* Vol. 59, No. 2 (March–April 1971), p. 250, citing E. Athayde, "Incidencia de abôrtos e mortinatalidade nas operarias da industria de fumo," *Brasil Med.,* Vol. 62 (1948), pp. 237–39; P. Bernhard, "Sinchere Schaden des Zigarettenrauches bei der Frau," *Med. Woch.,* Vol. 104 (1962), pp. 1826–31; C. S. Russell, R. Taylor, and R. N. Maddison, "Some Effects of Smoking in Pregnancy," *J. Obstet. Gynaec. Brit. Comm.,* Vol. 73 (1966), pp. 742–46; and G. S. Hudson and M. P. Rucker, "Spontaneous Abortion," *Journal of the American Medical Association,* Vol. 129 (1945), pp. 542–44.

[37] J. Frederick, E. D. Alberman, H. Goldstein, "Possible Teratogenic Effect of Cigarette Smoking," p. 529, citing N. R. Butler and E. D. Alberman, *Perinatal Problems* (Edinburgh, 1969). Alton Ochsner, "The Health Menace of Smoking," p. 250, citing E. Athayde, "Incidencia de abôrtos e mortinatalidade nas operarias de industria de fumo," pp. 237–39; and C. S. Russell, R. Taylor, and R. N. Maddison, "Some Effects of Smoking in Pregnancy," pp. 742–46.

four weeks of life.[38] The risk increases with women in the lower socioeconomic groups who have had several babies and who are older than thirty-five years of age.[39] His chances of having congenital heart disease are possibly greater.[40] He is more likely to weigh too little.[41] Even at the age of seven, the child whose mother smoked during her pregnancy may be smaller and slightly (four months) retarded in reading ability.[42] His chances of being rated "significantly less well adjusted" at that age are greater than children born to nonsmoking women.[43] Fortunately, reassessment at age eleven shows encouraging results. After a long pull, the child born to the smoking woman usually catches up to his contemporaries, but the cost to both mother and child has been high.[44] As yet incomplete studies suggest that seven-year-old children born to women who smoked during pregnancy were 40 percent more prone to epileptiform convulsions than children of the same age born to nonsmoking women. Whether this persists is now being studied.[45]

Why is the unborn child so adversely affected? Smoking causes a decrease in the blood flow through the placenta, thus decreasing the supply of oxygen and other nutrients to the fetus. Also, it increases the poisonous carbon monoxide content of the placental blood. In addition, the nicotine has a directly detrimental effect on the unborn child.[46]

Some women do not smoke during pregnancy, but begin after their children are born. How do the birth weights of their babies compare with those born of mothers who smoke throughout their pregnancies? Interestingly, a recent statistical study suggests that the incidence of low-weight babies born to "future smokers" is just as high as that of infants born to women who smoked all during their pregnancies.[47] Moreover, the incidence of low-birth-weight infants

---

[38] J. Frederick, E. D. Alberman, and H. Goldstein, "Possible Teratogenic Effect of Cigarette Smoking," p. 529, citing N. R. Butler and E. D. Alberman, *Perinatal Problems.* Alton Ochsner, "The Health Menace of Smoking," p. 250, citing C. R. Russell, R. Taylor, and R. N. Maddison, "Some Effects of Smoking in Pregnancy," p. 250.

[39] Neville Butler, "Seminar on Smoking," *Midwives Chronicle,* Vol. 85, No. 1007 (December 1971), p. 415.

[40] J. Frederick, E. D. Alberman, and H. Goldstein, "Possible Teratogenic Effect of Cigarette Smoking," pp. 529-30.

[41] Ibid., p. 529, citing N. R. Butler and E. D. Alberman, *Perinatal Problems.* "Effect of Smoking on Infant Birth Weight Confirmed," *Ob. Gyn. News,* Vol. 6, No. 23 (December 1, 1971), p. 10.

[42] J. Frederick, E. D. Alberman, and H. Goldstein, *From Birth to Seven* (in press). "More on Smoking in Pregnancy," *Briefs: Footnotes on Maternity Care,* Vol. 34, No. 8 (October 1970), pp. 120-21, citing "Gravida's Smoking Seen Handicap to Offspring," *Ob. Gyn. News,* Vol. 5, No. 12 (June 15, 1970), p. 16.

[43] "More on Smoking in Pregnancy," p. 121.

[44] Ibid.

[45] The work of E. M. Ross as described at the "Third European Symposium on Epilepsy" is cited in "Smoking During Pregnancy is Linked to Convulsions and Fits in Offspring," *Medical Tribune,* Vol. 11, No. 40 (July 20, 1970). The work of Ross is also cited in Alton Ochsner, "The Health Menace of Smoking," p. 250.

[46] Alton Ochsner, "The Health Menace of Smoking," p. 250.

[47] J. Yerushalmy, "Infants with Low Birth Weight Born Before Their Mothers Started to Smoke Cigarettes," *American Journal of Obstetrics and Gynecology,* Vol. 112, No. 2 (January 15, 1972), p. 277.

born to both categories of smokers was significantly higher than the incidence of low-birth-weight infants born to women who never smoked. Thus, the differences in the incidence of low-birth-weight infants may be due to the individual rather than to smoking. Further studies in this area are being conducted.

Cannabis   Marijuana may be a hazard to the unborn child. Studies with animals have shown that the active principle of marijuana, tetrahydrocannabinol, does cross the placenta. It may concentrate in the fetus in sizeable amounts.[48] The effect on the fetus is not yet known. This has a special meaning for the pregnant woman.

LSD   Does LSD harm the fetus? In 1971, much of the pertinent scientific literature relating to this question was reviewed by several California workers. They examined sixty-eight studies and case reports that had been published over a period of four years. They concluded that "from our work, and from a review of the literature, we believe that pure LSD ingested in moderate doses does not damage chromosomes in vivo [within the living body], does not cause detectable genetic damage, and is not a teratogen or a carcinogen in man."[49] (A *teratogen* is an agent or factor that causes physical defects in the developing embryo. A *carcinogen* is a cancer-causing agent.)

They also noted that "in a study of human pregnancies, those exposed to illicit [probably impure] LSD had an elevated rate of spontaneous abortions."[50] These investigators, therefore, suggested that "other than during pregnancy, there is no present contraindication to the continued controlled experimental use of pure LSD."[51] They further noted that a review of fifteen other studies had revealed conclusions similar to their own.[52]

Opiates (heroin)   There has been much concern about the heroin dependency of the very young in this culture; the youngest of all are the newborns whose mothers are heroin dependents. In 1970, New

---

[48]"Marihuana and Health," Second Annual Report to Congress of the Secretary of Health, Education, and Welfare (Washington, D.C., 1972), p. 173, citing R. I. Freudenthal, J. Martin, and M. E. Wall, "The Distribution of Delta-9-Tetrahydrocannabinol in the Mouse," *Journal of Pharmacy and Pharmacology* (1972); R. D. Harbison, "Maternal Distribution and Placental Transfer of C^{14} Delta-9-Tetrahydrocannabinol in Pregnant Mice," *Journal of Pharmacology and Experimental Therapeutics* (1972); and J. Idanpaan-Heikkila, G. D. Fritchie, L. F. Englert, B. T. Ho, and W. M. McIsaac, "Placental Transfer of Tritriated (1) Delta-9-Tetrahydrocannabinol," *New England Journal of Medicine,* Vol. 281 (1969), p. 330.

[49]Normal J. Dishotsky, William L. Loughman, Robert E. Mogar, and Wendell R. Lipscomb, "LSD and Genetic Damage," *Science,* Vol. 172, No. 3982 (April 30, 1971), p. 439.

[50]Ibid.

[51]Ibid., citing William H. McGlothlin, Robert S. Sparkes, and David O. Arnold, "Effects of LSD on Human Pregnancy," *Journal of the American Medical Association,* Vol. 212, No. 9 (June 1, 1970), pp. 1483–91.

[52]Ibid., citing B. K. Houston, "Review of the Evidence and the Qualifications Regarding Effects of Hallucinogenic Drugs on Chromosomes and Embryos," *American Journal of Psychiatry,* Vol. 126, No. 2 (August 1969), p. 251.

York City municipal hospitals reported 489 instances of children born with heroin dependence due to the drug use of the pregnant mothers. In 1971, the number rose to 706.[53] In addition, numerous heroin-dependent babies are born in private hospitals; their condition is not reported. The peculiar high-pitched cry and the intense irritability of the heroin-dependent newborn are danger signals to every experienced physician; prompt treatment is necessary to save the child's life. "Worse still, many of these babies will grow up to be addicts—although they are detoxified before they leave the hospital—because they are brought up in 'addict households'," says William Papenty, administrator of the family disease and maternity department at Kings County Hospital Center in Brooklyn. "In a family, it's very contagious. We're seeing third- and fourth-generation addicts now."[54]

THE EXTENT OF BIRTH DEFECTS

More babies die of defective development before they are born than after. Such defective embryos account for most of the million miscarriages in this country every year. Most occur early in pregnancy—the period of greatest vulnerability of the developing child. Some miscarriages occur so early that the woman may never have known she was pregnant. Others occur after a few months. "Many [of such deaths] are nature's way of getting rid of an abnormally developing fetus in order that a new and better one can be started."[55] Of every sixteen babies born alive in this country, one is found to be defective within the first year. (Some birth defects, such as gout and diabetes, may not be apparent for years.) This amounts to about a quarter of a million babies a year. Eighteen thousand of these die in the first year of life.

> *It may be estimated conservatively that 15 million persons in the United States have one or more congenital defects which affect their daily lives. Included are an estimated 4 million with clinical diabetes, 2,900,000 with mental retardation of prenatal origin, 1 million with congenital orthopedic impairments, 500,000 who were born blind or with serious loss of vision, 750,000 with congenital hearing impairment, at least 350,000 with congenital heart disease, and more than 100,000 with speech defects of prenatal origin.*[56]

[53] "Heroin-Addicts Estimates Soar," *Medical World News*, Vol. 13, No. 7 (February 18, 1972), p. 20.
[54] Ibid.
[55] Edith L. Potter, "Defective Babies Who Die Before Birth," in Morris Fishbein, ed., *Birth Defects* (Philadelphia, 1963), p. 46.
[56] V. Apgar and G. Stickle, "Birth Defects: Their Significance as a Public Health Problem," *Journal of the American Medical Association*, Vol. 204, No. 5 (April 29, 1968), pp. 79–82.

As the population grows, the number of babies born with birth defects increases. Moreover, modern surgery, newer drugs, and more research combine to keep many defective children alive to adolescence and maturity. Though this kind of effort will always be a basic purpose of medicine, such survival, nevertheless, means problems.

For too long birth defects have been associated with stigma and superstition. "If a woman gives birth, and the abdomen of the child is open, there will be a dwindling of the suburbs." So predicts an ancient Babylonian tablet. Greek mythology makes frequent reference to half-human, half-animal centaurs and minotaurs. Believing fertility between species to be possible, and birth defect the result, many Greeks were contemptuous of malformed children. In early Judeo-Christian cultures, the parents of defective children were ostracized. Even today, the word *harelip* is used. Mothers of such children were once thought to have been frightened by a rabbit. But modern science has brought mankind a long way from such ignorance.

how to avoid some birth defects

1. A physician should be seen as soon as pregnancy is suspected because (a) the baby is most vulnerable during early pregnancy (the first twenty weeks), and (b) delay increases the chances of premature birth and a defective child.

2. No medication, not even vitamins, should be taken unless prescribed by the family doctor. Drugs may pass through the placenta and the child may be injured (see also the discussion of drugs above, pages 172-76).

3. Except in emergencies, abdominal X-rays early in pregnancy should be avoided. Any physician about to X-ray a female patient, therefore, will want to know if she is pregnant.

4. Cigarette smoking should be discontinued. At the very least, excessive cigarette smoking must be avoided. Recent studies show that nicotine injected into a pregnant monkey swiftly crossed the placental barrier. In the monkey fetus the nicotine level declined slowly. Both the heart rate and blood pressure of the monkey fetus were depressed. Potentially harmful disturbances in the unborn monkey's acid-base state and oxygen supply were noted[57] (see also the discussion of drugs above, pages 172-76).

5. If possible, elective surgery should be delayed until after pregnancy. Abrupt changes to high altitudes should be avoided. In both instances, even temporary oxygen depletion might injure the embryo. In commercial airliners this is not ordinarily a problem.

[57] Karlis Adamsons et al., "Effects of Nicotine on the Unborn," cited in *Briefs: Footnotes on Maternity Care,* Vol. 33, No. 7 (September 1969), pp. 99-100.

TABLE 5-5 the more common birth defects

TYPE OF DEFECT	APPROXIMATE FREQUENCY	DESCRIPTION	CAUSES AND TREATMENT
Birthmarks	Very common.	The disfiguring ones are red or wine-colored patches of small dilated blood vessels.	Cause unknown. Treatments include plastic surgery, skin grafts, or tattooing of normal skin colors over the purple area.
Cleft lip (harelip)	About 1 in 1,000 babies born in the U.S. has a cleft lip; two-thirds of these also have cleft palate. Frequency seems lower in blacks than in whites.	If embryonic swellings that will become the upper lip do not fuse at the right time, the gap remains and the baby will have a cleft lip.	Sometimes related to genetic defects. Influence of intrauterine environment and of some drugs given during pregnancy are being studied. Harelip can be repaired in the first few weeks after birth, and cleft palate before age fourteen months in most cases.
Cleft palate	About 1 in every 2,500 babies has a cleft palate without cleft lip. The two conditions are not genetically related.	A cleft palate is a hole in the roof of the mouth.	
Clubfoot	1 in 300.	The foot turns inward (usually) or outward and is fixed in a tip-toe position.	Possibly due to position of child in uterus or to maldevelopment of the limb bud. Treatments include shoe splints, braces, corrective shoes, plaster casts, or surgery. Tends to recur, so treatment must begin early and is often prolonged.
Congenital heart disease	1 in 125.	Some are so slight as to cause little strain on the heart; others are fatal. In some abnormalities, the baby appears blue.	German measles during pregnancy is one cause. Many heart conditions can now be repaired by surgery, saving lives and preventing invalidism.
Congenital urinary tract defects	1 in 250.	May involve kidneys, ureters, bladder, and genitalia. Organs may be absent, fused, or obstructed.	Causes include certain hormones given during pregnancy. Some hereditary tendency. Most conditions are correctable by surgery.

Table 5-5 Continued

TYPE OF DEFECT	APPROXIMATE FREQUENCY	DESCRIPTION	CAUSES AND TREATMENT
Diabetes	The prevalence of diabetes increases with advancing age, varying from about 1 case per 625 persons under age 25 to 1 in 15 persons age 65 to 75.	A metabolic disorder. The body cannot handle sugar normally, and high glucose levels in the blood and urine result. This familial condition is related in some unknown way to abnormal utilization of insulin. Long-standing diabetics may develop complications involving blood vessels, kidneys, heart, eyes, and peripheral nerves. Obesity predisposes individuals to the disease.	Marked hereditary tendency. Persons with family history of diabetes should seek periodic check-up. Doctors can recognize symptoms, make positive diagnosis, and prescribe specific treatment. Special diets, oral medication, and injections of insulin are measures that will usually keep condition under control and permit normal activity. Good prenatal care is especially important for known or suspected diabetics.
Erythroblastosis fetalis (see also pages 169–71)	Prior to use of Rh immune globulin, hemolytic disease of the fetus and newborn occurred in 1 in every 150 to 200 pregnancies. About 15 percent of whites and 5 percent of blacks in the United States are Rh negative.	Without Rh immune globulin—and among infants of mothers sensitized during previous deliveries—baby is often yellow soon after birth. Anemia is a common symptom. Mental retardation may be severe. Erythroblastosis is a common cause of stillbirth.	Baby inherits Rh-positive gene from his father, and the mother is Rh negative. Red blood cells of fetus reach mother's blood, causing her blood to form antibodies that pass back through the placenta to the baby and destroy his red cells in varying degrees. First pregnancy is usually uneventful. Rh immune globulin prevents sensitization of mother, if given soon after birth of each baby. Intrauterine or exchange transfusion, replacing baby's blood with compatible blood right after birth, prevents severe damage to babies of sensitized mothers.
Extra fingers and toes (polydactyly)	Extra digits are twice as frequent as fused digits. Incidence is 1 in 100 among blacks; 1 in 600 among whites.	Extra fingers or toes.	Cause unknown; frequently hereditary. Cure is amputation of the extra digits. This can often be done at birth or at about age three.
Fused fingers and toes (syndactyly)	Fused digits do not have such racial variation.	Too few digits.	Surgery can improve the function and appearance of the hand or foot.

Table 5-5 Continued

TYPE OF DEFECT	APPROXIMATE FREQUENCY	DESCRIPTION	CAUSES AND TREATMENT
Fibrocystic disease (cystic fibrosis)	About 1 in 1,000 births. Rare among blacks; infrequent in Orientals.	A sickly, malnourished child with persistent intestinal difficulties and chronic respiratory problems. Death usually due to pneumonia or other lung complications.	Hereditary. New tests detect carriers. Mucus blocks the exit of digestive juices from the pancreas into the intestinal tract. Excess mucus is also secreted by lungs. Treatments have extended life.
Galactosemia	Somewhat more rare than PKU (see below).	Causes eye cataracts and severe damage to liver and brain, resulting in mental retardation.	Hereditary. Caused by absence of an enzyme required to convert galactose to glucose. Experiments show that early recognition and dietary treatment can arrest the disease. Diagnosis can be made at birth.
Hydrocephaly (water on the brain)	1 in 500.	Enlargement of the head due to excessive fluid within the brain. Fluid's pressure often causes compression of the brain with resulting mental retardation.	Cause unknown. May result from prenatal infection or abnormality in development. Treatment is an operation to lead fluid from brain into blood stream or some other body cavity. Frequently fatal if not treated.
Missing limbs	Very rare.	One to four limbs missing or seriously deformed.	Cause unknown. A recent international outbreak was due to thalidomide used by pregnant mothers. Great strides have been made in prosthetic (artificial) devices.
Mongolism (Down's syndrome; see also page 153)	1 in 600. Women twenty-five years old have about 1 chance in 2,000 of producing a Mongoloid child. Women of forty-five have about 1 chance in 50.	Short stature, slightly slanted eyes, and varying degrees of mental retardation.	All patients have an extra chromosome or its equivalent. Causes can be hereditary or environmental. No known cure, but IQ can be improved by special training.

Table 5-5 Continued

TYPE OF DEFECT	APPROXIMATE FREQUENCY	DESCRIPTION	CAUSES AND TREATMENT
Open spine (spina bifida)	Approximately 1 in every 500 births. More common among whites than blacks. About half of the patients are also victims of hydrocephaly (see above).	Failure of the spine to close permits the protrusion of spinal cord or nerves; often leads to total dysfunction of legs, bladder, and rectum. Often the child has other serious defects.	Cause unknown. Sometimes surgery in the early months of life can correct or arrest the condition, preventing other complications. Several new surgical techniques are being used on the bladder, rectum, and spinal cord.
Phenylketonuria (PKU)	Approximately 1 in 20,000 whites. Extremely rare in blacks.	Child appears normal at birth, but his mind stops developing during the first year. Retardation is severe. One-third never learn to walk; two-thirds never learn to talk. Pigment of skin and hair is decreased.	Hereditary metabolic defect. The liver enzyme that changes the protein phenylalanine to tyrosine is inactive or absent; phenylalanine accumulates. PKU can be detected within the first few days of life. Treatment is special low-phenylalanine diet for the infant, which can prevent further retardation. Early treatment important. Some experiments show that after a few years PKU children can be fed normal diets.
Sickle cell anemia	One in 10 American blacks has trait; one in 400 has anemia. Low among whites.	Red blood cells of people with this disease periodically become crescent or sickle-shaped, clump together, and prevent transport of needed oxygen to body organs, causing painful sickle cell "crises."	Hereditary. When both parents have the trait, each child has 1 chance in 4 of inheriting sickle cell anemia. Careful management can help prevent crises; research to develop medications is promising.

Source: Adapted from a booklet published by The National Foundation–March of Dimes, White Plains, New York.

6. An adequate diet must be followed.

7. Relatives should never marry. Even rare hereditary disorders occur much more commonly among the children of such unions. Except in Georgia, state laws forbid a person from marrying a parent, grandparent, child, or grandchild. In Georgia a man may marry his daughter or grandmother. Generally, marriages between persons with a relatedness equivalent to first cousins or closer are not legally sanctioned.[58]

8. Many physicians feel that the relationship between the older mother and the occurrence of Mongolism (and a few other rarer abnormalities) should never alone deter childbearing.

9. Under some circumstances, the advice of a genetic counselor is indicated. The family physician will know if such help is necessary.

SOME INTERESTING RELATIONSHIPS

Is there any relationship between survival of a fetus and a child and the spacing of pregnancies? What, if any, are the relationships between fetal and child survivals and the age of parents? In attempting to find answers to these questions, Richard L. Day[59] surveyed the statistical literature. Although his findings by no means necessarily apply to individual cases, they are nonetheless of significance.

1. The ideal age for maternity seemed to be between the ages of twenty and thirty.

2. An interval of about two years between the end of one pregnancy and the beginning of another was associated with the lowest incidence of late fetal and newborn (up to one month of age) mortality as well as prematurity. Since prematurely born babies have a higher mortality than those born with a normal weight, this finding takes on added significance.

3. If pregnancy intervals are three years or more, survival through childhood is statistically more likely.

4. If the mother is over thirty-five, the first-born is more likely to be a stillbirth than if she is younger. On the other hand, the very young mother also shows a higher rate of stillborn babies. Very young mothers present special problems, as was noted earlier.

5. Children of small families grow taller and weigh more than children of large families.

6. It is the young mother, who has already had at least one child and whose baby is at greatest risk from preventable conditions, who is apparently most likely to profit from medical care (including contraceptive advice). Special efforts to improve her health, particu-

[58] Michael G. Farrow and Richard C. Juberg, "Genetics and Laws Prohibiting Marriage in the United States," *Journal of the American Medical Association*, Vol. 209, No. 4 (July 28, 1969), p. 534.
[59] Richard L. Day, "Factors Influencing Offspring," *American Journal of Diseases of Children*, Vol. 113, No. 2 (February 1967), pp. 179–85.

larly if she is poor, would result in a great improvement in statistics that are used to describe the outcome of pregnancy.

7. An older father, regardless of the age of his wife, is statistically more likely to beget a stillborn child than a younger father.

8. Certain birth defects seem to occur more frequently in children with older parents than in those whose parents are young.

GENETIC COUNSELING

Second cousins want to marry. They share three diabetic parents. What are the genetic dangers? A couple have a second child that is Mongoloid. Can they hope for a normal child? A young man's sister has been incapacitated for ten years with severe muscular dystrophy. He is engaged and deeply troubled. An agency brings a pretty child, the product of an incestuous union. What are the risks to adopting parents? Parents bring their baby. They have been putting it off, but something is wrong. Their family doctor has suggested that they come here.

Such are some of the intensely human problems brought to the genetic counselor. He can help as no one else can. He may discuss risks with those who inquire. In the event a diagnosis of a possible genetic illness is required, more detailed work is necessary. *The International Directory of Genetic Services,* 3rd ed. (September 1971), compiled by Henry T. Lynch, has been published by the National Foundation. It is of great professional value.

At this point, it would be well to differentiate between two frequently confused terms. The word *congenital* does not have the same meaning as *genetic. Congenital* means only "present at birth." It does not signify the cause of a condition. Some congenital conditions are not genetic, and many genetic conditions are not congenital. Huntington's chorea is an illness marked by irregular movements, speech disturbances, and mental deterioration. Although a genetic disease, it is not manifested until adulthood. However, maternal infection with German measles (rubella) virus in the first trimester of pregnancy may result in the infection of the unborn child. The child may then manifest the congenital rubella syndrome.

The mere fact that an illness occurs in more than one member of a family is not necessarily an indication that it is hereditary. Family members often share similar environments and habits; more likely, a combination of environment and genetic predisposition is responsible. During a person's first visit to a geneticist (who is usually, but not necessarily, a physician), a complete family history is taken. In order to obtain a complete family history, more than one family member may have to be interviewed. The geneticist must obtain information about both the paternal and maternal grandparents, parents, siblings, uncles, aunts, and first cousins. Miscarriages, stillbirths, and infant deaths are carefully noted. The inquiry may, but usually does not, extend beyond the first cousins.

From the history the geneticist constructs a *pedigree chart.* Blood samples provide cells for study. These are taken from the patient, both parents, and other relatives likely to be carrying the abnormality. Other procedures besides blood studies are helpful. A few cells scraped from the inside of a patient's mouth can help determine the number of X-chromosomes a patient has. Normal females have a dark area called the *Barr body* in these cells. It is absent in the male. The greatest number of Barr bodies in a buccal cell equals the number of patient's X-chromosomes minus one. Thus abnormal females with no Barr body have only one X-chromosome and abnormal XXY males have one Barr body. Since bone marrow provides most of the circulating blood cells, it also may provide much valuable information.

genetic disorders: the hope in research

It was not until 1956 that scientists discovered that the normal human cell contained forty-six (and not forty-eight) chromosomes. Since then, a whole new era in genetic counseling has taken place. Among the most significant advances have been in three major areas. One has to do with the ability to grow cells in culture and to fuse together cells of different origins. The second involves magnificent new staining techniques that reveal hitherto unknown facts about the chromosomes of mankind. The third is a procedure known as *amniocentesis,* in which the amniotic fluid (see page 193), in which the fetus floats, is withdrawn; both the fluid and the cells within it that are shed by the fetus can reveal the age, sex, some genetic defects, and other valuable information about the unborn child. Many of these discoveries have come to fruition within the past few years.

Man-mouse cell hybrids   For over half a century scientists have been able to grow cells in culture. Live cells are placed in a container of specially prepared "soup." There they are nourished and multiply. As waste collects some of the cellular growth is transferred to another container of fresh nourishment. These transferred cells multiply in turn. Another transfer is made and still another. In this way chicken heart cells were kept functioning for more than thirty years. Other cells derived from various tissues have grown in culture, outside and independent of the organism of their origin, for sixty years. In all that time they lost neither vitality nor reproductive power. Some years ago, cancer cells from a patient's uterine cervix were obtained and, by transfer, repeatedly cultured. Tons of cells, originating from this one person's original cervical cancer cells, have been distributed to virus laboratories throughout the world. (Viruses are grown in them for a variety of technical purposes.)

Laboratory-cultured cells are a basic genetic tool. Long before the microscope was invented, medieval scientists imagined that each human sperm contained a whole, but tiny, person who was just waiting to grow big enough to be born. Today, it is known that each normal body (somatic) cell contains a full set of inherited chromosomes. Thus, the existing genetic differences between entire organisms can be studied from cultured cells gained from those different organisms. When human beings mate, a genetic event takes place. Scientists now know how to mate cells. Such cell fusion was first accomplished between living mouse cells. A third new cell type arose from the fusion; it contained a total number of chromosomes equal to the sum of the chromosomes of the parent cells. Such a cell is called a "hybrid cell"—a hybrid being an animal or plant produced from parents different in kind, such as parents belonging to a different species. In 1967, scientists reported the successful fusion of human and mouse cells. A human-mouse hybrid cell had been obtained. For a public, long fed a scary diet of mad scientists in monster movies, this was alarming news. To the geneticist interested in studying chromosomes to prevent untold human suffering, it was a landmark achievement.

Why? Suppose a human being has a genetic illness. Is it due to the lack of an enzyme the presence of which is normally dependent on a certain gene? Cells of the individual lacking the gene can be grown outside the body in a culture medium. They can then be taken from the culture and mated (hybridized) with cells of a mouse that do not contain that gene. The hybrid cells are then grown in culture. As the hybrid human-mouse cells go through mitosis they lose human chromosomes. Human chromosomes seem to be eliminated preferentially. Finally the hybrid cells stabilize; they lose no more human chromosomes. If one human chromosome is retained in the cells of the final hybrid cell culture, then one may regard that entire stabilized culture as a mouse cell culture with one human chromosome. That one human chromosome can be identified. Then the geneticist can test the cell culture for the missing enzyme. If it is not present in the mouse cells, and is, indeed, absent in the entire culture, then one can point to the possible failure of the single human chromosome in the culture in making the critical enzyme. This procedure can be carried out in a variety of ways. Does cell hybridization have practical use today? Not yet. Then why is it being carried out and perfected? For the answer to this question one may refer to the reply of Louis Pasteur when, a century ago, he was asked if certain of his experiments had any practical value.

"No," replied the great bacteriologist.

"Then of what use is it?"

"Of what use is a newborn baby?" was the reply.

Staining for chromosomal stripes   The elucidation of the human karyotype (see page 158) spurred the study of both normal and abnormal chromosomes. Many genetic conditions became better understood. It was demonstrated that some genetic diseases were due to an additional chromosome, for example, the Klinefelter's (see pages 154-55) and XYY syndromes (see pages 155-56). In addition, it was found that a chromosomal deficit accounted for some genetic disorders; among these were most cases of Turner's syndrome (see page 154). However, as has been pointed out, there are more subtle errors of the human karyotype that can result in serious illness. These include small deletions and translocations (see page 152) of one portion of a chromosome to another. Until very recently, classification of these disorders was very difficult because the geneticist was unable to consistently identify each chromosome of the normal human karyotype. He was forced to base his identifications on the relative size of the chromosomes and on the position of the clear region where the arms of the chromosome meet (*centromere*).

Now that has changed. Today, newly developed staining techniques permit the accurate identification of every chromosome in the human karyotype. Fluorescing compounds have been discovered that bind to chromosomal DNA. (A fluorescent substance has the property of emitting light after exposure to light.) When treated with the fluorescent substance and placed under a special fluorescent microscope, chromosomes are seen to have a banded appearance; it is as if they had stripes. Certain bands exhibit more fluorescence than others, and the pattern of banding is specific for each chromosome. In addition, not only are the banding patterns characteristic for each pair of the twenty-two autosomes, and for the X- and Y-chromosomes as well, but they are also consistent from cell to cell and from person to person. Thus, in its middle phase of mitosis (metaphase), each chromosome can be identified by its distinctive pattern of fluorescence. The production of bands at specific locations, by bringing out unique chromosomal patterns, will help identify structurally abnormal chromosomes, determine their origins, and provide a means of earlier and more accurate identification of abnormalities. Easy identification of subtle changes, such as extra or missing chromosomal segments, is now feasible. But the banding technique promises to do more. It provides another tool for the gigantic task of "mapping" human chromosomes. The goal of mapping chromosomes is to locate each gene in relation to others and to determine which of the twenty-three pairs of chromosomes carries it. When one considers the many thousands of genes in each chromosome and the significance of each, the size of the task becomes more apparent. But it will be worth the labor. For among the many future possible benefits of chromosome mapping will be the possibility of earlier diagnosis and treatment of genetic disease.

Diagnosis of the unborn   Amniocentesis is a procedure in which a needle is inserted through the walls of both the abdomen and the pregnant uterus in order to withdraw amniotic fluid (see page 193) and the cells suspended in it, for examination. As pregnancy advances, the amniotic fluid becomes a rich source of information about the unborn child. Enzymes, amino acids, and a variety of other normal and abnormal products may be added to the fluid as a result of the child's excretion of urine. Among the sources of cells in the amniotic fluid may be the amnion itself, the fetal skin, urine, trachea (windpipe), bronchi, and the lining of the gastrointestinal system. Cells from the fluid proliferate in cell culture. Examination of connective tissue cells from cultured cells of the amniotic fluid can then be examined for chromosomal abnormalities. The cells may also be studied for enzyme activity, or the presence (or absence) of various substances.[60]

Thus, the amniotic fluid is useful for diagnosing and possibly preventing a variety of conditions. In a test that requires only an hour of laboratory work, the amniotic fluid, drawn after the thirty-fourth week of pregnancy, can be tested for the maturity of the lungs of the fetus. In this way the physician can determine the likelihood of a serious condition called the respiratory syndrome of the newborn.[61] After the twentieth week of pregnancy, the cells of amniotic fluid may be tested for Rh blood disease (erythroblastosis fetalis, see pages 169–71). The cells of the amniotic fluid inform the geneticists of the genetic sex of the fetus,[62] while both the fluid and the cells within it are useful in determining the age of the unborn child.[63] In addition, amniocentesis provides a valuable procedure for the diagnosis of a considerable number of genetic disorders. Before the fourteenth week of pregnancy the amount of amniotic fluid is small; thus, amniocentesis before the fifteenth week of pregnancy increases the risk of damage to the mother or child. But the diagnosis of serious genetic disorders is a race against time. If abortion is to be contemplated, it must be done as early as possible. To diagnose genetic disorders, amniocentesis is performed at about the fifteenth week of pregnancy.

Amniocentesis has been performed thousands of times. Although in the hands of a trained operator the risk is slight, it is never done unless absolutely necessary. Amniocentesis for the determination of genetic sex, for example, is never done to satisfy parental curiosity about whether their child will be a boy or a girl. It may be done so that a woman who is a carrier of an X-linked disorder can elect to

[60] "Diagnostic Amniocentesis," *Medical Letter on Drugs and Therapeutics,* Vol. 14, No. 15, Issue 353 (July 21, 1972), p. 53.

[61] "Prenatal Test Developed for Respiratory Distress," *Journal of the American Medical Association,* Vol. 220, No. 12 (June 19, 1972), p. 5.

[62] M. E. Ferguson-Smith, M. A. Ferguson-Smith, N. C. Nevin, and M. Stone, "Chromosome Analysis Before Birth and Its Value in Genetic Counselling," *British Medical Journal,* Vol. 4, No. 5779 (October 9, 1971), p. 69; and Melvin Gertner, Lillian Y. F. Hsu, Joan Martin, and Kurt Hirschhorn, "The Use of Amniocentesis for Prenatal Genetic Counselling," *Bulletin of the New York Academy of Medicine,* Second Series, Vol. 46, No. 11 (November 1970), p. 916.

[63] "Assessment of Gestational Age from Amniotic Fluid," *Lancet,* Vol. 1, No. 7742 (January 15, 1972), pp. 132–33.

permit abortion of a male fetus. Such a woman will transmit the X-linked disorder to only one-half of her sons. Should an abortion be done, a normal as well as an abnormal male fetus could be sacrificed.[64] Unfortunately, the more common X-linked disorders, such as hemophilia, still cannot be diagnosed before birth.

The same is true of genetic disorders that result in abnormal body metabolism. The diagnosis of cystic fibrosis, for example, the greatest killer of white children, cannot be diagnosed before birth. This difficult disease affects the sweat glands and those ductal glands that empty into organs leading to the outside of the body. The clear, usable fluid usually produced by these glands is replaced, in cystic fibrosis, with a sticky, thick material. Widespread clogging of the ducts leads to a host of dangerous symptoms. Nor is sickle cell anemia (see pages 161–63) yet among the metabolic genetic disorders that can be diagnosed by amniocentesis. (Recent studies, however, suggest that a blood sample obtained from the placenta may provide the material necessary to diagnose this condition, which afflicts and kills so many thousands of black children every year.)[65] An important metabolic genetic disorder that can be diagnosed by amniocentesis is Tay-Sachs Disease. This tragic condition, characterized by blindness and severe mental retardation, can be diagnosed as early as the sixteenth week by the detection of the absence of an enzyme. It is most commonly found among this country's Ashkenazi Jews, that is, those Jews who originally settled in northern and central Europe (as distinguished from the Sephardic Jews, who settled in Spain and Portugal). Preliminary results of a recent survey suggest that one of twenty-five U.S. Jews may be a carrier of Tay-Sachs Disease.[66]

The most common chromosomal aberration that can be detected by amniocentesis is that causing Down's syndrome (Mongolism, see page 153). The frequency of this disorder increases with the mother's age; between ages thirty-five and thirty-nine, the risk is about 1 in 300; between forty and forty-four, 1 in 100; the risk is 1 in 40 at age forty-five or older. Although only 13 percent of all pregnancies occur in women over thirty-five years old, over one-half of all Mongoloid children are born to women in this age group. Aside from the suffering and the anxiety that amniocentesis may avert, it is well to mention the economic benefits. About four thousand children with Down's syndrome are born in this country every year. Institutional care for each child that is placed costs about $250,000.00.[67]

[64] "Diagnostic Amniocentesis," pp. 53–54.
[65] Yuet Wai Kan, Andrée M. Dozy, Blanche P. Alter, Frederic D. Frigoletto, and David G. Nathan, "Detection of the Sickle-Cell Gene in the Human Fetus," *New England Journal of Medicine,* Vol. 287, No. 1 (July 6, 1972), pp. 1–5; see also in the same issue Haig H. Kazazian, Jr., "Antenatal Detection of Sickle-Cell Anemia," pp. 41–42.
[66] "Estimates of Tay-Sachs Gene Carriers May Be Low," *Journal of the American Medical Association,* Vol. 220, No. 7 (May 15, 1972), p. 915.
[67] Gerald H. Prescott, R. Ellen Magenis, Neil R. M. Buist, "Amniocentesis for Antenatal Diagnosis," *Postgraduate Medicine,* Vol. 51, No. 3 (March 1972), pp. 216–17.

Even with the best care, the possibility of a miscarriage always exists. One study of fifty women who lost their babies at or shortly after birth showed that they exhibited typical grief reactions.[68] None, however, developed severe emotional problems. Data as to the development of sexual problems as a result of suffering a miscarriage are unavailable. Several interviews with the family physician or another professional person can help resolve the grief of a miscarriage and, hopefully, bring the couple closer together.

[68] John R. Wolff, "Emotional Aftermath of Miscarriage," *Medical Aspects of Human Sexuality,* Vol. 5, No. 12 (December 1971), p. 103, citing R. Wolff, P. Nielson, and P. Schiller, "The Emotional Reaction to a Stillbirth," *American Journal of Obstetrics and Gynecology,* Vol. 108 (1970), p. 43.

on continuing the human beginning

6

pregnancy

The ovum is one of the body's largest cells; the sperm, the smallest. Alone, they are just potential. Together, they can fuse, and the product of their fusion can multiply to form a creature that can wonder. But even in the earliest phases this product is already remarkable. "Every child starts as an invisible unit with a weight of only $5/1000$ of a milligram and gains during the first weeks of life more than a million percent in weight. Which industry, whatever direction or planning boards there may be, can claim such an increase in output?"[1]

THE DURATION OF A PREGNANCY

Counting from the time of fertilization of the egg by the sperm (*conception*), the duration of the pregnancy is $9\frac{1}{2}$ lunar months (38 weeks or 266 days). A "lunar" month is 28 days because there is a full moon every 28 days. Counting from the first day of the last menstrual period, the average pregnancy lasts 10 lunar months (40 weeks or 280 days).

In calculating the expected date of confinement (birth), three months are subtracted from the date of the beginning of the last normal menstrual period. Then seven days are added. For example, if the first day of the last normal period was June 17, the expected date of confinement would be March 24.

But these calculations are only based on averages. Perhaps 10 percent of all pregnancies end 280 days after the beginning of the last menstrual period; less than 50 percent end within one week of the 280th day. The time required for the fetus in the uterus is individual. Extreme but normal variances of 240 days to 300 days in the uterus occur. The calculated expected date of confinement is

[1]G. M. H. Veeneklass, cited in *Physicians Bulletin,* Vol. 24, No. 8 (November 15, 1959), p. B/8.

not often exact. There is less than a 50 percent chance that the child will be born within a week of that date and a 10 percent chance that labor will occur about two weeks later.

THE CHILD WITHIN THE UTERUS

Before pregnancy the uterus weighs one ounce. At the end of pregnancy, the empty uterus weighs 2.2 pounds and its capacity has increased more than 500 times. (A short time after delivery, it returns to almost its original size.) The remarkable events occurring during the development of the child in the uterus are described in the science of *embryology*—the story of a new individual.

The new individual is the zygote—the fertilized egg. It is unique and no larger than the tiniest sand speck. It does not wait long in the uterine tube. While on its two- to four-day, four- to five-inch journey to the uterus, the zygote cleaves daily. When it arrives the uterus is not yet ready for it. About two to four more days pass as the small, continuously multiplying cell mass floats in the uterus. Meanwhile, as described in Chapter 2, the uterine lining continues to prepare for it. At last, as early as day eighteen and as late as day twenty-three of the menstrual cycle and as much as eight days following fertilization, implantation occurs.[2]

When implantation occurs, the cellular mass (*blastocyst*) is a fluid-filled sphere of cells. Cell multiplication continues until, on the internal surface of the blastocyst, a layer of cells separates; this is the *endoderm*. It will contribute heavily to such inner body parts as the digestive and respiratory systems. Cells of the outer layer also multiply. These comprise the *ectoderm* destined for outer structures such as the skin, hair, and nervous tissue. A middle layer of cells multiplies to push in between ectoderm and endoderm. This intermediate *mesoderm* will be muscle and bone, marrow and blood, kidney and gonad. These three layers will further differentiate to become the organized human creature. After the first week of development following fertilization, the cell mass is called an *embryo;* the youngest human embryo is about seven-and-one-half days old. Not until the beginning of the third month will the embryo be a *fetus*.

the firm establishment of the new life

But not all of the fertilized egg becomes an embryo. Some is destined to be auxiliary embryonic equipment that will not only protect the embryo but will also provide a means of nourishment, excretion, and respiration. Even in the blastocyst two cell masses differentiate: the

[2] The American College of Obstetricians and Gynecology considers implantation and conception to be synonymous. The reason for this is that implantation cannot be diagnosed unless conception has occurred.

inner cell mass, which is to become the embryo, and an outer cellular wall, the *trophoblast,* which is the beginning of the auxiliary tissue. (Later in pregnancy the trophoblast is called the *chorion.*) The cells of the trophoblast have the ability to digest or dissolve both the wall of the uterine endometrial lining and the walls of small blood vessels in that area. The multiplying and digesting cells of the trophoblast extend into the endometrium and around them occur slight uterine bleedings. From the little lakes of mother's blood seepages of nutriments feed the growing cellular mass. Via these early maternal blood lakes, then, the mother offers the first food to the parasitic cell mass imbedded in the lining of the uterus. Then the inner layer of the trophoblast grows out to push fingerlike projections into the endometrium. These are the *villi;* their encroaching cells continue to digest the cells of uterine endometrium and small adjacent blood vessels.

Some villi extend not only into the endometrium but also into the maternal lakes in which they float free. Soon the maternal lakes are so crowded by villi that there are now only *intervillous spaces.* It is primarily in these intervillous spaces that the physiological exchanges occur between mother and child during pregnancy. Each mature villus eventually contains fetal blood vessels connected with the circulation of the child.

By a month after fertilization, the inner cell mass that is the embryo is encircled by a *chorionic membrane* and this membrane is surrounded by *chorionic villi.* A fluid-filled sac, or vesicle, has been created. The embryo is attached to the wall of this *chorionic vesicle* by a *body stalk,* which will elongate to become a cable containing blood vessels, the *umbilical cord.* As the last part of the second month of pregnancy approaches, many of the villi on the surface of the chorionic membrane begin to degenerate. Only about 20 percent of the villi remain as the *fetal placenta.* It is apparent that the mother contributes to the placenta and, via her placental arteries, the mother brings oxygen and nourishment to the blood lakes. The placenta is attached to the fetus by the umbilical cord. Within the umbilical cord are two arteries and one vein. Through the arteries waste-laden blood is carried from the fetus to the villi of the placenta. From the villi, these fetal waste products are then lost to the blood lakes. (The mother will take them up into her placental veins and excrete them with her own venous wastes.) At the same time, oxygen and nourishment are taken up into the villi from the blood lakes. The single umbilical vein carries these from the villi of the placenta to the fetus. At no time will there normally be a direct connection between maternal and fetal blood. The fetal circulation of blood in the placenta is a system that is closed to the mother.

Other extraembryonic equipment is also formed. At the age of two weeks the embryo is tucked beneath the surface of the uterine lining. A hollow beneath it will enlarge to a fluid-filled cavity surrounded by a sac called the *amnion*. This sac is filled with *amniotic fluid;* by the fifth month the fetus is swallowing some amniotic fluid. As long as the fetus remains within this sac in the uterus, it lives the aquatic life of a fish. Also during early development, the extra-embryonic membranous *yolk sac* and *allantois* appear. After the second month the yolk sac begins to wither and becomes quite useless, but not until it has contributed to the gut as well as early blood cells and vessels. The allantois becomes the blood vessels in the umbilical cord. It is well to now summarize the functions of the placenta and the amnion.

A versatile temporary organ, the placenta (Figure 6-1) is derived, then, from a fertilized ovum, but the mother contributes too. It serves as a gland, intestine, kidney, lung, sieve, and barrier. Also, the placenta separates two genetically different individuals. When the placenta is by-passed in laboratory animals, the fetus is rejected.[3] This is not unlike the process that occurs when a recipient rejects a transplanted heart. From the maternal side of the placenta, projections branch into the endometrium and into the mother's blood. By osmosis, nutrients from the mother's blood ooze through the placenta. In a reverse manner, the child eliminates wastes. Attached to the fetal surface of the placenta is an umbilical cord and fused membranes. Through the cord circulation, exchanges are made to and from the placenta. Together, the membranes form a bag or sac, completely encompassing the child. In the bag are the "waters" or amniotic fluid. Throughout intrauterine life the child is submerged in these waters. Like an astronaut in a space capsule, the fetus within the amniotic sac is in a state of weightlessness. Therefore, the child is able to move about without expenditure of energy that is needed for growth and development. In addition, the fluid protects delicate tissues, provides a stable temperature, and is of some help in the dilatation of the cervix in early labor.[4] It is not true that a baby born in the membranes of the amniotic sac is lucky. Unless unassisted by a doctor, this does not happen. To enable the baby to breathe immediately at birth, the doctor will, if necessary, rupture the membranes.

The month-by-month changes in the human being during intrauterine residence are now related.

End of the first lunar month   By the end of the first lunar month, the embryo is about one-quarter of an inch long (about the size of a pea) and resembles a sea urchin. About one-third of the embryo is the head, which almost touches the tail. The bulging, beating heart propels blood through primitive vessels. From a devel-

[3] Joseph Dancis, Symposium on "Homeostasis of the Intrauterine Patient," cited in "The Purpose of the Placenta," *Briefs: Footnotes on Maternity Care,* Vol. 33, No. 4 (April 1969), pp. 54-55.
[4] Peter J. Huntingford, "The Fetus in Its Aquatic Environment," cited in "Amnion: Protector of the Unborn Baby," *Briefs: Footnotes on Maternity Care,* Vol. 32, No. 9 (November 1968), pp. 131-32.

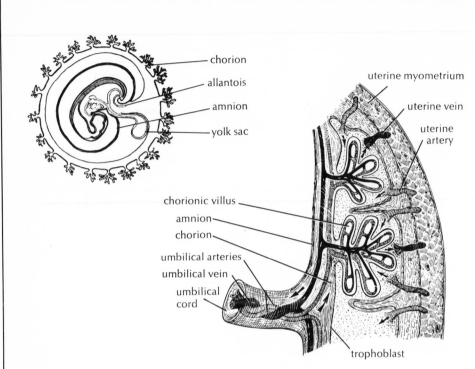

6-1 The development
of human embryonic membranes

Two stages of embryonic development, showing
the interrelationship of embryo and membranes (*top left* and *bottom*)
and a cross section of the placenta (*right*).

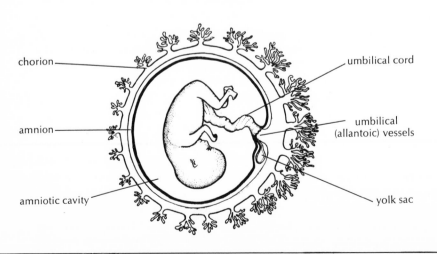

oping mouth leads a tube that will become the digestive tract. Rudiments of eyes, ears, and nose appear, and buds that will become extremities are all visible. Soon the umbilical cord will develop, not as an outgrowth from the baby's body but from accessory tissue.

End of the second lunar month   Every week the embryo has grown one-quarter of an inch and is now a fetus weighing one-thirtieth of an ounce. Sex organs are apparent, but the sex of the fetus is difficult to determine. The developing brain causes the head to be disproportionately large. Pawlike hands have appeared. The half-closed eyes will soon close completely; they remain closed until the end of the seventh month. A few muscles are developing and the feet may kick a few times (but much too feebly to be felt by the mother). The tail begins to regress. At the end of two months, almost all the internal organs have begun to develop. The changes now are mostly related to growth and tissue differentiation.

End of the third lunar month   The three-inch fetus weighs about an ounce but the placenta weighs more. The ears rise to the level of the eyes and the eyelids are fused. Soft nails appear on the stubby fingers and toes. Gender sex can be discerned. From rudimentary kidneys, small amounts of urine are excreted into the amniotic fluid. Tooth sockets and buds are apparent. Now the mother's enlarging uterus can be felt below the umbilicus.

End of the fourth lunar month   The four-ounce fetus is not quite seven inches long. On the scalp a few hairs may sprout. Soon there will be a fine downy whorl-like growth of hair called *lanugo* covering the whole body. The mother may feel the first subtle movements of the fetus at the end of this period (quickening) but usually these do not occur until the following month.

End of the fifth lunar month   The ten-inch fetus weighs about eight ounces. The heart can be heard through the stethoscope. The baby moves actively. Later in pregnancy movements may become quite vigorous but they do not hurt. Since the lungs are not sufficiently developed, babies born prematurely at this time do not survive; they may live but a few minutes. Many states require legal notification of the delivery of a fetus at this age.

End of the sixth lunar month   Now the fetus weighs a pound and one-half and is about a foot long. The fetus is not idle. Sucking an available thumb, swallowing amniotic fluid, exercising developing muscles, even an occasional spasmodic chest movement—these are some activities. Noise startles the child in the uterus. When the mother rocks, the child may go to sleep. The child's activity may waken the mother. Intrauterine quarters are crowded and some children are more restless than others. The sebaceous glands and cells that are shed from the wrinkled skin combine to provide a protective *vernix caseosa* or "cheesy varnish." At birth this may be one-eighth of an inch thick. At the end of this month, the eyelids separate and eyelashes form. If born at this stage, the child is still too undeveloped to survive. The medical literature has recorded the rare case of a thirteen-ounce child born at this age who lived three months.

End of the seventh lunar month   The two-and-one-half-pound fetus is about fifteen inches long. The eyes are open and the child can appreciate light. The testicles are usually in the scrotum. Fat begins to flatten out a few wrinkles. Every day in the uterus at this stage is vital. A baby born at this time has only a fair chance of survival because the lungs and intestinal canal are incompletely developed.

End of the eighth lunar month   The fetus now weighs about four pounds and measures some sixteen-and-one-half inches. The bones of the head are soft. The fetus looks like a little old man. If provided with good nursing and medical care, a baby born now has a much better chance of surviving than one born in the previous month.

End of the ninth lunar month   The fetus, weighing about six pounds and measuring about nineteen inches, begins to make ready to leave the weightless watery ecosystem within the uterus. As if to prepare for the new environment, the fetus gains half a pound a week and wrinkles now disappear. The fingernails need cutting and the fetus may be born with harmless scratch marks. If born prematurely during this month, the chances for survival are good.

The tenth lunar month   By about the middle of the tenth lunar month, the full-term twenty-inch fetus is born, weighing about seven pounds (girls) or about seven-and-one-half pounds (boys). The umbilical cord is about as long as the baby. The placenta weighs about one-and-one-quarter pounds; it is a disc that is about six to eight inches in diameter. There is from one-half to two quarts of amniotic fluid. Most of the lanugo is gone, although some may remain about the shoulders. The vernix caseosa remains and has to be wiped away. The hormones that cause the mother's breasts to enlarge cause the unborn child's breasts to protrude a little. The newborn may secrete milk ("witch's milk"). Within a few days after birth, the breast enlargement subsides and there is no further secretion of milk. The final hue of the slate-colored eyes cannot be predicted.

THE MOTHER

Some married women, perhaps too long denied, eagerly await a first child. Many others want a baby, but not at the moment. Some feel a trifle taken in by their pregnancy. Frequently, a first-time mother may need time to accept the idea. She has about three months to do so. During that time, she weighs herself often. But the scales say little. Her pregnancy is not very real. Nothing much changes.

In the second three months, she grows, and not just physically. The emotional preparations may be more profound than the physical ones.

For many a woman, the last three months of pregnancy drag. A dozen discomforts plague her. This ordeal, she thinks, will be capped by still another. She may wish to be rid of her pregnancy. Yet, she may fear its end. She is weary of glossy magazine pictures of over-joyed women hurrying to the hospital without a care in the world. She wishes she could control her urinary bladder better. And she may worry that her husband, too, is tiring of her pregnant condition.

During pregnancy, some women (not all) are somewhat less responsive to sex. Knowing this, the husband will not feel rejected. The sensitive husband will, moreover, understand that his wife's emotional state profoundly affects the pregnancy. It is here that his responsibility is so considerable. As never before, she needs his love, patience, and confidence.

about some changes, pregnancy tests, and rules

A regularly menstruating woman's first, most common, sign of pregnancy is a missed menstrual period. The breasts are sensitive. The nipples enlarge and become pigmented. More than one-half of all pregnant women experience nausea. Vomiting is infrequent. This is not necessarily "morning sickness." It may occur at any time of the day. It may never occur at all. It is much less frequent than formerly. Serious vomiting during pregnancy hardly ever occurs anymore.

Within days after the first missed menstrual period, laboratory tests indicating pregnancy are over 95 percent accurate.[5] Following implantation, a hormone is found in the woman's urine. Injection of that urine into immature female mice or rabbits causes ovarian

---

[5] Before the days of pregnancy tests "imaginary" or "unconscious" pregnancy was not uncommon. Young brides hoping for a baby or older ladies who worried about having one often developed many of the symptoms of pregnancy without actually being pregnant. At thirty-nine, "Bloody" Queen Mary Tudor was so anxious for a child by her husband Phillip II of Spain that she developed many signs of pregnancy including milk-filled breasts. Counting the months, she sewed baby clothes, fitted out a royal cradle, and had announcements made of the birth of her child. Her expected due date was calculated to be between May 23 and June 5, 1555. Surrounding her at Hampton Court were physicians, midwives, and wet nurses who were dismissed when, two months after her expected due date, she failed to deliver. (*M.D., Medical Newsmagazine*, Vol. 13, No. 3 [March 1969], p. 282.)

changes. With a male frog, the hormone causes spermatozoa to occur in the urine. Other such biological pregnancy tests are constantly under study. Several nonanimal chemical tests are also being used to diagnose pregnancy. Opinions as to their accuracy vary somewhat. However, they do have the advantage of enabling the laboratory to provide a reading within a matter of hours after receiving the specimen. One disadvantage of the standard urine pregnancy tests is that they do not work until about twelve days after the first missed menstrual period. The most recent advancement in this field is a test that can detect pregnancy before the mother-to-be is aware that she has missed a period. In some cases the pregnancy can be determined within approximately fourteen days of conception. Still another pregnancy test is being tried in Sweden. It gives positive results before implantation into the womb's wall occurs. (Such implantation occurs before the first missed period.) The woman who has a tendency to miscarry will be particularly benefited by such early information about her pregnancy. She can then avoid those activities that may bring about a miscarriage.

Pregnancy has some cosmetic effects. Skin blemishes abate. The complexion glows. But pink stretch marks (*striae*) may appear, mostly on the abdomen. Neither massage nor costly oils prevent them. Most (but not all) will disappear. There is also, temporarily, increased pigment on the abdominal midline, around the nipples, and on the face. The breasts fill. By three months, *colostrum,* the precursor to milk, is secreted. During pregnancy, an average of twenty pounds is gained. Much of this occurs in the last two months. The pregnant woman who, as a girl, ate intelligently and exercised, and continues these habits under a physician's direction during and after pregnancy, has the best chance of keeping her figure. Walking is good for her. During the first four months, she may, if she likes, play golf. In the first few months, she may be permitted to swim. Some physicians permit swimming in later months. Surf bathing, horseback riding, and tennis are not advisable. Activities that involve bumping and compression are ill-advised. Only absolutely necessary long trips should be made. Nonfatiguing employment is acceptable. In considering the amount and kind of activity that is best for the patient, the physician always considers the individual. Some pregnant women seem able to do more than others. One recent Olympic swimmer was not much handicapped by her three-and-one-half-month pregnancy; she placed third in her class. It has been reported that of the twenty-six female Soviet Olympic champions of the Sixteenth Olympiad, in Melbourne, Australia, ten were pregnant.[6]

Extra rest is essential. Although showers are preferable in the last month, a daily tepid bath adds to comfort. The teeth, although more

---

[6]Michael Bruser, "Sporting Activities During Pregnancy," cited in "Sports and Pregnancy," *Briefs: Footnotes on Maternity Care,* Vol. 33, No. 4 (April 1969), pp. 51–53.

vulnerable, are not demineralized. "For every pregnancy a tooth" is an untrue old wives' tale. The kidneys need special attention. The doctor will examine the urine often. Constipation may be relieved by fruits and vegetables; prunes, dates, and figs help.

prenatal care

Two or three weeks after the first missed period, a doctor should be consulted. This marks the beginning of a relationship that, as much as any other single factor, has made pregnancy so safe. Compared to just a generation ago, decreased maternal (and infant) mortality rates in this country have been spectacular.

The pregnant woman must visit her doctor regularly. This *prenatal* (before-birth) *care* is essential to her well-being. The whole complex of physical examinations, laboratory examinations of the blood (for syphilis, blood types, Rh factor, and anemia), urine tests —all these, and more, create a constancy of communication between patient and doctor that has brought security to mother and child. Problems can be prevented. If trouble threatens, the doctor can then avert it.

Unless special problems arise, visits to the doctor are scheduled every three or four weeks during the first six months. In the next two months, these are usually increased to every two or three weeks. Visits thereafter are usually weekly.

sexual intercourse and masturbation during pregnancy[7]

An increasing number of physicians permit their pregnant patients to have sexual intercourse throughout the entire period of pregnancy up to the time of the onset of labor. However, not all cases are alike and there are valid reasons for exceptions. The decision must be made by each physician on an individual basis. Some women experience increased sexual desire during the second three months of pregnancy. During the last three months of pregnancy the woman's sexual interest may wane. (The same may be true of her husband.) Some physicians are legitimately concerned that the contractions of the uterus resulting from orgasm might initiate labor. Although definitive data regarding this risk are still unavailable, there are a few small studies that indicate this as a definite risk. Thus, some physicians believe that "while there is no proof that coitus in the second and third trimester induces premature labor, it is undoubtedly safest to abstain from intercourse in the last four weeks of gestation [child-

---

[7] Much of the material in this section is based on Chapter 4, "Sexual Relations During Pregnancy and the Post-Delivery Period," in *Sexuality and Man,* compiled and edited by the Sex Information and Education Council of the United States (New York, 1970).

bearing]."[8] Similarly competent physicians disagree. They believe that the harm done by forbidding intercourse during the last three months of pregnancy is greater than that done by the unproved risk of uterine contractions resulting from orgasm. Of course, the orgasm resulting from masturbation also causes uterine contractions. These contractions are often more intense than those consequent to sexual intercourse. Therefore, concern about uterine contractions would also logically indicate the prohibition of masturbation during the last three months of pregnancy. There is no longer much concern that sexual intercourse during a normal pregnancy will cause infection. Should it occur (which is rare) it can usually be easily treated. Moreover, infection of this sort could occur at any time during pregnancy and not just during the last three months.

There are times during pregnancy in which sexual intercourse should be avoided. Abdominal or vaginal discomfort or pain are always reasons to avoid coitus during pregnancy and at any other time. (When the discomfort can be relieved by the physician's care coitus may sometimes be resumed.) Uterine bleeding during pregnancy is also a valid reason to abstain from coitus. In addition, the pregnant woman should avoid all genital play as well as sexual intercourse after the membranes have ruptured. Inattention to this problem is dangerous. When the membranes are ruptured the hazard of infection from coitus is greater than at any other time during pregnancy. Infection that occurs from intercourse after the membranes rupture may harm both the mother and the child. There is general agreement among physicians that these three conditions are definite contraindications of sexual intercourse during pregnancy: abdominal or vaginal discomfort, vaginal bleeding, and ruptured membranes. In some cases, other hazards may be defined. These are always the concern of the responsible physician in charge.

One form of precoital play that is safe during the nonpregnant state has been proved dangerous during pregnancy. Oral-genital contact by the male may result in his blowing air into the vagina. This air may enter the uterus through the cervical opening. Then the air enters the dilated blood vessels of the uterus surrounding the pregnancy. Air in the maternal blood circulation is dangerous. A few maternal deaths have been reported as a result of this tragic accident.[9]

As pregnancy progresses, the couple may have to adjust their coital position. The purposes of this adjustment are to make intercourse easier as well as insure the wife's comfort. Some couples

[8] Leonard L. Hyams, "Coital Induction of Labor," *Medical Aspects of Human Sexuality,* Vol. 6, No. 4 (April 1972), p. 90.

[9] P. K. Nelson, "Pulmonary Gas Embolism in Pregnancy and the Puerperium," *Obstetrics and Gynecology,* Vol. 15 (August 1960), p. 449, and M. E. Aronson and P. K. Nelson, "Fatal Air Embolism in Pregnancy Resulting from an Unusual Sexual Act," *Obstetrics and Gynecology,* Vol. 30 (July 1967), p. 127, both cited in *Sexuality and Man,* p. 55. Although this could also happen during menstruation, no such accidents have been reported as having occurred during this time.

ordinarily prefer the male-superior position. As the pregnant woman's abdomen progressively protrudes and she nears delivery, this position may have to be temporarily abandoned because of the man's weight. For those couples who have already experimented with a variety of positions, a change at this time is no innovation. A face-to-face position with both husband and wife on their sides may be tried during the later period of pregnancy. Also recommended is a position in which the wife is on her side while the husband's penis enters the vagina from behind.

LABOR

A few days before the onset of true labor, "false labor" may occur. However, it is the onset of regular, rhythmic contractions that heralds true labor. Discomfort, beginning in the lower abdomen, spreads to the back and thighs. The bag of water may break. (A "dry birth" does not prolong labor. Indeed, it may shorten it.) The "show" is another common sign of early labor. This pink vaginal discharge occurs with the onset of cervical dilation. Most first-time mothers may start for the hospital when contractions occur every ten minutes. Others should pay no attention to timing. When contractions are regular, they should go to the hospital. Long before, several reliable ways of transportation should have been arranged.

the stages of labor

There are three stages of labor (see Table 6-1). The first stage is the longest. The upper part of the uterus contracts. The lower cervix dilates. To allow passage of the infant into the vagina, dilation of the cervix must be complete (four inches). In this stage the baby, assisted by uterine contractions, does the work. Both mother and doctor must await dilation of the cervix and the descent of the baby into the

TABLE 6-1 stages of labor

| STAGE | TASK | DURATION | | WHO DOES THE WORK* |
		FIRST BABY	SECOND OR LATER BABY	
First stage	Dilation of cervix	8 to 20 hours	3 to 8 hours	Baby
Second stage	Delivery of infant	20 minutes to 2 hours	20 minutes to 2 hours	Mother
Third stage	Delivery of placenta	5 to 20 minutes	5 to 20 minutes	Obstetrician

* In some cases the physician may decide to do a Caesarean section during the first stage or to apply forceps during the second.
Source: Adapted from M. Edward Davis and Reva Rubin, *De Lee's Obstetrics for Nurses,* 18th ed. (Philadelphia, 1966), p. 273.

proper position. To minimize possible infection, the pubic hair will have been shaved. To increase the space in the pelvic cavity, an enema may have been given. As the first stage progresses, the uterine contractions become more frequent and of longer duration. When the cervix is fully dilated, the mother is taken from the labor room to the delivery room. If for any reason the child cannot do his job, if he cannot adequately act as a wedge, the doctor will perform a *cesarean section*. By this safe surgical procedure, the infant is removed through an incision in the abdomen and uterus.

It is in the second stage of labor that the mother works. By bearing down only with each contraction, the mother adds her fifteen pounds of pressure to the twenty-five pounds of the uterine contraction. Very occasionally, for special medical reasons, such as a premature baby, the physician will shorten this stage. For the mother who desires to see her baby born, a mirror can be arranged.

After the birth of the baby, the *afterbirth* (placenta) is delivered. This is the third stage. A drug is then given to further contract the uterus.

about the pain of childbirth

It was 1561. The place: Castle Hill overlooking what is now Princes Street in Edinburgh, Scotland. At the top of the hill a stake had been driven into the ground. Around it had been piled firewood. Up the hill and to the stake was dragged a lovely lady named Eufame Mac Layne. Only a few moments before, her newly born twin babies had been torn from her arms. Now she was chained to the stake. Within an hour she was ashes. Her crime? She had employed "one Agnes Sampson to administer unto her a certain medicine for the relief of pain in childbirth contrary to divine law and contempt of crown." [10]

Labor pain is as old as humanity. As the Bible says: "in sorrow thou shalt bring forth children" (Genesis 3:16). Surely it is life's most rewarding sorrow. However, few people today interpret any part of the Bible as meaning that sorrow and pain are not to be relieved.

The human is the only mammal that has pain with the expulsion of the fetus.[11] Uterine contractions do not hurt. What does hurt is the pressure of the descending baby on lower pelvic structures and the stretching of the cervix. In 1857, Queen Victoria was given the anesthetic chloroform for childbirth. A resultant controversy about the morality of this was largely limited to men. Today, most women expect, and receive, relief from the pain of childbirth. No woman need endure more than she can bear. Today, there are adequate safe pharmaceuticals to control pain.

Dr. Grantly Dick Read correctly taught that ignorance breeds fear

[10] Donald T. Atkinson, *Magic, Myth and Medicine* (New York, 1956), pp. 271-72.
[11] Dorothy V. Whipple, *Dynamics of Development: Euthenic Pediatrics* (New York, 1966), p. 74.

and fear impedes labor. Although fear is not responsible for all the pain of childbirth, it can cause much of it. The pregnant woman is not helped by those who exaggerate those pains, which, in any case, vary greatly with the individual. Read's concepts of natural childbirth include education, plus exercise in relaxation and breathing. All this is commendable. Pain may occur. Drugs may be used. For some couples, there is much in favor of natural childbirth. Not only the mother but also the expectant father may derive considerable psychological benefit from the experience. There is a long overdue, growing awareness of the father's opportunities to participate in the birth experience.

The past few years have seen an increasing acceptance of the Lamaze method of childbirth, commonly referred to as natural childbirth. Both the pregnancy and the actual childbirth process become a family affair. Together, husband and wife attend prenatal classes to learn the facts about pregnancy, labor, and delivery. The mother-to-be is given breathing and muscle exercises that are useful during labor and delivery. The husband is taught to monitor them correctly. The husband is with his wife during labor and in the delivery room, and he puts his knowledge to good use. Not all physicians approve of this method of childbirth. They believe that childbirth is a surgical procedure with which the father-to-be may interfere.

THE "PREGNANT FATHER"

An increasing amount of attention is finally being paid to the "pregnant father." He, too, is expecting. He, too, must adjust to the birth of a baby. One manifestation of this need is the ethnic custom known as *couvade*. According to the custom the husband feigns illness before, during, and after the birth of his child. In the fifth century B.C. the Greek historian Herodotus described couvade among African tribes; in the Middle Ages Marco Polo described couvade among the mountain tribes of China. The custom still exists today among some primitive peoples. During the pregnancy the husband complains of a variety of discomforts, such as nausea and abdominal pain. But it is during the birth of the child that his expressions of discomfort reach their height. "When the woman gives birth, the man goes to bed sobbingly, writhes with ostensible pains, moans, has warm compresses applied to his body, has himself nursed attentively, and submits to dietary restrictions for days, weeks, or, in exceptional cases, even for months. Until his first bath, he is considered unclean, just as though he had himself given birth to the child."[12]

---

[12] Helen Diner, *Mothers and Amazons* (New York, 1965), p. 113. An extremely rare case of false pregnancy, complete with morning sickness, distended abdomen, and a feeling of movement within the abdomen, has been reported in a male. He was delighted with his "condition," took vitamins, and decided he would have to be delivered by cesarean section. (James A. Knight, "Unusual Case: False Pregnancy in a Male," *Medical Aspects of Human Sexuality*, Vol. 5, No. 3 [March 1971], pp. 58, 63-64, 69.)

But couvade is hardly limited to primitive cultures. Certain aspects of it are known to many expectant fathers in industrialized societies. Nausea, diarrhea, constipation, and backache are all common complaints of the father-to-be. In one study of U.S. servicemen it was found that 60 percent of the expectant fathers had some symptoms of pregnancy. Some even went through the "baby blues," the postnatal depression exhibited by some mothers[13] (see page 206). This has been confirmed by other studies. "Some men experienced the pregnancy as a severe test of their masculinity. Some expressed their envy of pregnancy all the way from vigorously denying it to almost fusing with the wife in an attempt to experience the pregnancy biologically."[14]

Thus the birth of the baby is accompanied by a wide variety of stresses for both parents. It is a time when both husband and wife have to draw from their deepest wellsprings of mutual understanding.

NOT ALL HUMAN MILK IS MOTHER'S MILK

Not all the signs and symptoms usually attributed to the pregnant state occur with pregnancy, nor are they invariably limited to the female. The ancients were aware of this as can be seen in the biblical observation: "His breasts are full of milk" (Job 21:24). *Prolactin* is the primary hormone responsible for *lactation,* which is the period of milk secretion. As the hormone that stimulates the production of milk in lactating women, it is but one of the several potent products of the anterior lobe of the pituitary gland (see page 30). However, lactation can occur in a wide variety of conditions and situations other than pregnancy. The prolonged use of some tranquilizers and other drugs that influence the hypothalamus may produce lactation. Mechanical trauma, chest or breast burns, herpes zoster (shingles) of the chest wall, are among other conditions that occasionally stimulate lactation. Breast milk may also occur as a result of poorly fitting garments or manipulation of the breasts. Lactation has been noted, along with amenorrhea (absence of menstruation), in young women who have never borne a child and who are taking birth control pills. This may theoretically be due to a temporary loss of the hypothalamic control of some aspects of the anterior lobe of the pituitary gland in a certain percentage of women.[15] The occurrence of breast milk has been noted with childless and postmenopausal women who undergo the sucking stimulus. Men who experience a prolonged

---

[13] *Sexuality and Man,* p. 59.

[14] B. Liebenberg, W. H. Trethowan, and M. F. Conlon, "The Couvade Syndrome," *British Journal of Psychiatry* (March 1965), and Illinois State Medical Society, "Expectant Fathers Experience Pregnancy Symptoms Too," Release No. 249 (November 2, 1966), both cited in *Sexuality and Man,* p. 59.

[15] Robert B. Greenblatt, "Inappropriate Lactation in Men and Women," *Medical Aspects of Human Sexuality,* Vol. 6, No. 6 (June 1972), p. 33, citing R. D. Gambrell, R. B. Greenblatt, and V. B. Mahesh, "Post-Pill and Pill-Related Amenorrhea-Galactorrhea" (in press).

sucking stimulus may, in time, also lactate. And not only lactation, but also breast enlargement, has been occasionally observed on refeeding severely malnourished prisoners of war.[16]

POSTNATAL CONCERNS

Before leaving the hospital the mother is examined. In six to eight weeks she should be examined again. Of particular interest to the physician are her weight, blood pressure, and the condition of her breasts, uterus, cervix, vagina, and genitalia. He advises her that the first menstruation may normally be somewhat profuse. Some women are troubled by a vaginal discharge. This is easily treated. The busy mother may forget or defer the examination. This is unwise. She cannot adequately take care of anyone else unless she also takes care of herself.

mother love: not always at first sight

It is widely believed that the moment the mother beholds her baby for the first time she feels an immediate love for the child. For many women this is not true. Some mothers apparently love their new babies immediately, but many good mothers do not. During labor the woman usually limits her thoughts to completing the job entailed in the birth process. After the birth many mothers want to see their

---

[16] Ibid., p. 33, citing C. Klatzkin et al., "Gynecomastia Due to Malnutrition: Clinical Studies," *American Journal of Medical Science,* Vol. 213, No. 19 (1947); R. E. Hibbs, "Gynecomastia Associated with Vitamin Deficiency Disease," *American Journal of Medical Science,* Vol. 213, No. 176 (1947); and E. C. Jacobs, "Effects of Starvation on Sex Hormones in Males," *Journal of Clinical Endocrinology,* Vol. 8, No. 227 (1948). Investigators have recently studied the effect of breast and nipple stimulation on the level of prolactin in the blood serum of seven men and eight nonlactating women. All were healthy; the ages of the men ranged from twenty-eight to thirty-three years; the women were between twenty-one and twenty-eight years old. Three of the women had a history of nursing a child; the time intervals between nursing the children and the study were forty, seventeen, and fourteen months. Among the findings:

1. A woman who stroked her own breasts and nipples for five minutes induced at least a ten-fold increase in the output of prolactin by the anterior lobe of her pituitary gland. Self-stimulation of the breast, without direct stimulation of the nipple or areola, resulted in a lesser rise in prolactin blood-serum level.

2. When the husband of the woman stroked her breasts, the increase in her blood-serum prolactin level was about the same.

3. Self-stimulation by men of their nipples produced no increase in prolactin output by the anterior pituitary.

4. The prolactin level in the blood serum of men rose markedly when their wives stimulated their nipples.

5. Although male nipple stimulation is often an effective form of foreplay, these particular men experienced no sexual arousal with such stimulation either by themselves or their wives. None of the women reported sexual arousal by breast stimulation alone; three of the women reported sexual arousal when their breasts and nipples were stimulated either by themselves or their husbands.

A nerve reflex via the hypothalamus of the brain (see page 30) is believed to account for the increased prolactin levels. The significance of the psychological aspects of physical breast and nipple stimulation is particularly emphasized by the results with the males. (Robert C. Kolodny, Laurence S. Jacobs, and William H. Daughaday, "Mammary Stimulation Causes Prolactin Secretion in Non-Lactating Women," *Nature,* Vol. 238, No. 5362 [August 4, 1972], pp. 284-85. The references in this article include some that discuss lactation in the nonpregnant state.)

babies to make certain they are healthy, or simply out of curiosity. A recent study of fifty-four mothers from the middle and upper socioeconomic levels of Washington, D.C. revealed some interesting information in this regard.[17] Thirty-three percent of the mothers reported having no particular feelings upon seeing their babies for the first time. Seven percent had negative feelings. Fifty-nine percent reported positive feelings that were, nevertheless, quite impersonal. Most of the mothers did not note the beginnings of positive feelings until the third week following childbirth. With the return of her strength, a growing sense of competence, and a reciprocating baby, the mother's attachment to her child grew. By the end of the third month the attachment had become powerful. Although there is no data, it must be assumed that love for the child evolves at least as slowly for the father as for the mother. For most parents, then, mother love and father love grows slowly; it is not mature upon the birth of the baby. Many parents feel a totally unwarranted sense of guilt for not loving their babies immediately.

sexual intercourse following childbirth

Most women do not desire sexual intercourse for some days following childbirth. This is understandable. The new mother may experience fatigue resulting from delivery. A new baby, moreover, means adjustments for the mother, especially if the child is her first-born. This may be a difficult period for the husband too. A house that was once organized around him may now be organized around the baby. During the first month or so following childbirth, the stresses of motherhood may cause his wife to be less interested in coitus. Her desire for sexual intercourse may be further lessened by postpartum depression. The cause of this ordinarily transient depression is not clear. It may be associated with the return of the menstrual cycle following pregnancy. A profound series of endocrine gland readjustments occur. It would be surprising if the woman did not experience some emotional changes.

Added to all these new stresses is a certain amount of discomfort about the anus and vagina. Incisions and small tears must heal. There may be some vaginal bleeding. When healing has occurred and the bleeding has stopped, sexual intercourse may be resumed. A small

[17] Kenneth S. Robson and Howard Moss, "Patterns and Determinants of Maternal Attachment," *The Journal of Pediatrics,* Vol. 77, No. 6 (December 1970), p. 976. In many U.S. hospitals, newborns are taken from their mothers after a brief initial visit, and the mother-child relationship is continued only at feeding times. Some research has been done to find out if more prolonged contact would result in any changes in the mother. It did. One month after leaving the hospital with their babies, mothers whose early contact with them had been extended "were more reluctant to leave their infants with someone else, usually stood and watched during the examination, showed greater soothing behavior, and engaged in significantly more eye-to-eye contact and fondling." (Marshall H. Klaus, Richard Jerauld, Nancy C. Kreger, William McAlpine, Meredith Steffa, and John H. Kennel, "Maternal Attachment: Importance of the First Post-Partum Days," *The New England Journal of Medicine,* Vol. 286, No. 9 [March 2, 1972], p. 460.)

amount of brown vaginal discharge may persist for a while, but this is no reason to defer coitus. After the birth of a baby, a woman usually wants to resume sexual intercourse as soon as possible. There is no reason to discourage her if she is comfortable with it; by that time the bleeding usually has stopped. Some women defer sexual activity for an unduly long period of time following childbirth. This may be associated with their own needless fears and misconceptions. In these instances the physician can and will do much to allay apprehensions and correct misapprehensions.

conception during breast feeding

Contrary to popular notions, sexual intercourse during the time a woman is a nursing mother can result in pregnancy. Breast-feeding tends to prolong the period following childbirth during which the woman does not menstruate (*postpartum amenorrhea*). During this period, conception usually will not occur. But the extent of the prolonged amenorrhea and the delayed conception cannot be accurately estimated in the individual woman. As soon as ovulation occurs, conception can take place, and a woman may ovulate before her first menstrual period following childbirth. About one in twenty women do start another pregnancy without having resumed menstruation following the birth of a baby. It is not known if breast-feeding following the return of menstruation reduces the likelihood of conception.

not all mothers should nurse

By no means should every mother nurse her child. There are medical contraindications to breast-feeding. Some drugs that are prescribed for the mother for a variety of reasons may pass into the breast milk in doses sufficient to harm the child. Breast infections may also make breast-feeding unwise. By early autumn of 1972 no human cancer had been proved to be caused by a virus. Nevertheless, viruslike particles have been detected in human milk and in tissue specimens of breast cancers; these are known to cause leukemia and breast cancer in mice. For this reason, there is competent medical opinion that "women with a personal or family history of breast cancer should not nurse, since it is possible that the viruslike particles in milk may induce breast cancer or other malignancies later in the life cycle of the nursling."[18]

Various methods have been used to inhibit lactation. Among these are the restriction of fluid intake and the use of a breast-binder or well-fitting brassiere. During this period the breasts should not be

[18]Helmuth Vorherr, "Suppression of Postpartum Lactation," *Postgraduate Medicine,* Vol. 52, No. 1 (July 1972), p. 145.

manipulated. Sometimes breasts do become painfully engorged; for this condition the physician may recommend the application of an ice pack and, perhaps, judicious use of medication to relieve the pain. Using these procedures, lactation usually stops within a week. Many women who have had more than one child do not do well with these procedures. To avoid painful breast engorgement and the discomfort due to milk leakage, some physicians may wish to administer a single injection of an androgen-estrogen combination toward the end of labor or immediately after delivery. A woman who has had a spontaneous or therapeutic abortion after the sixteenth week of pregnancy, or whose child was stillborn, will usually require help for suppression of lactation.

parental anxiety

A distraught young mother presented her dilemma to her family physician this way:

"It's my fault," she said, her voice trembling. "I should have breast-fed my baby." Suddenly she was angry. "But I hated it. I couldn't stand it. I never liked it, and I can't hide not having liked it any more. Last month I read an article in this magazine." She held a popular woman's journal. "Is it really that unnatural not to breast-feed the baby? My doctor told me to forget about it. But a friend of mine read that unless you breast-feed your baby, you have Lesbian tendencies or something. Is that somebody's idea of a joke?" She wiped her eyes. "I'm beginning to hate this whole thing." She was crying. "I hate it. I hate having a baby. Everybody says something different."

Some women want to breast-feed their babies. They enjoy it, and do it easily. Others, just as well adjusted, do not enjoy breast-feeding. They should not do so. A guilt-ridden mother, resentfully holding her child to her breast, will do that child no good. It is the total experience of dining, of human comfort and tenderness, that is essential to the baby in this, the stage that Erikson calls basic trust versus mistrust. And, as has been pointed out above, not every mother should breast-feed her child.

The young woman described above is still another victim of an endless barrage of conflicting advice. Don't pick up Billie when he screams. Pick up Billie when he screams. Exclude Susie from the bedroom. What if she does feel left out? Don't exclude Susie from the bedroom. She'll feel left out. Never take Willie's hands away from his penis; if you do he'll masturbate in public. Always divert Willie when he's doing his exploring; if you don't, he'll masturbate in public. And so on, ad infinitum. The result is a confused parent, doubtful of every action, suspicious of his own love, convinced of his inadequacy, and suffering parental guilt. This very anxiety and confusion may distress the child more than anything else. The child needs a relaxed and comfortable parent.

THE CHILD'S NEED FOR MOTHERING

Observe a newborn calf. Shakily it struggles to its trembling legs. Still wet, listing, it totters to its mother's teat. Such is its early independence. The dependence of the human newborn, however, is complete. Even the purpose of the breast must be shown him. To completely deprive the human newborn or infant of mothering is catastrophic.

At birth, threats promptly beset the utterly vulnerable human infant. The respiratory center of the brain, the respiratory muscle (diaphragm) separating the chest from the abdomen, the respiratory muscles between the ribs in the newborn—all these need further development. To meet his consequent threat of inadequate respiration, the newborn human must breathe two or three times as fast as the adult. To the respiratory threat is added a gastrointestinal threat. The gut lining is incomplete. For a time, it functions poorly. A third threat is that of an inadequate relationship between the infant and his mother or mother-substitute. And still a fourth threat is that the infant might not be able to satisfy his needs for pleasure, for example, the oral pleasure of enough sucking. For all people, to a varying degree, these threats become realities.

The infant feels hunger. Hunger hurts. He is threatened, anxious. He cries and he is fed. His tension is relieved. But sometimes he cries and the breast (or bottle) does not come. All he can do is cry more. He hurts more. His stress grows. He suffers more anxiety. About six months of a small amount of frustration will teach him how to deal with frustration. Too much frustration, however, will teach him that his most important person cannot be counted on. He loses his basic trust. At the breast the infant learns, for the first time, love and hate (see pages 5-6).

The effects of prolonged maternal deprivation have long been studied. In 1801, the "wild boy" of Aveyron was found in a French forest. Attempts to help him laid the foundation for present treatment of the mentally retarded. For more than thirty years, reports of children completely deprived of mothering have described their sad expression, pitiable dejection, rigidity, mental and social deterioration, stupor, and even unduly high sickness and death rates.

Animal infants also develop emotional problems from maternal deprivation. Laboratory monkeys bred without mothers grieve piteously. At times they clasp their heads in their arms and rock. Some pinch the same patch of skin hundreds of times daily or develop other compulsive mannerisms. Others fail to mate successfully.

One experiment separated young monkeys from their mothers and raised them with mother-substitutes constructed of wire. One wire substitute incorporated a bottle containing warm milk from a mother monkey. The other substitute was covered with terry cloth. The young monkeys turned to the bare wire effigy only to feed. Otherwise they clung to the soft terry cloth mother-substitute. This study indicated "that contact comfort is a variable of overwhelming importance in the development of affectional response, whereas lactation is a variable of negligible importance."[19] Monkeys reared with the never scolding, always warm terry cloth "mother" nevertheless did not mature properly.

Observations such as these, combined with highly defensible, if theoretical, schema of personality development (see page 4), correctly emphasize the critical importance of the mother to the growth of the child. The fact that most psychiatrists vigorously emphasize this has not helped to diminish the widespread sense of guilt and anxiety among many working mothers of young children. And an anxious mother means an anxious child.

THE WORKING MOTHER

The life of the average mother today is not like her grandmother's used to be. Her grandmother was not isolated with a runabout child in a huge uncaring pile of rock. Her grandmother was not locked up in a carefully measured, stingily allotted, two-room space, a three-dollar telephone call away from her nearest relative. Her grandmother lived among a retinue of relatives and neighbors, all interfering but caring. Her grandmother's time was a time of *Kirche, Kinder, Kochen* (church, children, cooking). Bread was baked at home, not bought practically odorless and neatly sliced. It was a time of the "superhome," not the supermarket. Her grandmother had a single gadget—a music box given her as a wedding present. And when her grandmother bade farewell to her son, who was leaving to be on his own, she had another child at her breast. When her grandmother died at forty-three, and the child died too, it was very sad. Sad, but not unusual. Most grown people died of some infection before they reached the age of fifty; and, in those days, countless babies died of summer diarrhea.

Today's average mother will live well past seventy. She will have borne her children (two) by the age of twenty-seven. She will have raised them before she is fifty. Production of basic services outside the home (education, recreation, food), combined with laborsaving automation, add perhaps as much as ten more years during which child-raising can be a reasonable part-time job. Even a woman who

[19] Harry F. Harlow, "The Nature of Love," *American Psychologist,* Vol. 13, No. 12 (December 1958), p. 676. Lactation refers to the period of milk secretion.

manages to keep busy at home throughout all the childbearing years can count on only about twenty years of complete occupation. These are interim years. They come out of the middle of her life. What is more, some 80 percent of married women become widows—many at a young age. If they hope to remarry, they must become involved in activities outside the home. And they must compete with the growing number of divorcees and other unmarried women.

These potential problems do not contribute to the modern woman's desire to consider domesticity a full-time lifetime occupation. Child-rearing is now a temporary full-time job. Since 1950 the number of married working women in the United States has exceeded the number of single working women. Moreover, the acceptance of women by industry testifies to their success in the business world. Twenty percent of mothers with children under six years and over 40 percent of mothers with children between six and seventeen years work away from home. Millions of these must work because of financial reasons. In the past ten years, however, an increasing number of working mothers have been working because they are unhappy at home. For them, the horizons of home are too limited. They make poor full-time mothers and dull, nagging wives. At work they are happier. But many working mothers are anxious that they are failing their children. They feel guilty. Need they be?

The mother who is content at home need not be defensive about it. A happy full-time mother always will be best for children. But an unhappy mother, resentfully brooding over her missed life outside the home, is best outside that home. An outside job may well improve her performance with her children. And a smaller amount of high-quality mothering is better than a massive amount of poor mothering.

A job, then, may relieve the guilt she feels about being a dissatisfied mother. But what can she do about her new guilt—her feeling that she has deserted the home? Recent studies have amply indicated that the vast majority of modern young women choose careers that will not lead them into later serious conflicts with their desire to be successful wives and mothers.[20] However, there is little doubt that the choice of occupation is the result of countless cultural pressures—a learned phenomenon.[21] The greatest problem for the working mother is the care of the infant and preschooler. The care of older children is more easily arranged. People who care for other people's children must have enormous sensitivity, patience, and tenderness. Such people are very hard to find. The degree of the average working mother's guilt depends in part on her success in meeting the critical problem of substitute care. Also, she must honestly ask herself if she is physically and emotionally able to handle both complex, demanding

[20] Harold L. Wilensky, cited in "Woman's Work Is Never Done: Roundup of Current Research," *Transaction*, Vol. 6, No. 7 (June 1969), p. 8.
[21] Jean Lipman-Blumen, "How Ideology Shapes Women's Lives," *Scientific American*, Vol. 226, No. 1 (January 1972), pp. 34-42.

aspects of her life. The care and feeding of a business executive for eight hours a day, for example, may be just as taxing as caring for any child. (It is possible that experience with one is helpful with the other.) A woman who is exhausted and tense from a high-pressure business or professional life may find it difficult to be the feminine mother of a child waiting at home. Not only in dress, but also in manner she will have to be a quick-change artist. Children thrive on love, not ticker tape.[22] A child will reject a mother who is masculine in dress or behavior. For this reason and despite "heavy investment in preparing their chosen careers, [she] must impose self-limitations after marriage and children."[23] The guilty working mother who tries to "make it up" to the child for being absent will not mother, but overprotect the child. In the end, the child will fight her off.

What about the father? Without his support, the working mother will fail. The husband of the working mother has added responsibility. He will do well to help his working wife in every way possible. But if the wife is prone to constantly remind him of her contribution to the family income, she will receive not support but hate. Work will become for each of them an escape from the other. And the child at home will live on a deserted island threatened by the stormy seas of dissension.

Finally, do not the studies of mother-deprived children mentioned above provide adequate evidence that a mother's absence deprives and sickens a child? One must guard against glib conclusions. To begin with, the absent mothers in the studies were usually completely absent. Moreover, maternal deprivation was not the only misfortune of these children. Other factors—such as bitter family dissension, poverty, and racial discrimination—also contributed to the mental illness of children without mothers. Recent evaluations point to little or no direct correlation between working mothers and childhood instability. Children raised in kibbutzim (the cooperative agricultural communities of Israel) are kept in nurseries. The nursery workers are carefully selected to provide affection and warmth for the children. Every day the children are visited by their own parents. A degree of family life is thus part of each child's day. Some investigators claim that the absence of continual parental attention plus the kibbutz emphasis on the community welfare in some ways enhance the child's development.

In summary, many working mothers and fathers succeed in raising emotionally healthy children. But they must work at it.

[22] "Where I come from," Fiorello La Guardia used to shrewdly say, "we knew the difference between ticker tape and spaghetti." The Little Flower was reflecting even deeper feelings than a social conscience. He was saying: "Society should care like a mother."

[23] Louise Sandler, "Career Wife and Mother," *Archives of Environmental Health,* Vol. 18, No. 2 (February 1969), pp. 154-55.

THE SUDDEN INFANT DEATH SYNDROME[24]

Each year, some twenty-five thousand to thirty thousand[25] U.S. babies are put to bed at night and unexpectedly found dead in the morning. Typically, the child is between two and four months old (90 percent are between one and nine months; the average age is 2.8 months).[26] The child had previously been in good health and had given no warning of the tragedy. There may have been some minor symptoms of an upper respiratory infection. This situation is now known as the Sudden Infant Death Syndrome (SIDS).

The agonized parents ask why this has happened.[27] Research has proved the following about the SIDS: (1) it is in no way related to the adequacy of parental care and occurs among the best loved and cared for babies; (2) it is not hereditary; (3) it does not cause the afflicted child to suffer; (4) it cannot be predicted by even the most competent physician, much less by the watchful parent; it presents no warning symptoms; at this time, it is in no way preventable; (5) it is not caused by vomiting, nor by regurgitating and choking from the last feeding; and (6) it often occurs under conditions in which there is no possibility of smothering.

What, then, causes the Sudden Infant Death Syndrome? One distinguished physician has suggested that "the most convincing hypothesis at this time would tend to suggest that the baby's first experience with respiratory viruses may be overwhelming and that a 'cold of the lungs' is sufficient to interfere with vital and essential ventilation, leading to sharply reduced supplies of oxygen and sudden unexpected death."[28] This conception is somewhat strengthened by recent research. It has been found that during normal sleep the infant may not breathe 5 to 10 percent of the time. During a virus infection, the spells during which the child does not breathe may increase to between 25 and 30 percent of the time. In addition, it has been shown that the reactivity of the autonomic nervous system (which controls involuntary body functions) varies among infants. This division of the nervous system does not mature until the second or third month of life.[29] A mild infection plus an immature nervous system not yet

[24] Also called "cot deaths" and "crib deaths."
[25] R. J. Wedgewood and E. P. Benditt, *Proceedings of the Conference on Causes of Sudden Death in Infants.* Public Health Service Publication No. 1412 (Washington, D.C., 1965), pp. 1-9.
[26] Frederick B. Hodges, "Sudden Infant Death Syndrome," *California Medicine,* Vol. 116, No. 1 (January 1972), p. 85.
[27] Only too often parents mistakenly blame themselves for the sudden death of their child. To increase public education about the problem, the National Foundation for Sudden Infant Death, Inc. (NFSID) was formed. The address of its national headquarters is 1501 Broadway, New York, New York 10036. Chapter members, themselves SIDS parents, devote many hours talking to and helping other parents learn to cope with the sudden death of their infant. Recent SIDS families are also often referred to professional help. ("The National Foundation for Sudden Infant Death, Inc.," *Clinical Pediatrics,* Vol. 11, No. 2 [February 1972], p. 83.)
[28] John M. Adams, *Viruses and Colds: The Modern Plague* (New York, 1967), pp. 103-04.
[29] Frederick B. Hodges, "Sudden Infant Death Syndrome," p. 86.

competent to protect the child may be part of the picture. An added bit of evidence leading to the notion that infection is one of the causes of the SIDS is that the deaths occur more frequently during cold weather.

Nevertheless, attempts at isolating viruses and bacteria from afflicted children have not been routinely rewarding. "If infection plays a part it appears as a trivial affliction rather than as a frank one."[30] Since some investigations reveal the highest risk to be at night, it may be that body metabolic changes during sleep hinder the ordinary response to respiratory difficulty in some children. Crib deaths have occurred in babies who have been breast-fed all their lives; however, breast-feeding may have some role in preventing such deaths because human breast milk does contain components that "have positive antiviral and antibacterial activity in the baby, and human milk is believed to be nonallergic to man."[31] Nevertheless, there is considerable dispute about whether slowly developing milk allergy causes the respiratory distress leading to crib deaths.

One physician suggests that not all reported crib deaths actually occur in the crib. A considerable number occur in the parents' bed. Smothering occurs when a parent accidentally lies over the child. Today, this accident is called "overlying"; such a tragedy was first reported in the Bible by the woman who tells King Solomon that "this woman's child died in the night; because she overlaid it" (I Kings 3:19). "Parents must be informed that to sleep in the same bed with an infant is to invite disaster which is as ancient as the Temple of Solomon."[32]

SUBFERTILITY

How long should it take before a normal couple may expect conception? Usually six months of ordinary cohabitation results in pregnancy. If conception does not occur within a year of marriage, the couple would do well to seek the advice of the family doctor.

Among the married, the threat of childlessness often begins with suspicion, which may grow to anxious doubt, and end in sad resignation. Fully 20 to 25 percent of couples in this country fail to have as many children as they wish. Only 10 percent seek adequate help.

In this culture, many people incorrectly consider subfertility[33] to be primarily a fault within the woman. In the Bible, it is the sterile woman who is regarded with pity, if not scorn. The "adversary" of

[30] "Cot Deaths," *British Medical Journal,* Vol. 4, No. 5782 (October 30, 1971), p. 250.
[31] Ibid.
[32] J. J. Francisco, "Smothering in Infancy: Its Relationship to the 'Crib Death Syndrome'," *Southern Medical Journal,* Vol. 63, No. 10 (October 1970), p. 1114.
[33] *Subfertility* refers to a state of being less than normally fertile. It is relative sterility. *Sterility* refers to the inability to conceive or to induce conception.

Hannah "provoked her sore, for to make her fret, because the Lord had shut up her womb" (I Samuel 1:6). Of course, the problem occurs just as often within men.

The cause of subfertility may be easily discovered, or it may require a long investigation. Sometimes it is necessary to consult various medical specialists.

Severe nutritional deficiencies have been known to cause reduced fertility. Both ovulation and menstruation may be impaired in this way. Alcoholism, other drug abuse, chronic infections—all may contribute to a subfertile marriage. Physical problems may range all the way from excess obesity of both marital partners (interfering with actual consummation of the marriage) to an occluded uterine tube. Malfunction of the uterine tube accounts for no less than 25 percent of all cases of subfertility. A kinked tube, or one blocked as a result of an infection, may be unable to receive the ovum and permit its passage to the uterus. Or it may stop the sperm's ascent to the ovum.

Emotional problems may impede conception. A young wife, forced to live with an interfering mother-in-law, may learn to bide her time. But, while she is biding her time, her vagina, uterus, and tubes tense. She may be unable to conceive. Moving to her own apartment might cure her. Spasm of the vagina and tubes may disappear. The quality of her cervical mucus improves and becomes more receptive of her husband's sperm. She will then more likely conceive. A prolonged sense of guilt over a previous sexual misfortune, such as a venereal infection, combined with lack of knowledge, has resulted not only in subfertility but in serious marital problems. The erroneous idea "VD germs kill sperms" has, at times, been eradicated by showing a husband his own spermatozoa darting about under the microscope.[34] Too many girls, subjected to exaggerated and lurid stories by "well-meaning" mothers and acquaintances, fear both intercourse and childbearing. Resultant tensions may well interfere with fertility. Knowledge of the reassuring facts about both will help her. The husband who is sensitive to his wife's sexual needs will enrich his marriage. He is also more likely to enhance her fertility.

The physician usually first investigates the man, since the cause can often be more easily established in the male. After a thorough physical examination, there are several tests to be done. Spermatozoa are examined for numbers, motility, appearance, and other features.

The search for the cause of female subfertility is usually more complex. It may be a persistent, simply treated, vaginal inflammation. Or the physician may find that his patient encourages intercourse but once every month or two and then without attention to her ovulation cycle. Some physicians feel that *coitus interruptus* establishes a reflex that results in withdrawal just before male ejaculation.

[34] For a discussion of the venereal diseases, see pages 60–78.

The causes of a woman's inability to conceive may be multiple and complex, and patience is needed in investigating them. Only with the discovery of the cause of the problem may rational approach to its solution be made. When the cause is failure of the woman to ovulate, "fertility drugs" may be considered. However, as has been pointed out, failure to ovulate is not the major cause of subfertility. Approximately 33 percent of all problems of subfertility are due to male dysfunction. Factors involving the uterine cervix account for approximately 20 percent of the cases of infertility, disorders of the Fallopian tubes for 33 percent, and hormonal factors for about 15 percent.

the sometimes overefficient "fertility drugs"

Gonadotropins are substances that have an affinity for or stimulate the gonads (ovaries and testes). In recent years several have been used to stimulate the ovary to ovulate. Among these is the luteinizing hormone (LH, see page 31). These are the so-called fertility drugs.

A major problem with their use has been their control. Some women become pregnant with more than they bargained for. Not long ago a twenty-nine-year-old Australian woman who had been given a fertility drug gave birth to nine infants. They were twelve weeks premature. None survived. In the winter of 1970, a New Jersey woman who had also received fertility drugs gave birth to quintuplets. Such multiple births should not condemn the use of fertility drugs. For example, the New Jersey woman had become pregnant twice before with the aid of fertility drugs, and both were single pregnancies. To prevent excessive ovulation, fertility specialists are developing new techniques to regulate dosage. Moreover, the recent discovery of the chemical structure and the synthesis of the luteinizing hormone-releasing factor of the hypothalamus (LH-RH, see page 31) may well revolutionize infertility therapy.[35] (It will be remembered that the luteinizing hormone controls the release of the ovum from the ovary.) The synthesis may result in the production of safe and inexpensive fertility stimulators.

Already some success has been reported in this area. In one woman, egg production was induced by an injection of follicle-stimulating hormone (FSH, see page 31) followed by an injection of natural LH-RH. Not only did she ovulate, but she also had a healthy baby. Single ovulations have also been induced in two women by giving each of them two injections of LH-RH ten days apart. In these two cases, no FSH was used beforehand.[36]

A wide variety of procedures that do not involve drugs that

[35] For a discussion of the possibilities of LH-RH as a contraceptive, see page 32, footnote 2.
[36] "Correcting Infertility Without Multiple Births," *Science News*, Vol. 101, No. 2 (January 8, 1972), p. 24.

stimulate ovulation are being perfected. Among these are the correction of uterine defects, surgical procedures to reconstruct the Fallopian tubes, and the increased use of artificial insemination. This last procedure offers some hope. Within present limits, improved freezing techniques may make it more possible for newly established semen banks to help solve problems caused by male infertility.

ON PLANNING A CHILD'S GENETIC SEX

"Throughout antiquity, it was believed that boys were the products of the right testicle, and that girls were the products of the left one."[37] The ancient Hebrews improved on this notion; in the Talmud they apparently appreciated the significance of the time of orgasm and conception in influencing the sex of the offspring.[38] Is it indeed possible to influence the genetic sex of a child? Some interesting (and curious) correlations have been noted that lend credence to the notion that prediction of whether a child will be born a boy or a girl is possible. A few years ago, a U.S. statistician noted that early summer seemed to favor the birth of boys.[39] Also, an English investigator has suggested that couples who have intercourse more frequently are more likely to have boys.[40] His investigation was stimulated by earlier German data showing that more male than female babies are born if intercourse is engaged in earlier in the menstrual cycle. The observation that more males are born during the usually more active first eighteen months of marriage, and that women under twenty-five years of age have more boys than women over thirty-five further supports this theory. Such a hypothesis may explain why more boys are born after wars, when sex-starved soldiers return to

[37] Helen Diner, *Mothers and Amazons*, p. 71. It is further noted that the notion that females were the product of the left testicle may well have been part (or the result) of a male chauvinism that found its way into both language and behavior. Thus, just as the word *black,* in another context, meant "dirty" or implied gloom, so does *left* imply something sinister or clumsy. In French, *gauche* means either "left" or "awkward," and *Les Gauches* refers to the Radical Party. In English, the word *sinister* means "left," but it also signifies evil; a U.S. politician whose philosophy is considered "to the left" has a hard time getting elected. The Spaniards use *siniestro* as an adjective, meaning either "on the left" or "disastrous," and, in German, *links* means "left," but, as slang, it (or *linkstrum*) can also signify homosexual behavior, and *linkisch* means "awkward." In many primitive cultures, the woman serves the man's food from his right, but she eats at his left, even as is often good etiquette in civilized societies. Also, before the days of modern psychology, an attempt was made to train left-handed children to eat and write with their right hands because it was more acceptable socially. And "it seems worth noting that practically all the Madonnas painted or sculptured in the period of real feeling, that is, approximately in the Christian centuries prior to the Renaissance, held the Christ child on their *left* arms." (Helen Diner, *Mothers and Amazons*, p. 71.)

[38] Landrum B. Shettles, "Predetermining Children's Sex," *Medical Aspects of Human Sexuality,* Vol. 5, No. 6 (June 6, 1972), p. 178.

[39] "Early Summer Favors the Birth of a Boy," *New Scientist,* Vol. 45, No. 691 (March 5, 1970), p. 448.

[40] "Why Marital Enthusiasm Upsets the Sex Ratio," *New Scientist and Science Journal,* Vol. 49, No. 735 (January 21, 1971), p. 104 and "Make More Love, Make More Boys," *Canadian Medical Association Journal,* Vol. 104, No. 11 (June 5, 1971), p. 975, both citing William James, "Cycle Day of Insemination, Coital Rate, and Sex Ratio," *Lancet,* Vol. 1, No. 7690 (January 16, 1971), p. 112.

their wives. Still another British researcher has noted a correlation between the ingestion of hard (high mineral content) water and an increased sex ratio; that is, the ratio of boy/girl births increases markedly.[41]

Landrum B. Shettles, of Columbia University's College of Physicians and Surgeons, has studied various factors that might be considered to influence the sex of offspring at fertilization. These factors include the timing of intercourse with respect to the female cycle, the timing and type of douche used, whether or not the woman achieves orgasm, the depth of penile penetration, and the quality of the spermatozoon and ovum. A male offspring is more likely to be conceived if intercourse takes place as close as possible to the moment of ovulation with prior abstinence during a given cycle. This more likely provides a fresh spermatozoon and a fresh ovum. Male offspring are favored by the use of an alkaline douche (two tablespoons of baking soda in one quart of water) immediately preceding intercourse, by the woman's achievement of orgasm, by deep penile penetration, and by the union of a fresh spermatozoon and a fresh ovum. A female offspring is more likely to be conceived if intercourse takes place no later than two to three days before ovulation, and the occurrence of intercourse ceases at that time. This more likely provides a fresh ovum and an older spermatozoon for fertilization. Female offspring are favored by the use of an acid douche (two tablespoons of white vinegar in one quart of water) immediately preceding intercourse, by the woman's failure to achieve orgasm, by shallow penile penetration, and by the union of a fresh ovum and an older sperm.[42] On what basic principles do his suggestions rest?

Human male spermatozoa (those carrying Y-chromosomes) seem to be more efficient at fertilization than the X-spermatozoa resulting in females. Why? The heads of the X-spermatozoa are bulkier because they contain 3 to 4 percent more DNA than do the heads of Y-spermatozoa. This is equivalent to a 1 percent difference in the radius of a sperm head. Thus, the lighter Y-sperm is more efficient in moving against gravitational pull than an X-sperm.[43] In addition, X- and Y-spermatozoa do not occur in approximately equal numbers. Y-spermatozoa greatly outnumber X-spermatozoa. (The reason that more females than males are born is that after fertilization the male nucleus containing the chromosomes is less likely to survive to full term.[44])

To favor the birth of a boy, it would thus seem logical to create an environment in which the smaller, more numerous Y-spermatozoa

[41] W. R. Lyster, "Sex Ratio and Hard Water," *Science Journal,* Vol. 6, No. 11 (November 1970), pp. 61–63.

[42] Landrum B. Shettles, "Predetermining Children's Sex" pp. 172, 177, 178.

[43] "Slimmer Males Win the Race to Self-Perpetuation," *New Scientist,* Vol. 55, No. 807 (August 3, 1972), p. 228.

[44] W. R. Lyster, "Sex Ratio and Hard Water," p. 61.

can outdistance the larger X-spermatozoa. Indeed, conditions favoring conception (fertilization) favor male offspring. Conditions impeding conception favor the birth of a girl. The age (viability) of the spermatozoa and ova are also important factors in determining whether conception occurs. Therefore, the availability of a fresh spermatozoon and a fresh ovum (as near to ovulation as possible) favors a male birth. A fresh ovum and an older spermatozoon would favor a female birth; this is more likely if sexual intercourse occurs two to three days before ovulation. Deep penile penetration during emission results in the deposition of spermatozoa near the favorable alkaline secretions within the cervix. This, combined with the alkaline orgasmal secretions and an alkaline douche that is salubrious for spermatozoa, makes it possible for the Y-spermatozoa to outdistance the X-spermatozoa in the competitive race to the awaiting ovum. The lack of the female orgasm adds no alkalinity to a sperm's environment. An acid douche promotes its acidity. (It should be noted, however, that douches should not be used without a physician's advice.) Shallow penile penetration results not only in the emission of the spermatozoa-containing ejaculum into the more hostile acid vaginal environment, but it also increases the distance that the spermatozoa must travel to fertilize the ovum. By using these concepts, it has been reported that couples can select the genetic sex of their children with an 80 to 85 percent chance of success.[45] Not all scientists accept Shettles' suggestions. Nevertheless, they certainly merit trial.

ADOPTION

The ancient Greeks and Romans adopted children to assure continuance of the family line, thereby protecting property. The child was secondary. Today, he is primary. He needs a secure home and love. The adopting parents must be able to give both.

The depth of relationship between adopted child and parents is no less profound than that with the biological parents. The risk is mutual.

Unfortunately, many an unmarried mother is unaware of the strict privacy available at social welfare agencies. Her child is then placed through a "black market" agency. In this way, she disadvantages both herself and her child. There is yet another problem. There are twice as many nonwhite illegitimate children as white. Yet, most adopted children are white.

A couple considering adoption should seek help from the social welfare agency in their community. They will further profit from conferences with the family attorney and physician.

[45] Landrum B. Shettle, "Predetermining Children's Sex," p. 178.

In this country between 1 and 2 percent of the population is adopted; however, this includes only those children who are brought into families in which neither parent is the biological one. A similar number of children are adopted into families in which one parent is the child's biological parent.[46] It has been observed that adopted children are brought to psychiatric treatment with considerable frequency. This may be due to the greater anxiety of the adopting parents, or to their increased awareness of the psychological problems of an adopted child. Some psychiatrists believe that such problems are somewhat more frequent among adopted children.[47]

Before the adoption takes place, the parents are frequently under stress. During the nine months of pregnancy, natural parents have time in which to build a basic beginning and basic emotional structure for parenthood. For the adopting parents, however, the waiting period may be long and filled with anxiety, rather than one of much pleasurable anticipation. Most adopting parents are, moreover, older than natural parents; they are more set in their ways and may find a new personality in their midst a demanding trial. For some parents, the adopted child may even be a symbol of infertility, which creates an unconscious hostility toward the child. In addition, an errant adopted child may be too severely judged by the parents. His childish transgressions may stimulate the parents into unconscious or even conscious condemning thoughts, such as "bad blood will tell."

The adopted child also has his problems. The need for answering the question "Who am I?" and the difficulties inherent in the search for self-identity, have already been discussed (see pages 10-11). For the adopted child the whole process may become a veritable travail. To the natural child, for example, the parents are powerful and beautiful—for a while at least. During this time (when such a child, as Erik Erikson has written "hitches his wagon to nothing less than a star") his fantasies about his parents help him to establish his own uniqueness as a person. For the adopted child, however, the fantasy has a measure of reality. He, indeed, does not know who his real parents are. The child's inability to fuse his image of the unknown parents with that of his adopted parents may fill him with anxiety. In an effort to establish continuity in his life, as well as some identity, the adopted child may even run away in search of his real parents. However, this is not common.

What are the risks, to the adopting parents, that drug abuse by the natural parents may adversely affect a child? A study of one thousand infants who were relinquished for adoption, which included chromosomal analysis of forty-one, revealed that "parental use of

[46] Marshall D. Schechter, "Is Adoption a Handicapping Condition?" *Medical Insight,* Vol. 3, No. 8 (August 1971), p. 18.

[47] Henry H. Work and Hans Anderson, "Studies in Adoption: Requests for Psychiatric Treatment," *American Journal of Psychiatry,* Vol. 127, No. 7 (January 1971), pp. 124-25.

illicit drugs does not in itself constitute a valid reason for the refusal to accept or place an infant relinquished for adoption."[48]

When should the child be told of the adoption? There is no exact time for all children; it should be individualized. There are those who insist that the child should be told as soon as possible and that the information should be affectionately, but consistently, reiterated in a variety of ways. For example, the child could routinely be introduced as one's adopted child. The theory to support this advice is that, in this way, the adopted child becomes desensitized to the knowledge. Later, the theory holds, when the child learns the meaning of adoption, he finds it more acceptable. Others dispute this; they believe that the concept of adoption means little to the very young child. The period between six and ten years of age has been suggested as the best time to tell the child about his adoption; during those years most children are usually less beset by emotional difficulties.[49] To develop a sense of identity, the adopted child will need the opportunity to develop a strong sense of self-esteem. Then, together, child and parent can come to see how they have helped one another while meeting one another's needs.[50] In this, they are like all parents and children. And that they succeed is borne out by the hundreds of thousands of happily adopted children in the United States.

THE LONELIEST ONES

Sitting up straight in her chair, almost primly, a little defiant, tightly clasping ringless fingers, she tells the social worker her name. She is nineteen and came to town eight months ago. It has been five months since she has menstruated. She is not sure who the father is. And then, suddenly, she begins to cry.

"I don't care," she says, "I hate him anyway."

Scenes like this are twice as common in this country today as they were twenty years ago. Over three hundred thousand out-of-wedlock babies were born in the United States in 1970; that was over 9 percent of the total number of births.

What do we know about the unwed mother? Who is she? What are some of her problems?

One anxiety of many an unwed mother is in her sense of being unloved. Yet often she cannot love. She may come from an over-coercive home. Perhaps her parents do not respect the person in the girl. Her individual speed and pattern of doing things are faults to be constantly corrected. She is directed and overdirected. Little do her parents realize the significance of this poetic advice:

[48] Kenneth W. Dumars, "Parental Drug Usage: Effect on Chromosomes of Progeny," *Pediatrics,* Vol. 47, No. 6 (June 1971), p. 1037.
[49] Marshall D. Schechter, "Is Adoption a Handicapping Condition?" p. 21.
[50] American Academy of Pediatrics: Committee on Adoptions, "Identity Development in Adopted Children," *Pediatrics,* Vol. 47, No. 5 (May 1971), pp. 948–49.

You may give them your love but not your thoughts,
For they have their own thoughts.
You may house their bodies but not their souls,
For their souls dwell in the house of tomorrow, which
*   you cannot visit, not even in your dreams.*
You may strive to be like them,
*   but seek not to make them like you.*[51]

Constant coercion causes anxiety in the child. It is met in various ways. The child may dilly-dally, daydream, and develop a fine "forgettory." Or the anxiety may be manifested by rebelliousness. Any parental advice then becomes a tyranny to be ignored. Moreover, the child feels unworthy. She may think everything she does is wrong. She feels rejected. She is thrown back on herself.[52] She loses the ability to give love to others. How can she again risk giving love when the people who mean the most to her, her parents, think her very existence a wrong? Out of rebellion, out of desire to retaliate, or in a desperate search for appreciation, she has sexual intercourse. But this arises from a feeling of rejection, not love.

Other girls are the victims of the opposite extreme. The parents are oversubmissive and overindulgent. No whim of the child is denied. The child is showered with unneeded gifts in such profusion that their meaning is lost. Such a girl is bored. She need consider nobody but herself. A severe anxiety about her health (hypochondriasis) may develop. As an attention-getting mechanism, it is useful. She may, moreover, fix all her expectations on the all-powerful, always sacrificing parents. Her ability to love anyone else is diminished. Even the very thought of loving someone else may be threatening. She is without discipline, without the ability to love, for to love requires discipline. Passion requires compassion. Her doting parents have impoverished her with indulgence.

The disadvantages of the unwed mother are considerably more than emotional. Some are socioeconomic. Others are manifested by an increased risk to health, even to life.

Relatively few unwed mothers give birth in private hospitals. More than 50 percent of unmarried mothers get late or no prenatal care. Eighty percent of married women, on the other hand, receive prenatal care in the first six months of pregnancy. In the first three months of pregnancy, less than 10 percent of unmarried mothers get prenatal care. But almost 50 percent of married mothers get this crucial early care in the first three months.

The poorer care of the unwed mother is apparent in the greater threat to the life of both herself and her child. Eclampsia (a toxic condition of pregnancy, once common) and syphilis are both more

---

[51] Kahlil Gibran, *The Prophet* (New York, 1923), p. 18.
[52] Percival M. Symonds, *The Dynamics of Human Adjustment* (New York, 1946), p. 552.

frequent in unmarried mothers than in married mothers. Unmarried-mother maternal death rates are over three times higher than those of married mothers. The life of the unmarried white mother is at tragic risk. Her pregnancy ends in her death eight times more often than the married white mother's. Both black and Puerto Rican unmarried mothers have a better chance of surviving pregnancy than the white unmarried mother.[53]

The reasons for this are cultural. Black and Puerto Rican unmarried mothers are generally more accepted by their families. The white unmarried pregnant girl is cruelly cast out of her milieu. Often she cannot share her great burden with those who brought her into the world. She must skulk on the perimeter of society. Former friends shun her. By delaying prenatal care as long as possible, she risks her life. Despite liberalized abortion laws, she still submits to a dangerous, illegal abortion more often than the Puerto Rican or black woman. And, much more often than they, she is killed by it.

Compared to the baby of the married mother, the baby of the unmarried mother is twice as likely to be premature, is twice as likely to die in the first month, and is twice as likely to be stillborn.

Maimed by emotional maldevelopment, more than three hundred thousand young girls of this wealthy country every year experience hazards that alienate them still further. They need help. Their help must start with the education of parents.

Moreover, too often only the plight of the unmarried mother has been considered. Whenever possible, the unmarried father should be helped.[54] The popular idea of the elderly, uneducated, totally maladjusted seducer is not accurate. In one study, most unmarried fathers were found to have at least a high school education, were but a few years older than the mother, and functioned quite adequately in school or work. Delinquency patterns were not usual. Nor is the relationship between unmarried parents so casual as has often been assumed. On the other hand both young people may be suffering emotional inadequacies established in childhood. Deferment of personal gratification for the more lasting satisfactions of societal approval is difficult enough for the mature, let alone the immature. Thus "when neither sexual partner possesses any strong identity, and when neither one is strong in the area of responsibility and maturity, each reinforces the other to satisfy personal needs, with little regard for the consequences of the act."[55]

[53]National Council on Illegitimacy, *Illegitimacy: Data and Findings for Prevention, Treatment and Policy Formulation* (October 1965), pp. 34-36.
[54]Not uncommonly, a man may question or vigorously deny that he is the father of a child. If wrongfully named, paternity blood tests may prove him right. They are not always conclusive. Only about 60 percent of men who are improperly accused may be cleared by paternity tests.
[55]Reuben Pannor, Fred Massarik, and Byron W. Evans, *The Unmarried Father,* Final Report, Children's Bureau, Welfare Administration, U.S. Department of Health, Education, and Welfare (February 1967), pp. 230-31.

some premarital 7 considerations and advisements

courtship and conquest:
animal instinct, human learning

"The snail is a hermaphrodite: male and female are incorporated into one; there is no he and no she. Perhaps that is why snails are so sluggish; they have nothing to stir them, nothing to fight for, nothing to pursue, nothing to win."[1] Almost all other creatures, however, actively differentiate between the sexes and engage in elaborate mating rituals too. The index of neither Kinsey volume on human sexual behavior contains the word *courtship*. In a discussion of animal sexuality, such an omission would be impossible. For elegance and variety, nonhuman love-planning is both instructive and humbling. The fighting fish of Siam do an underwater courtship ballet, of which the color, grace, and timing would delight the most exacting choreographer. And the female cricket knows true devotion. Responding to a phonograph record playing the ardent chirp of a long-dead male cricket, she will desert locally available swains. Hurrying a considerable distance, she will lovingly seek an approach into the record player.[2] Gift-giving, too, is not unknown to creatures that go courting. Indeed, with some species of spider, an empty-handed male may become a snack. So, instinctively, he often arrives with a fly, carefully gift-wrapped in silk. Dancing a specific pattern and carefully displaying his markings, he can only trust to luck. As for higher animals, the complex courtship that goes on among penguins, for example, or among monkeys and apes, has long fascinated zoologists.

And so, all in season, the nonhuman world is a rhythmic maneuvering of love, a pervasive, instinctive planning for new life. Instinc-

---

[1] James Kemble, *Hero Dust* (London, 1936), p. xiii. *Hermaphrodite* derives from the names Hermes (the Greek god who served as messenger to the gods) and Aphrodite (the Greek goddess of love and beauty).
[2] R. H. Smythe, *The Female of the Species* (London, 1960), p. 58.

tive, not learned. But people need to be taught the art of love. One classic "textbook" is the third-century novel by the Greek romancer Longus, *Daphnis and Chloë*. It tells the story of two innocent child lovers, a goatherd and a shepherdess, who needed instruction in the art of love. In his Introduction, Longus holds out this promise to his readers:

> For this will cure him that is sick, and rouse him that is in dumps; one that has loved, it will remember of it; one that has not, it will instruct. For there was never any yet that wholly could escape love, and never shall there be any, never so long as beauty shall be, never so long as eyes can see.[3]

Among earth's creatures, man is almost alone in becoming confused by such matters. His confusion is created by his culture, for in no other aspect of his life are his self-imposed regulations more rigid.

on the establishment of marital codes

Three hundred years ago, John Garland and his wife stood at the bar of justice in Suffolk County, Massachusetts. They had come all the way from Salisbury County to appeal their conviction by the local court, of a crime against man and God. Mrs. Garland had been delivered of a child eleven weeks too early. For this event, unblessed by their community, they had been fined five pounds.

"I and She had parents Concent to marry," John Garland protested, "had any Such Act been comited by us we could haue preuented it by marrying sooner." The untimely birth, he insisted, was due to a fall.

The prosecutor pointed a scornful finger. Garland, he rasped, hid his guilt behind a learning hardly suited to him. His contemptible quotes from "Aristottle" to prove that a child could come in the seventh month were mere deceptions. "Please to Cast an eye vpon John garland," the prosecutor exhorted the court, "they will judge Him to be no deepe man in philosophie."

The judge pondered. This was his decision:

> It was well known to the Honored Court at Salisbury that the usuall time of woman was a set time As in genesis the 18 and the 10 compared with 2 of kings the 4th & the 16 verse, the Honored Court likewise knew that that time was aboue seaven month as is the first of luke the 36 vers compared with the 39 & 40 & 57 verse of that chapter.[4]

[3]Longus, "Proem," *Daphnis and Chloë*, translated by George Thornley (New York, 1906), p. 9.
[4]From the manuscript *Early Court Files of Suffolk* (1675), No. 1412, quoted in George Elliott Howard, *A History of Matrimonial Institutions*, Vol. II (Chicago, 1904), p. 187.

The decision of the lower court at Salisbury was reversed. John Garland paid no fine. Today, despite having more accurate biological knowledge than the judge in the Garland case had, most members of this culture still live by biblical codes. Why did they develop and persist?

STABILITY AND DECAY AS SOURCES
OF MARITAL CODES

Family life of this culture is based on Judeo-Christian traditions. These can be traced to the age of the biblical Hebrew patriarchs. The family was established as an institution to provide stability and protection for the group. In the home of the ancient Hebrews, the father was the head and the mother the heart.

From the Hebrews, the early Christians got a model for building a stable family structure. From the Romans, they learned the price of excessive societal laxity and disruption of normal family life. Three Punic Wars against Carthage (in the second and third centuries B.C.) occupied Rome for over a century. These had made many Roman families enormously rich. Roman sons were constantly off at war. Fathers consequently placed their daughters in positions of wealth and indirect power. Roman women of leading families began to vie among one another and with men for power. The Elder Cato complained bitterly: "All men rule over women, we Romans rule over all men, and our wives rule over us." Even the Roman mother reflected the times. "Return with your shield, or on it," she sternly told her war-bound son. The new preoccupations of women led them to neglect their families. Contemptuously, Roman men rejected marriage. "Why do I not marry a rich wife?" asks a Roman writer. "Because I do not wish to be my wife's maid."[5] Laws penalizing celibacy were to no avail. The upper classes, remaining childless, customarily adopted children for purposes of inheritance. Divorce, previously rare, became widespread. Marriage became a cynicism. Slaves cared for children. Children were spoiled. "Expressions which would not be tolerated even from the effeminate youths of Alexandria," wrote Quintilian, "we hear from them with a smile and a kiss."[6] With the family structure crumbling, morals declined. Rome underwent a sexual revolution. Luxury and sloth replaced the formerly strict family life. The public amorality of the highborn also became a way of life for the middle classes. Other factors, such as widespread malaria and an overextended economy, certainly helped to enfeeble the once mighty empire. But a basic flaw marred Rome. The vitality of the family had been wasted. Rome collapsed. On its ruin, Christianity began to build.

[5] Quoted in Willystine Goodsell, *A History of Marriage and the Family* (New York, 1934), p. 136.
[6] Ibid., p. 152.

WHY THE RIGIDITY?
WHY THE GUILT?

The year 312 saw Christianity legally recognized by the decaying Roman Empire. Observing the social disarray about them, the early Christians were determined not to repeat the errors of their predecessors. Polygamy, practiced by the Hebrews, was rejected. Roman sexual laxity was anathema. The abortion and infanticide, the divorce and adultery of the Greeks and Romans were condemned. In this atmosphere, sexual permissiveness was out of the question. Sexuality was sin. Centuries passed before even marital coitus became more than a base need, to be tolerated only because it provided children.

This is not to say that rigid sexual regulations immediately took hold in the Christian world. Controls developed gradually. Before the end of the first millenium A.D., and during the Middle Ages, the feudal lord often was obliged to deflower the bride. In some societies all the male guests preceded the husband. This was meant to relieve the husband of the onus of causing the bride the first pain of intercourse. This custom probably originated in an earlier day. Centuries before the Christian, era, a Mesopotamian girl was obliged to visit a temple before her marriage. There she gave herself to the first male who threw a coin in her lap. Some historians suggest that the modern custom of kissing the bride is but a happy, albeit less vigorous, remnant of these practices.

This custom is not the only example of the liberal sexual attitudes of the past. In the premedieval period, trial marriage was common; it was not until 786 that the Anglo-Saxon Synod passed a decree ensuring permanence to marriage. Indeed, up to the time of the Reformation, trial marriage of one year was practiced in Scotland. In early Europe, adultery, nudity, premarital sexual intercourse, trial marriage were all freely practiced. William the Conquerer was proud of being known as William the Bastard, as illegitimacy was often no shame, but something that added an aura of importance to a person. "Bastardy was a mark of distinction because it often implied that some important person had slept with one's mother."[7] The Church, however, held fast. Gradually its precepts took hold. Yet, even as sexuality gradually became a sanctified part of marriage, restrictive rules were retained. Those who took short cuts found society harsh indeed. Why? Because their actions threatened the family as the basic unit of society and, therefore, threatened society itself. If men were to survive, it was essential that sexual expression and mating be controlled.

The Judeo-Christian culture, then, established basic marriage codes that have endured for the Western world. Often, these codes

[7]Judd Marmor, "'Normal' and 'Deviant' Sexual Behavior," *Journal of the American Medical Association*, Vol. 217, No. 2 (July 12, 1971), p. 165.

have been supported by threat and guilt, two powerful tools of Western society. "In the last analysis, guilt feelings, for most people, are simply a realization that they have failed to follow societal convictions of right and wrong."[8]

But guilt promotes anxiety. Many people who ignore marital codes may reject their own sense of guilt, but it does not go away. Prolonged, unresolved guilt may become a disease—a disease that may impair the ability of a person to function effectively, not only sexually, but in other areas of life as well.

the lover, whom all the world does not love

PRIMITIVE COURTSHIPS

The tribulations of love and courtship vary from culture to culture. Among the Macusis of Guyana, a young swain may not choose a wife until he has proved his courage. One way to demonstrate it is by allowing himself "to be sewn up in a hammock full of fire ants."[9] The hopeful Arab bridegroom of Upper Egypt displays his valor by undergoing a severe whipping by the bride's relatives.[10] The romantic maneuvering among the young of one Bolivian Indian tribe is no less hazardous:

> Ordinarily young people of nubile age are supposed to be shy of one another, and while tending herds pass one another by many times without apparently seeing each other. Around Camata, if a boy in such a situation wishes to take notice of a girl, he picks up a handful of fine earth or dust and throws it at her. This is a first step of courtship in the Jesús de Machaca region. The next time they meet, the boy picks up some fine gravel, and the girl may do likewise. If they continue to be interested this goes on until finally they throw rocks at each other. Informants told me that there were two cases of deaths in Camata during the last four years from such a cause; one woman received a fractured skull and the other a broken back.[11]

YESTERDAY'S COURTSHIPS

In 1700, the British Parliament enacted the following:

> That all women of whatever age, rank, profession or degree, whether virgin maid or widow, that shall from and after such

[8] William M. Kephart, *The Family, Society, and the Individual* (Boston, 1961), p. 117.
[9] Edward Westermarck, *The History of Human Marriage*, 5th ed., Vol. I (New York, 1921), p. 49.
[10] Ibid., p. 51.
[11] Weston La Barre, "The Aymara Indians of the Lake Titicaca Plateau, Bolivia," *American Anthropologist*, Vol. 50, No. 1, Part 2 (January 1948), p. 129.

Act impose upon, seduce and betray into matrimony any of His Majesty's subjects by means of scent, paints, cosmetic washes, artificial teeth, false hair, Spanish wool, iron stays, hoops, high-heeled shoes or bolstered hips, shall incur the penalty of the law now in force against witchcraft and like misdemeanors, and that the marriage upon conviction shall stand null and void.[12]

It was perhaps such legislation that prompted the degree of cautious honesty, if not outright optimism, so often proclaimed as proper in eighteenth-century English books on model letterwriting. One such volume, the *New London Letter Writer,* includes a model letter entitled, "From a Young Lady After Having Smallpox to her Lover." Apparently, the young man had led her to believe that "the beauties of my person were only exceeded by the perfection of my mind." She was, therefore, not regretting too much the loss of her good looks, for "it gives you a happy opportunity to prove yourself to be a man of truth and veracity."[13]

Many years later, in the nineteenth century, English lovers, for reasons of their own, were wont to go skating. Since chaperones rarely skated, they were benched on the sidelines. In 1876, *Punch* published a cartoon of these scandalous goings-on.[14] Not all was raucous humor, however. A Mrs. Burton Kingsland, composing for the *Ladies Home Journal* (*circa* 1900), prepared this brief, but presumably effective, speech to be made by a young lady whose debauched swain had slipped his arm about her waist: "Don't you think it rather cowardly for a man to act toward a girl as you are doing when she has trusted him and is in a measure powerless to resist such familiarity?"[15]

Things have changed.

MODERN COURTSHIP

In this culture, basic training for mating begins early, with group dating. This is followed by random dating. Perhaps it is during a shopping tour with their mothers that modern children gain the first unconscious tips for random dating. Random dating is just shopping around. One does not have to buy. There is time for window-shopping. If one chooses, one may come in and browse. Sometimes, a small investment is made. By telephone, one learns a lot and overcomes much. Everybody gets stung a little, some more than others. But one gets to know the game. And, in the end (hopefully), one sees enough and adds up enough experience to get some idea of what

[12] Quoted in Henry A. Bowman, *Marriage for Moderns* (New York, 1960), p. 129.
[13] E. S. Turner, *A History of Courting* (London, 1954), p. 121.
[14] Ibid., p. 178.
[15] Ibid., p. 195.

one needs, what to look for, and what commitment may be safely made. People of some other countries view random dating with astonishment. For them, the sheer number of dates per teen-ager is fickleness amounting to immorality. And the absence of a chaperone—an open invitation to family dishonor.

Admittedly superficial and often hurtfully competitive, random dating is instructive as a prelude to the next stage of mating, "going steady" (a status often anxiously sought both by high school and by many college students). Since the random dater is but a recent graduate of the shy group-dating system, his sexual behavior is usually not a problem. It is not until the going-steady stage that the problems associated with sexual relationships arise. Fearful that their children will drift or be forced into a poor marriage, many parents who regarded random dating with tolerance are suspicious of the going-steady stage of courtship. Nevertheless, going steady does relieve the competitive pressures of random dating. Moreover, it gives priceless training in such virtues as tolerance, patience, and gentleness that will be useful in the married state.

Characteristic of a few college attachments is a form of trial engagement called "pinning." Many, probably most, students do not consider pinning of significance. For some, however, it does provide an opportunity to become better acquainted before the more formal social step of an engagement is made. Since the commitment is not as binding, most girls will remove a pin without embarrassment. On the debit side, pinning provides an opportunity for sexual or other exploitation. A "big man on campus," for example, may trade his pin for sexual privileges with an otherwise unnoticed girl. He is like the lover described in Shakespeare's *Taming of the Shrew,* "who wooed in haste and means to wed at leisure." Today, whatever the commitment may be, a great many young people have replaced the pin with some other symbol—a bracelet, an Indian charm, or the like. Some have dispensed with all outward intent and, indeed, with the traditional courtship period as well. Others use the period formerly devoted to courtship for experimentation in living together. The extent of these arrangements, and their effect on the individual and on society, are being studied.

It is in the turbulent, searching years of adolescence that a person must begin learning the mating game. In this anxious time of searching for a self-acceptable self, of trying to settle on a life's work, of attempting to cope with overwhelming bodily changes, and of beginning a separation from one's parents—it is in these years that the dating dilemma occurs. The dilemma is this: without being clearly told what is expected of him, the teen-ager is nevertheless given to understand that much is expected of him. "Grow up," he is told, yet he is forbidden to do what he sees grownups do. Driven by urges he has not yet learned to understand or control, he attempts to answer them as grownups do. With the paraphernalia of sexual activity, such as cars and condoms, readily available, what is missing? A chaperone? In this society, she is all but extinct.

premarital sexual standards

Strephon kissed me in the spring,
   Robin in the fall,
But Colin only looked at me
   And never kissed at all.

Strephon's kiss was lost in jest,
   Robin's lost in play,
But the kiss in Colin's eyes
   Haunts me night and day.[16]

This poem tells of emotions of a distant day. But is also tells something about people. In this age of laboratory-observed sexual intercourse and a welter of sexual statistics, it has its place. People, not numbers, do the loving. No matter how informative the numbers seem to be about people, each person has a secret heart. Discussions of premarital sexual activity are incomplete without an exploration of individual answers to a variety of questions. In what context does the premarital sexual experience occur? What does premarital sexual intercourse do to the relationship of the participants? How much love is involved? Uses and abuses of sexuality are numerous. Valid uses of sexual intercourse vary from reproduction and pleasure to deep desires to share and cooperate with and to give and belong to someone. Its abuses range from destructive domination to sheer revenge. How much premarital sexual activity is based on emotional problems having little to do with love needs? How much results from genuine mutual caring and how much from attempts to rebel or to escape anxiety or other problems, such as loneliness or a sense of personal worthlessness? How often does a young person engage in a premarital sexual experience because of the conviction that any pain or humiliation must be endured to get love? When is premarital sexual intercourse an exploitation of one person by another? Does it relieve these nonsexual problems or merely accentuate them? Is the young person who has just terminated a first premarital sexual experience more vulnerable to becoming promiscuous? Is the decision to engage in a premarital sexual experience based on a realistic appraisal of the self, or is it part of a glamorized view of a constantly shifting "scene"? Statistics of coital rates among the unmarried

---

[16] Sara Teasdale, "The Look," in Marjorie Barrows, ed., *The Quintessence of Beauty and Romance* (Chicago, 1955), p. 151.

hardly reveal adequate information about the actual causes or significance of these rates. Moreover, although this discussion is primarily concerned with premarital coitus, premarital sexual experiences include varying degrees of petting that stop just short of coitus. More research is needed in all these areas. And that research must be tempered with the understanding that premarital sexual experiences, like all experiences, affect different people differently.

PREMARITAL SEXUAL INTERCOURSE: A DIFFERENCE OF OPINION

One study[17] of college students and their parents indicates that a majority of girls (66 percent) and boys (52 percent) considered sexual intercourse between engaged couples acceptable. This compared with only 20 percent of their fathers and 17 percent of their mothers approving. That so many of the boys—48 percent of them—considered premarital intercourse unacceptable is not surprising. Some young men still expect to marry a virgin yet attempt to seduce every girl they date. In *Hamlet*, Ophelia notes this male paradox in a little song that relates a lovers' conversation:

> *Young men will do 't, if they come to 't,*
>
> · · ·
>
> *Quoth she, "before you tumbled me,*
> *You promised me to wed."*
> *He answers:*
> *"So would I ha' done, by yonder sun,*
> *An thou hadst not come to my bed."*[18]

Another college study[19] of the late 1960s emphasizes the apparent difference in opinion between the generations. Only 55 percent of coeds questioned considered virginity at marriage very important. (In recent years this percentage may have diminished in some parts of the country.) Eighty-eight percent of the coeds' mothers considered it very important.

WHY THE DISPARITY?

the parental dilemma

Why are mothers generally less tolerant of premarital sexual intercourse than their daughters? One reason is that although mother and

---

[17] Seymour L. Halleck, "Sex and Mental Health on the Campus," *Journal of the American Medical Association,* Vol. 200, No. 8 (May 22, 1967), pp. 684-90.
[18] William Shakespeare, *Hamlet,* IV.v.61-66.
[19] Seymour L. Halleck, "Sex and Mental Health on the Campus," pp. 684-90.

daughter share the same basic cultural values, their positions within that culture are quite different. So are the pressures to which they are exposed. It is much easier for an anthropologist to explain the benefits of premarital coitus among South Sea Islanders than it is for a mother to explain them in Dubuque, Iowa.

Maternal disapproval of premarital coitus may seem particularly incongruous in light of available data. Some studies indicate that women do not regret their own premarital coitus; others regret that they were virgins before they married.[20] But such data needs further analysis. For example, one should obtain some evaluation of the marital happiness of the women in either group. A woman who is sexually starved in an unhappy marriage might regret either premarital virginity or coitus. Among the other questions that would need answering are those that are relative to the religious faith of the woman as well as the place in which she grew to maturity. Feelings on the day after the first intercourse were reported to be much more negative among students at an unidentified Mormon university than those among students at Purdue. Men and women at the University of Copenhagen reported less negative feelings than either American group.[21] True, the data on which this report was made is a decade old. In some cases the figures may have changed. Yet this is further evidence that the effect of culture on the individual's feelings about premarital sexual intercourse is considerable. The mother's cultural exposure may be a decisive influence on her later evaluation of her own premarital coital experience as well as that of her daughter.

Moreover, the fact that the mother reports no regret of her own premarital coital experience is no indication that she will prefer it for her daughter. The reasons for this are as complex as they are various. Consider but a few of them. A woman may believe (rightly or wrongly) that her own mother failed to provide her with a firm sense of values. She may think (again rightly or wrongly) that she has successfully imparted this sense to her own daughter. Thus, the mother may feel her own premarital sexual experience to be understandable and not to be regretted but that of her daughter to be censurable. Another mother may think she does not regret premarital coitus, say so in a questionnaire, and yet unconsciously regret it nevertheless. A long hidden guilt may need to be released; this may result in restrictions on the daughter. A mother may rationalize her own episodes of premarital coitus in still other ways. In this culture, she was taught that premarital intercourse was bad. In her case, however, she only remembers that it was good. Why? Because she loved the man. Yet she still may not sanction such an experience

[20] Alfred C. Kinsey, Wardell B. Pomeroy, Clyde E. Martin, and Paul H. Gebhard, *Sexual Behavior in the Human Female* (Philadelphia, 1953), p. 316.

[21] Robert O. Blood, *Marriage* (New York, 1969), p. 148, citing Harold T. Christensen and George R. Carpenter, "Value-Behavior Discrepancies Regarding Premarital Coitus," *American Sociological Review*, Vol. 27 (1962), pp. 66-74.

for her daughter. She knows that boys are often taught that pre-marital sex is bad—for girls, that is. And some men are not above showing their own negative feelings to the unmarried girl with whom they have coitus without any commitment.

the young person's dilemma

The increasing percentage of college students sanctioning premarital permissiveness is emphasized by their frank approach to the discussion of sexuality. Their very openness gives young people an advantage over their elders. On many college campuses, subjects such as masturbation, homosexual behavior, and oral-genital sexuality are not taboo in group discussions. Nonetheless, many young people still receive much of their information about sexual behavior from the uninformed. This can be damaging. Those who desire to help the sexually ignorant must add informed reason to rules. An increasing number of young people, on and off campuses, recognize this as a responsibility of parenthood. Although it has been argued that increased knowledge about sexuality encourages premarital sexual experiences, Kinsey's studies indicate that premarital coitus was highest in the noncollege group. There is some evidence that these formerly noncollege attitudes toward premarital coitus are now being adopted by some college students, but this is true only to a degree, and this change in attitude is not necessarily due to increased education about sexuality, as will be indicated below.

There is evidence to indicate that the majority of today's college students do not carry out their permissive attitudes as much as is supposed. There is, in short, a difference between attitude and action. To some extent this disparity arises because of an honest respect for another person's decision. The tolerance of differing opinions that is traditional in this country now seems to be extending to other people's sexual behavior. It is in this area that increased knowledge has had a marked effect. Today a person may try to understand and be tolerant of both group sex and abstinence, yet accept neither as a personal code.

SOCIETAL CONFUSION ABOUT SEXUALITY

On January 13, 1668, the English diarist Samuel Pepys wrote that he had "stopped at Martin's, my bookseller, where I saw the French book which I did think to have had for my wife to translate . . . but when I come to look in it, it is the most bawdy, lewd book that ever I saw . . . so that I was ashamed of reading in it." By February 8, he had overcome his shame enough to buy the book. On the next evening, having fortified himself with "a mighty good store of wine," he read the "mighty lewd work, but yet not amiss for a sober man once to read over to inform himself of the villainy of the world." [22]

These entries are perhaps the first written references in English to what was then considered a pornographic work. They show Pepys to be a sexual man striving to fit well into his times. The conflict between what he felt and what he saw (and did) is reflective of human history. It has led to much inconsistency about sexuality.

In 1782 the president of Harvard successfully prevented the licensing of a tavern near the college so "that the morals of the youth educated here should, as far as possible, be preserved untainted." [23] Shortly thereafter, a brothel was opened at that very location. So, confusion about sexual matters is not new. The difference today is that this confusion is being questioned more openly.

Today young people see many incongruities in the sexual attitudes of their culture. [24] Most people in this country, including those who condemn premarital coitus, believe in free courtship. But free courtship encourages premarital sexual experimentation. Similarly, love is considered to be a prerequisite for marriage. There are studies that indicate that the majority of the young women do engage in premarital intercourse do so in a context of love. [25] Many people believe that contraceptive knowledge increases premarital permissiveness, but there is little evidence that this is generally true. Indeed, as will be seen, the so-called sexual revolution began over fifty years ago— long before sophisticated contraceptives, such as the pill, were common knowledge. These are but a few of the conflicting factors confronting the young person trying to make up his mind about premarital sexual behavior. What is happening?

THE PACKARD STUDY OF COLLEGE COITAL RATES

One investigator recently wrote:

Since approximately the time of World War I, there is no strong evidence that the rates of premarital coitus have been

---

[22] David Foxon, *Libertine Literature in England, 1660–1745* (New York, 1965), pp. 5–6.

[23] Item 231, quoted in Charles Hamilton Galleries, *Auction Catalogue*, No. 54 (December 9, 1971).

[24] Nor are many of these incongruities understandable. "The female body has now become acceptable matter for open discussion and viewing, even by the most prudish. Public service announcements recommend a Pap smear or suggest that once a month, while bathing, a woman should palpate her breasts as instructed by her physician. But the male body is still taboo. Cancer of the testes and penis, two of the most obvious and deforming of male neoplasms [new growths] (responsible for up to 3% of all male cancers, 18% to 20% in an uncircumcised population) and usually attacking those in the prime of life, are never mentioned to the public. Can you imagine the public ad: 'Look your penis over by pulling back the foreskin. Feel your testicles once per month to check their size and firmness'?" (Robert B. Sanford and Barton Tannenbaum, "Gonadal Liberation," *Journal of the American Medical Association*, Vol. 216, No. 3 [April 19, 1971], p. 511.)

[25] *Sexuality and Man*, compiled and edited by the Sex Information and Education Council of the United States (New York, 1970), p. 43, citing Ira L. Reiss, *The Social Context of Premarital Sexual Permissiveness* (New York, 1967), pp. 45–47, 87–88.

increasing. Therefore, the belief that premarital sexual experience is much more common, especially for girls, since the end of World War II, is not supported by available research evidence . . . For the female, premarital coitus usually depends on strong emotional commitment and plans for marriage. The Terman, Burgess and Wallin, and Kinsey studies reported premarital coitus only with men they eventually married.[26]

But it should be emphasized that this and other studies were made some years ago. They relate not to today's college students but to their parents and grandparents. Within limitations the sexual activities of young people today can be compared with data gathered decades ago by varying sampling techniques. They cannot, however, be logically measured by these data.

In a study reported in 1968 by Vance Packard, an attempt was made to ascertain premarital coitus rates among juniors and seniors from all regions of the United States. A "College Checklist" was distributed to twenty-one hundred junior and senior students at twenty-one U.S. colleges and universities. At each of the twenty-one institutions one hundred students received the checklist. If the schools were coeducational, fifty of the checklists went to males and fifty to females. Of the schools, seven were in the East, five in the Midwest, three in the South, four in the Southwest, and two in the Northwest. Two all-male and two all-female colleges were included. Although these were located in the East, all four drew their students from the entire country. Two schools were church-related—one Protestant, the other Catholic. Both were in the Midwest. The mean age of the students was just under twenty-one. Great care was exercised to respect privacy and insure accuracy of reporting. Sixty-seven percent of the questionnaires were returned—1,393 of the 2,100—of which 665 were from males and 728 from females. The work lacks much in method and as interpretative social science. Some results, to be viewed within these limitations, are:

1. The coital experience of today's college male seems to have increased little since earlier studies. In the 1940s, for example, 51 percent of Alfred Kinsey's group of college-educated "younger generation" had reported that they were coitally experienced by age twenty-one. In the Packard report, the percentage was only slightly higher, 57.

2. Among the junior and senior female respondents, 43 percent reported coital experience. Bearing in mind the hazard of comparing results of present and earlier studies, one can nevertheless suggest that this represents a 60 percent increase over any data gathered before 1960. Only 27 percent of the college-educated females in the

[26]Robert Bell, *Premarital Sex in a Changing Society,* quoted in Lillian Cohen Kovar, *Faces of the Adolescent Girl* (Englewood Cliffs, N.J., 1968), p. 30.

Kinsey group had reported coitus by the time they were twenty-one. Despite this, it should be noted that most junior and senior women in the group remained virgins, as did 43 percent of junior and senior men. This hardly supports the concept that promiscuity is a general practice among U.S. college students.

3. Coital rates by regions, as reported by this study, are as follows:

	MEN	WOMEN
South	69%	32%
East	64%	47%
West	62%	48%
Midwest	46%	25%
National totals	57%	43%

The variance by region is striking. The "double standard" in the South, for example, is apparent. In that region more than twice as many college men as women experience coitus. The relatively low rates in the Midwest support results from regional studies in that area. Several previous studies, wrongly applied by some to the entire U.S. college population, were merely based on regional results. The unreliability of such a procedure can be illustrated by comparing the regional percentages with the national percentages in the Packard report.[27]

THE "MYTH OF AN ABSTINENT PAST AND PROMISCUOUS PRESENT"[28]

Compared to previous generations, the prevalence of unwed teen-age mothers has risen markedly. This fact has often been used to support the idea that today's teen-agers experience more sexual intercourse than formerly. But this is disputed by an analysis of the changing nature of menstruation during the adolescent years. In both this

[27] Summarized from Vance Packard, *The Sexual Wilderness* (New York, 1967), Chapters 9–11 and Appendixes. Other more recent studies of the incidence of premarital coitus appear to substantiate Packard's findings. One recent review in this country resulted in the conclusion that "the best available data indicate that about 60 percent of unmarried college girls remain virgins throughout college. It is also noteworthy that, although young people are more likely today than previously to consider sexual intercourse within the context of a close, trusting, exclusive, and relatively enduring relationship, they continue generally to reject casual, indiscriminate, or promiscuous sexuality." (Irving B. Weiner, "Premarital Sex Among Coeds," *Medical Aspects of Human Sexuality*, Vol. 6, No. 5 [May 1972], p. 177, citing his review "Perspectives on the Modern Adolescent," *Psychiatry*, Vol. 35, No. 2 [February 1972], pp. 20–31.) The 1972 report by the Commission on Population Growth and the American Future cites a national study of unmarried teen-aged girls that "revealed that 14 percent of the 15-year-olds and up to 44 percent of 19-year-olds reported having sexual relations. Only 20 percent of these girls used contraceptives regularly. Such a low incidence of contraceptive use is particularly significant when less than half of these girls knew when during the monthly cycle a girl can become pregnant." (*Population and the American Future*, A Report of the Commission on Population Growth and the American Future [New York, 1972], p. 136, citing John F. Kanter and Melvin Zelnik, "Sexuality, Contraception, and Pregnancy Among Pre-Adult Females in the United States" [prepared for the Commission, 1972].)

[28] Phillips Cutright, "The Teen-Age Sexual Revolution and the Myth of an Abstinent Past," *Family Planning Perspectives*, Vol. 4, No. 1 (January 1972), pp. 24–31.

country and Europe, adolescents begin to menstruate (*menarche*) at a younger age than did the adolescents of previous generations. "The present mean age at menarche in the United States (12.54 years) implies that 94 percent of girls aged 17.5 years are fully fecund [fertile]. When the mean age of menarch was 16.5 years, around 1870 in Europe, only 13 percent of girls were fully fecund at age 17.5." [29] In the United States, the average age of menarche declined one year in the period from the 1930s to the 1960s. Thus, today's teen-ager has an increased risk of pregnancy. One reason for the earlier menarche and longer fertile period of the modern teen-ager is her improved preadolescent health and nutrition.[30] These factors also reduce the number of spontaneous abortions and, therefore, increase the number of illegitimate births.

> *In the past, relatively poor health conditions may have moderated the consequences of nonmarital teenage sex. Improved health conditions appear to have increased the chances that an out-of-wedlock conception will be carried to term (hence, become visible, and a problem), and have also increased the capacity of sexually active young girls to conceive . . . Aside from substantial increases in premarital sex among young whites with their future husbands, we find no evidence that a change in nonmarital sex of "revolutionary" proportions has occurred since 1940 among the white or nonwhite teenagers.*[31]

These conclusions are based on statistical analyses that also include the effects of such variables as fetal loss and contraceptive use.

AN ANALYSIS BY GAGNON AND SIMON

Does the increased proportion of nonvirginal college girls indicate a sexual revolution? A superficial glance at the statistics might bring a quick affirmative reply. Unfortunately this is the kind of affirmation that is all too characteristic of many anxious observers of sexual mores today. A careful analysis of the Packard data fails to support the prevalent notion that premarital coitus has materially increased in the past forty odd years. As Gagnon and Simon have written about the prevalence of premarital coitus:

> *It does not appear that there is any body of research evidence leading to a belief that the figures generated by Kinsey et al.*

---

[29] Ibid., p. 24.

[30] Research with mice has indicated that although dietary protein has an accelerating effect on the ovulation of prepubescent mice, the presence of mature male mice (or their odors) seems to have a much greater influence. The researchers observe, "[The fact that] social stimulation was more effective than protein intake may have relevance to the phenomenon of accelerated sexual maturation in human females." ("The Male Presence," *Scientific American*, Vol. 226, No. 6 [June 1972], p. 53.)

[31] Ibid., pp. 30–31.

*for the period 1925–45 from an admittedly limited sample have
radically changed. Data recently gathered for Mr. Vance
Packard indicate there may be an increase in the proportion
of college-going females who are not virgins. The ultimate
meaning of these figures, however, is still in doubt. The proportion of a population having coitus before marriage can only be
calculated from a population that has completed the premarital
period, that is, from interviews with those married. What
Packard's data do indicate is that for the college-educated the
arena for premarital coitus has moved from the post-college to
the college level.*[32]

Among girls who do engage in premarital sexual intercourse is
the actual frequency of coitus increasing, and is it occurring with a
greater number of different men? It would seem not. In this country
the average age at which girls first have coitus has not declined. The
average age at which girls first marry has declined, although it has
recently stabilized. Thus young people have, on the average, fewer
years in which to engage in premarital sexual activity. Gagnon and
Simon conclude that "the evidence that girls now have intercourse
with a larger number of males than in the past must also rest upon
very weak grounds."[33]

The very insignificance of the increase in the percentage of
coitally experienced college men (as revealed by the Packard data)
may well have a special significance. Kinsey found that young men
in the lower socioeducational levels engaged in premarital coitus with
a much greater number of girls and to a considerably greater extent
than did young men in the upper socioeducational groups. That was
more than twenty-five years ago. In the last two decades, the number
of men from the lower socioeconomic levels that go on to college
has increased. In an educational milieu that their fathers did not have,
they are meeting middle-class men (and women) with middle-class
values. It is reasonable to believe that the long-established middle-
class patterns, such as deferment of gratification, so characteristic
of a striving group, are being assimilated by a new population. "It
is therefore possible," write Gagnon and Simon, "that previously
discovered high rates of coitus on the part of lower class men may
be declining towards the lower middle class patterns . . . If middle
and lower class patterns converge, it will be far closer to the style
of the former than the latter."[34]

And so there is considerable reason to seriously question the
highly advertised notion that premarital sexual intercourse without
commitment is more prevalent than formerly, that it is occurring with
greater frequency among those who do practice it, and that promis-

[32] John H. Gagnon and William Simon, "Prospects for Changes in American Sexual Patterns,"
Medical Aspects of Human Sexuality, Vol. 4, No. 1 (January 1970), p. 103.
[33] Ibid.
[34] Ibid.

cuous sexual behavior without rules is the way of life among young people today. "What is observed is a continued development of a process which has continued for some forty years in American society . . . the mating process has become more and more one of exchanging increasing levels of sexual intimacy on the part of the female for increasing emotional commitments on the part of the male." [35] If a major change in the pattern of premarital coitus had occurred in the past forty years, two factors would have been recognized as contributing much to that change. First, unmarried women would be having sexual intercourse with a large number of men without marriage plans with any of them; second, it would be the woman's responsibility to prevent pregnancy. However, the reverse is true. When premarital coitus occurs, it is usually in the context of a marital commitment. And contraception has generally remained the responsibility of the male. The unmarried woman in this country who does engage in premarital coitus does not usually use contraceptives in order to have sexual intercourse with a variety of uncommitted men.[36]

Why, then, have so many people been led to think otherwise? First, there has been a delay in the recognition of the sexual revolution that began almost fifty years ago. Second, the open mind of the citizen is a great receptacle for gossip and exceptions. As was the case with their parents and grandparents, this generation of college students has not escaped the accusatory press. Some newspapers, conveniently ignoring the behavior of most students, publish the flamboyant opinions or actions of the smaller percentage. There is a relatively small group of unmarried young people whose sexual behavior has become strikingly less than ordinary. But as one student counselor of long experience recently noted:

> *The much-publicized growing sexual promiscuity is not general practice on the campus. Shyness, introversion, vestigial guilt, self-doubt, and the fear of rejection keep students from the practice of their preaching, even with pills and intrauterine devices to reduce their fear of pregnancy. Actually, premarital pregnancies are on the wane, "sleeping around" is not admired*

---

[35] Ibid.

[36] Sociologist Ira L. Reiss considers "the causal connection between birth control pills and participation in premarital sexual intercourse on the part of the young . . . quite difficult to establish." Pointing out that "starting in the late 1960's a rise in premarital sexual intercourse did seem to occur particularly among college girls," he nevertheless cautions that "this is not by any means fully substantiated." Nevertheless, "most of the small studies done since 1965 do seem to find that the proportion of 20-year-old college girls who are nonvirginal reaches about 40% . . . I would think," he continues, "that basic attitudes would have to change before a woman would participate in premarital intercourse and use the pill . . . The paths leading to these attitudes do not depend as much on the availability of the pill as they do on such factors as love experiences with men, exploration of one's own sexuality, and the general acceptant sexual attitude that prevails in close friends and elsewhere in the social context." (Ira L. Reiss, "The Pill and Adolescent Sexuality," *Medical Aspects of Human Sexuality*, Vol. 6, No. 6 [June 1972], p. 178.

and premarital sex is practiced most often in a semiresponsible and monogamous relationship." [37]

There are people in every culture who see a sexual revolution as mankind's salvation. Others see it as mankind's destruction. It is neither.

As one looks around, most young people, even those who protest, are busily going about the business of mate selection that will eventuate in marriage and children. Among the vast silent, but not necessarily happy, middle class that still dominates the landscape of American youth, getting married and getting a job and a house are still their central concerns. What else was really expected to happen? What was expected was that young people, when the constraints on freedom of all sorts were released, would do what adults thought they might do (but also would not have): go out and have a sexual ball. [38]

It did not happen, of course. And it is to the credit of young people that they are so patient with those elders who thought it would. Whether in Samoa or Dubuque, sexual behavior in a culture changes rather slowly.

FOUR PATTERNS OF PREMARITAL SEXUAL BEHAVIOR

It is unlikely that over 150 million people in this country will ever agree on a single standard of premarital sexual behavior. Not one, but several, patterns of behavior are inevitable. The Sex Information and Education Council of the United States has summarized the present premarital sexual standards of the people of this nation, and have classified these standards into four groups:

Abstinence, the formal standard forbidding intercourse to both sexes; the Double Standard, the Western world's oldest standard, which allows males to have greater access to coitus than females; Permissiveness with Affection, a standard growing in popularity, according to which intercourse is accepted for both sexes when a stable affectionate relationship is present; and Permissiveness without Affection, according to which coitus is accepted for both sexes on a voluntary basis regardless of affec-

[37] Robert E. Kavanaugh, "The Grim Generation," *Psychology Today*, Vol. 2, No. 5 (October 1968), p. 55.
[38] John H. Gagnon and William Simon, "Prospects for Changes in American Sexual Patterns," p. 110.

tion. This last standard has a quite small number of followers, but it is most newsworthy and thereby misleads the public as to the size of its following.[39]

promiscuity: sexual behavior without rules

In the present context, promiscuity refers to indiscriminate sexual behavior. Promiscuous men and women who have sexual intercourse do so without rules. As a chronic behavior pattern promiscuous sexual behavior is often seen among those who fear love. They are afraid to be committed, to be vulnerable. To them, love is not a fulfillment but a threat (see page 22). Promiscuity may be a symptom of deep-seated unmet needs. The promiscuous woman may have had an unresponsive mother. Hungry for affection, she turned to her father. As an adult she seeks other sources of affection. Her constant search involves her in numerous short-lived sexual experiences. Sometimes promiscuity is the unhappy result of severe childhood denigration. The man who has numerous liaisons with women whom he considers inferior to himself may be seeking revenge on an over-critical mother. Some college students, separated from their parents for the first time, attempt to relieve their anxiety through promiscuous behavior.

Some people are sexually promiscuous because they fear that abstinence is harmful to health. There is no doubt that, for some, prolonged sexual repression may give rise to emotional problems. However, an extremely high percentage of patients undergoing psychiatric care can hardly be considered to be repressed. A recent survey conducted of twenty-four psychiatrists caring for 107 unmarried female students at a Midwestern university revealed that "86 percent had had sexual relations with at least one person, and almost three-fourths (72 percent) had relations with more than one person . . . Patients may be promiscuous but the population is not."[40] In this respect, however, further study of some of the nonvirginal college women of the Packard report[41] might have been helpful. As was stated above, a considerable percentage had reported coitus with "several" or "many" males. Whether any of these young women were receiving psychiatric therapy is not known.

It is by no means here inferred that promiscuous sexual behavior inevitably leads to severe emotional distress for everyone. But neither does abstinence inevitably result in emotional illness. The former president of the American Academy of Psychoanalysis recently wrote: "There is no reason to believe that one will develop a mental or physical illness unless one's sex needs are satisfied, or that an

[39] *Sexuality and Man,* p. 40.
[40] Seymour L. Halleck, "Sex and Mental Health on the Campus" pp. 684-90.
[41] Vance Packard, *The Sexual Wilderness,* p. 163.

individual patient's sex life must be paramount in his emotional adjustment."[42] Still another psychiatrist supports this statement in these words: "The proposition that gratification of sexual needs is highly correlated with mental health seems to be at least questionable."[43]

SEX WITHOUT PASSION

In recently examining the causes of student despair, a Midwestern psychiatrist discussed the campus "elite" group. They are so named because of their considerable influence on other students. Devoted to the present, apprehensive of the future, the members of this group work actively, if intermittently, for political causes. Their attitude toward sexual expression is certainly more casual than that of the average student. Halleck writes of them:

> No one doubts . . . that the elite group (in contrast to the student population as a whole) are having intimate relations with a greater variety of partners than ever before. Elite students insist that they do so only if a relationship is meaningful. Sometimes this is true. More often, however, this is a pious rationalization . . . Rollo May, professor of graduate psychology at New York University, has described the new sexuality as sex without passion . . . There is reason to doubt the capacity of such students to make successful marriages . . . The student psychiatrist sees more and more recently married couples who find themselves unable to tolerate the possibility of loving one person intimately or remaining faithful to that person . . . The new era of promiscuity seems to have done little to enhance the female student's image of herself as a productive and responsible person. The elite female student shows little inclination to seek a career but seems to be trapped in a new feminine mystique which deprives her of meaningful goals and self-respect. Her status as a whole person is subtly degraded.[44]

Almost five hundred years ago, the Dutch theologian Erasmus may have best described the true pain of the promiscuous: "I ask you: will he who hates himself love anyone? Will he who does not get along with himself agree with another? Or will he who is disagreeable and irksome to himself bring pleasure to any? No one would say so, unless he were himself more foolish than Folly."[45]

[42]Leon Salzman, "Recently Exploded Sexual Myths," *Medical Aspects of Human Sexuality,* Vol. 1, No. 1 (September 1967), p. 9.
[43]Seymour L. Halleck, "Sex and Mental Health on the Campus," pp. 684-90.
[44]Seymour L. Halleck, "The Roots of Student Despair," *Think,* Vol. 33, No. 2 (March-April 1967), pp. 22-23.
[45]Erasmus, "The Praise of Folly," in Louis Kronenberger, ed., *The Pleasure of Their Company* (New York, 1946), p. 564.

searching for someone to marry

WHY MARRY?

"We who dwell in the heart of solitude are always the victims of self-doubt. Forever and forever in our loneliness, shameful feelings of inferiority will rise up suddenly to overwhelm us in a poisonous flood of horror, disbelief, and desolation, to sicken and corrupt our health and confidence."[46]

Thomas Wolfe could make the despair of solitude seem to be a stimulating episode. It may be. But as a way of life solitude is nothing to be desired. As the Creator observed: "It is not good that the man should be alone" (Genesis 2:18).

Basically, men who are alone seek wives, and single women husbands, so that they will not be alone. True, there are other reasons, such as societal pressure. But, by far the greatest majority of ordinary people seek a meaningful, sharing relationship with another person.

There are studies in which respondents rated "the relief of loneliness" last as a need they wanted satisfied. But to be loved, to have someone to confide in, to show affection—these were mentioned most often. Without these, one is indeed lonely. But marriage is not merely an escape from a self-centered downbeat emotion. It is a positive and creative way to work for self-realization. Successfully married people can take and give affection. They confide in one another without fear of harsh judgment. They can cry together and not be ashamed. They can disagree, even quarrel violently, and know it is not the end. They are busy, not only with one another, but with a variety of life's challenges. In no other human relationship can this kind of mutuality be developed. But the skills involved in building and sustaining such a relationship are not inherent, nor are they easily acquired. They require effort. So to conquer loneliness through marriage is to gain many things. One should seek not a person with whom to share loneliness but one to help dispel it.

COURTSHIP:

REFLEXIVE? REFLECTIVE? OR BOTH?

The right person means contentment. The wrong one can indeed entwine two lives in grief. "Though thou canst not forbear to love," wrote Sir Walter Raleigh to his son, "yet forbear to link."[47] The brilliant Elizabethan knight did not advise against marriage. He advised caution. Of the three most elemental events in human life—

---

[46]Thomas Wolfe, "God's Lonely Man," in *The Hills Beyond* (Garden City, N.Y., 1941), p. 187.
[47]Quoted in Alan C. Valentine, ed., *Fathers to Sons: Advice Without Consent* (Oklahoma City, 1963), p. 16.

birth, death, and marriage—marriage is most open to intelligent personal decision. Love has been too simply defined as a conflict between reflex and reflection.[48] Reflection can enrich the expression of love that molds a good marriage.

At twenty, one can hardly contemplate fifty years of living. A marriage choice is thus all the more difficult. It is not easy to make one decision do for half a century. The wonder is not that one of three marriages in this country ends in divorce. The wonder is that there are not more failures.

There are those, like H. G. Wells, who considered it foolhardy to leave so vital a decision "to flushed and blundering youth . . . with nothing to guide it but shocked looks and sentimental twaddle and base whisperings and cant-smeared examples."[49] Samuel Johnson grumbled that all marriages should be arranged by the Lord Chancellor "without the parties having any choice in the matter."[50] Some sixteen centuries ago, Father Tertullian (160?–230?) gloomily regarded the corrupt Roman society and its tottering empire. "Divorce," he said, "was now looked upon as one fruit of marriage."[51]

To avoid tasting of that bitter fruit, what thoughts and questions should occur to the person who is considering someone as a potential mate?

some general pointers

1. How confident are both members of the couple that their marriage will be successful? Studies show that lack of confidence in this respect is a good indicator of future failure.[52]

2. Does the relationship survive loss of glamor? In the moonlight most girls look lovely. In a similar light most young men get by pretty well. However, how do matters seem when one of the parties is miserable with a bad cold?

3. How is conflict handled? Do the inevitable problems that erupt during a disagreement always get buried only by mutual physical attraction? Or do conflicts teach insight and better understanding of each other? It is as important to learn from a quarrel as it is to make up. But the courting couple whose quarrelling is constant and unresolved will find little happiness in marriage.

4. Is conversation easy? Perhaps the pair have never really talked to each other. Can one endure the occasional long silence of the other when necessary?

---

[48] *Szpilki* (Warsaw, Poland), cited in *Atlas,* Vol. 16, No. 3 (September 1968), p. 58.
[49] H. G. Wells, *Tono-Bungay,* quoted in E. S. Turner, *A History of Courting,* p. 15.
[50] Boswell's *Life of Johnson,* quoted in Holbrook Jackson, *Bookman's Pleasure* (New York, 1947), p. 77.
[51] Willystine Goodsell, *A History of Marriage and the Family,* p. 145.
[52] Judson T. Landis, "Danger Signals in Courtship," *Medical Aspects of Human Sexuality,* Vol. 4, No. 11 (November 1970), p. 40.

5. What happens to the pair in a group? Does either of them embarrass or persistently criticize the other? Is one ashamed of the other? Do they avoid groups altogether? Why? Courting is a private affair, but most married people have get-togethers with friends.

6. How are decisions made? Does one member of the pair expect the other to "like it or lump it"? Some couples say that "we have been married for forty years and have never had a word of disagreement." When two people agree on everything, only one is thinking.

7. Is that knitting or stamp collecting or pro football or interminable chatter on the telephone going to be bearable for fifty years?

8. What is the home life of the possible life partner like? Repeated studies have shown that people from relatively happy homes are the best marriage risks. (There is the exception, of course, of the child of divorced parents who works all the harder to make a marriage succeed. Too, there is the occasional case of the marital partner who sacrifices an entire life to the wounding memory of a parental divorce. Fearful of marriage failure, he or she may scrupulously avoid all disagreement and never express his or her individuality.) Moreover, although it need not be decisive, the attitude of the family toward the prospective mate is important.

9. What are his or her best friends like? Off-beat? If so, it is well for the marriage partner to be a trifle off-beat too. Or are they all conservative Republicans who treasure their used Goldwater buttons? In that case, matters will be more pleasant if the other partner is, at least, an admirer of Richard Nixon.

10. What is the physical health of the potential marital partner? A slight anemia may add a bewitching pallor to the complexion, but it may become wearing after a few years of marriage.

11. How self-sufficient is the proposed mate? How dependent? How much dependency does one need of the other? The following excerpt from a case history is pertinent:

> She dreamed that she was holding her son in her arms and that suddenly he began to increase in size while she began to decrease in height. Within a few seconds her child was standing, holding her in his arms. This patient unconsciously wanted to continue to be the child, to prolong indefinitely the dependency relationship that she had with her father and the father image.[53]

Overdependency can become an illness. That it is an illness only when carried beyond a certain point is not well understood. It is degree that often determines emotional illness. To some extent almost all people are dependent. Marriage provides the individual with one way of satisfying this need. However, as is noted from the above case, dependency may be extreme and unresolved. Manifesting

[53] James A. Peterson, *Education for Marriage,* 2nd ed. (New York, 1964), p. 187.

itself in marriage, overdependency may cause one partner to unconsciously expect the other to be a substitute parent. This role the
second partner may summarily reject. Frustrated, the dependent
partner may seek attention by becoming a hypochondriac or an
alcoholic. When this happens, the marriage is endangered.

The knowledge that marriage must satisfy both unconscious and
conscious needs should stimulate some analysis of the unconscious
needs. "Lay yourself open to yourself." [54] So, in about 1654, wrote
William Russell to his son Frank. It is good advice that is difficult
to follow. But, in the seeking of a marriage partner, it is essential.
One man, for example, needs to be submissive. Unconsciously
ashamed of this need, he hides it. Consequently, he behaves domi-
nantly. And, worse, he does not realize it. It is in his unconscious
self-deception that he is confounded, that he betrays himself. Another
man is submissive. He is uncomfortable with domineering women
so he marries a girl as submissive as he. When each looks to the other
for the final word, who will make a decision?

12. What role does each potential marital partner expect the other
to play? There is the man who wants to marry a pretty girl who is
a good housekeeper. He understands and wants the responsibility
of making money to support his family. Other men have a less
traditional approach. They emphasize companionship and education.
Those who contemplate marriage need, then, to examine the role
they expect to play and the role they want their intended partner
to perform in the marriage situation.

13. Has the relationship been frequently broken and renewed?
"An on-again, off-again type of relationship is predictive of trouble
if the couple marries." [55]

SOME SPECIAL PREMARITAL CONSIDERATIONS

A paradox in this nation's culture is this: the attributes of which the
nation is proudest endanger an institution on which it depends—
marriage. Individualism is revered, yet marriage is hardly an individual enterprise. The people of this country draw strength from the
cultural melting pot. Yet from this same pot come mixed marriages.
And mixed marriages are risky.

There are, in this nation, at least a dozen Protestant denomi-
nations with memberships that total over 70 million people. The
Roman Catholic church includes in its membership forty-six million
people with an almost bewildering variety of tongues and customs.
Other Christians belong to such groups as the Eastern Orthodox
church and the Polish National Catholic church. The Jews—Orthodox,
Conservative, and Reform—number five-and one-half million. There

[54] Quoted in Alan C. Valentine, ed., *Fathers to Sons: Advice Without Consent*, p. 33.
[55] Judson T. Landis, "Danger Signals in Courtship," p. 41.

are also quite a few Buddhists and Mohammedans in this country. Then, there are those who do not believe in God or in any divine personality or meaning. It may be the opinion of some that when they die and lie in state, they are indeed all dressed up with no place to go. But they rightfully expect their opinions to be respected.

In 1967, the great majority (87.9 percent) of the U.S. population was white. There were over 20 million blacks, hundreds of thousands of American Indians, Chinese, and Japanese. Filipinos, Hindus, Koreans, Hawaiians, and Malayans all add spice to the melting pot. And total racial amalgamation is unlikely to occur during the lifetime of anyone alive today.[56]

In the past century and a half, some 42 million immigrants came to this country. Over that long period of time, Ireland, Germany, and Great Britain contributed the greatest numbers. However, in 1960, Italy was the leading country of origin of foreign-born U.S. inhabitants. Most countries of the world have added some stock to the mixture.

This wonderful conglomeration of people marry and reproduce in a society dominated by one belief—the sanctity of the individual. A clash of interests is inevitable. The demand for the satisfaction of individual needs is opposed by the demands imposed on each individual by his cultural background. Too often the resulting conflicts lead to divorce.

interfaith marriages

People of different religious faiths often fall in love. Rebellion or status-seeking by no means accounts for all interfaith marriages. But those who contemplate marrying someone outside their own faith should comprehend their chances of happiness. Unfortunately, there have been methodological problems in the study of this matter. Still, the following data do provide food for thought.

Interfaith couples are less likely to adjust well to marriage. One study showed the following percentages of low-adjustment scores for married couples:[57]

Protestant-Protestant 20%

Nonchurch marriages 29%

---

[56] David M. Heer, "Intermarriage and Racial Amalgamation in the United States," *Eugenics Quarterly,* Vol. 14, No. 2 (April 1967), p. 120.

Application of research results of animal behavior to human activity is, at best, hazardous; often it is poor science. Nevertheless, it is of interest to note that lower animals may exhibit distinct desires for some variety in mating. In this regard a provocative observation has been made with some inbred strains of a species of mouse. "Females from inbred strains of *Mus musculus,* in a state of induced oestrus [see page 265, footnote 20], when allowed to choose between a male of their own strain and another of a different strain, prefer to associate and mate with males of the different strain." (Joseph Yanai and Gerald E. McClearn, "Assortive Mating in Mice and the Incest Taboo," *Nature,* Vol. 238, No. 5362 [August 4, 1972], p. 281.)

[57] James A. Peterson, *Education for Marriage,* p. 223.

searching for someone to marry

| Catholic-Catholic | 39% |
| Protestant-Catholic | 50% |

To look at it the other way, only 50 percent of Protestant-Catholic marriages scored *high* adjustments in this study, while 61 percent of Catholic-Catholic marriages, 71 percent of nonchurch marriages, and 80 percent of Protestant-Protestant marriages scored high.

Another study indicates that, by marrying a non-Catholic, a Catholic woman increases her chances of divorce or separation by about 50 percent. A Protestant woman, by marrying outside her religion, increases her risks of divorce or separation by more than 300 percent.[58]

Other research gives similar results (Figure 7-1). Some 5 percent of unmixed Jewish and Catholic marriages end in divorce or separation. This increases to about 6 percent in unmixed Protestant marriages. However, some 15 percent of mixed Catholic-Protestant marriages end in divorce. The most hazardous of all is the marriage of a Catholic man to a Protestant woman. More than one in five, over 20 percent, end in divorce. The same study indicates too that the marriage of a Catholic woman to a man without a religion is only

[58]*4,108 Marriages of Parents of Michigan State University Students,* cited in Robert O. Blood, *Marriage,* p. 83.

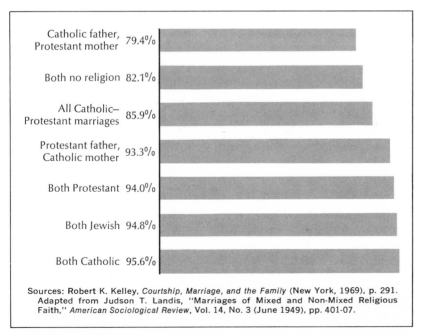

Sources: Robert K. Kelley, *Courtship, Marriage, and the Family* (New York, 1969), p. 291. Adapted from Judson T. Landis, "Marriages of Mixed and Non-Mixed Religious Faith," *American Sociological Review,* Vol. 14, No. 3 (June 1949), pp. 401-07.

7-1 Marriage stability: the religious factor.

half as risky as a Protestant woman marrying a man who does not profess a religion.[59]

A 1960 study also revealed a markedly higher (three times the average) divorce rate in Catholic-Protestant marriages. It is true that tolerance is growing in this nation. How far this will go to reversing figures pointing to the increased risk of Protestant-Catholic marriages remains to be seen. There are isolated signs of permissiveness among individual members of the major religious bodies. However, the general reaction of the religious leadership in the United States to interfaith marriage is negative.

Although the Jewish intermarriage rate is the lowest of the three major faiths in this country, it is certainly increasing. In 1963, Rosenthal[60] reported the Jewish intermarriage rate in the nation's capital to have risen from 1 percent with first-generation Jewish marriages to 10.2 percent for those of the second to 17.9 percent by the third generation. It is of interest that the number of children of these marriages raised in the Jewish religion fell spectacularly when compared to earlier generations. In 1964, Sklare[61] accepted the 17.9 percent figure as "probably very close to the current rate." Reform Jewish congregations are more tolerant of Jewish intermarriage than those of the Orthodox or Conservative tradition. Although a large number of such marriages are known to be successful, more adequate, and certainly more recent studies are indicated.

What are some major sources of disharmony in interfaith marriages? Despite ardent premarital agreements, conflicts often occur over the religious training of children. (This may account for the very high divorce rates of Protestant mothers from Catholic fathers.) Artificial birth control, a practice opposed by the Catholic religion, is another source of deep disagreement. Then, there are the multitudinous cultural differences. Religion is a way of life. Even those whose relationship to their own faith has been casual may find the rituals of another church an imposition.

Many interfaith marriages succeed. Nevertheless, it is well to remember that love alone does not necessarily conquer all.

interracial marriages

In 1967, the U.S. Supreme Court invalidated a Virginia law forbidding marriages between whites and blacks. That Virginia and sixteen other states had passed such laws testifies to the considerable hostility against such marriages. Nevertheless, they are increasing. In one

---

[59] Judson T. Landis, "Marriages of Mixed and Non-Mixed Religious Faith," *American Sociological Review*, Vol. 14, No. 3 (June 1949), pp. 401–07.
[60] Erich Rosenthal, "Studies of Jewish Intermarriage in the United States," *American Jewish Year Book* (New York, 1963), pp. 3–53.
[61] Marshall Sklare, "Intermarriage and the Jewish Future," *Commentary*, Vol. 37, No. 4 (April 1964), pp. 46–52.

study[62] of data from Hawaii, Michigan, Nebraska, and California, it was found that the rate of white-black marriages rose during the period studied. Hawaii had the highest reported incidence of black-white marriages, with California, Michigan, and Nebraska following. Interestingly enough, 1959 data, the latest available from California and Michigan, showed that the black-white marriage rate in Michigan was half that of California. Both are industrial states with similar proportions of black populations. An exploratory study in Indiana[63] indicated that such marriages generally occur among people who are, by and large, equals in education, economics, and culture. Kelley[64] suggests that those contemplating an interracial marriage would do well to carefully consider all the issues, varying from personal motivations to the possibilities of varying values, whether they be social, ethical, educational, or religious. Of course, these considerations, among others, are important in all marriages. As to the potential for marital success of these and other interracial marriages, adequate appraisal awaits more intensive study.

Not enough research attention has been given to the children born of interracial marriages. One group of investigators found that "interracial offspring of white mothers obtained significantly higher IQ scores at four years of age than interracial offspring of Negro mothers, suggesting that environmental factors play an important role in the lower intellectual performance of Negro children." [65] Preliminary results of a Los Angeles study suggest that the quest for identity of the child of a black-white marriage is even more difficult than that of the black child in this country. The child often resents both parents, is unable to identify with either, and also resents his siblings with characteristics that are racially different. These are among the problems of the small number of children who have been studied.[66]

interclass marriages

Numerous studies show that adjustment rates are poor in marriages in which the partners come from widely separated social classes. The wider the class difference between husband and wife, the lower is the percentage of good adjustment.[67]

Men are more likely than women to have a successful marriage with a partner slightly below their own class. The college English

[62] David M. Heer, "Negro-White Marriage in the United States," *Journal of Marriage and the Family*, Vol. 28, No. 3 (August 1966), pp. 262-73.
[63] Todd H. Pavela, "An Exploratory Study of Negro-White Intermarriage in Indiana," *Journal of Marriage and the Family*, Vol. 26, No. 5 (May 1964), pp. 209-11.
[64] Robert K. Kelley, *Courtship, Marriage, and the Family* (New York, 1969), pp. 270-71.
[65] Lee Willerman, Alfred F. Naylor, and Ntinos C. Myrianthopoulos, "Intellectual Development of Children from Interracial Matings," *Science*, Vol. 170, No. 146 (December 18, 1970), p. 1,329.
[66] Joseph D. Teicher, "Some Observations on Identity Problems in Children of Negro-White Marriages," *Journal of Nervous and Mental Disease*, Vol. 146, No. 3 (March 1968), pp. 249-56.
[67] Ruth Shonle Cavan, *The American Family*, 2nd ed. (New York, 1953), p. 232.

professor may marry the colorful truck driver and get away with it. She is more likely to end by criticizing his fingernails, and he will puzzle why she never noticed them before. Each will be right about the other and wrong for the other.

money

> *"My other piece of advice, Copperfield," said Mr. Micawber, "you know. Annual income twenty pounds, annual expenditure nineteen nineteen six, result happiness. Annual income twenty pounds, annual expenditure twenty pounds ought and six, result misery. The blossom is blighted, the leaf is withered, the god of day goes down upon the dreary scene, and—and, in short, you are for ever floored. As I am!"*[68]

In this, the most affluent of nations, countless couples attribute their marriage failures to "money problems." One major study[69] points out that it is not the amount but the manner of expenditures that is the major cause of marital friction. Tearfully, one young wife tells this story:

> *It's twenty years ago, but it's like yesterday. I was seven. I knew my father had just lost his job, but I pretended I didn't. He came out of the bedroom and told my mother, "I don't know. I just don't know where our next piece of bread is coming from." Sometimes, I can still hear him. His voice was quiet. In two years he was dead.*
>
> *What's this got to do with my husband? He doesn't understand. He'll go out and spend two hundred dollars on a suit. Or he'll buy white-wall tires. He just doesn't know that being poor can kill a person like it killed my father. He doesn't know what it's like not to know where your next piece of bread is coming from.*

It is true; he does not know. And the danger to their marriage is that he does not want to know. He has never known a day of financial want. His side of the story is typical:

> *We've been married eleven years. I've never made less than twenty thousand a year. We've got money in the bank. Even if we didn't, my folks could help. They have always had more than they need. What's she so scared about?*

---

[68] Charles Dickens, *David Copperfield* (London, 1849-50), Chapter 12.
[69] Lewis M. Terman, *Psychological Factors in Marital Happiness* (New York, 1938), pp. 167-71.

The problems of this couple spring from their widely disparate economic pasts. Spending patterns are learned in childhood from family experience. She will forever tighten the purse strings that he will forever loosen.

Similar tensions overtake the rich girl–poor boy marriage. The woman who once drove her own expensive car may well find a crowded bus irksome. The early fun of making a budget work often becomes a weary trial. Sadly, she may soon see the sum of her expenditures as the dreary sum of her marriage.

How can these pitfalls be avoided? One should know not only the financial behavior pattern of the proposed mate, but also his or her ability to plan expenditures. How one fits finances into married life is often critical.

age

In no other Western country do people marry so young as in the United States. Prosperity, the income of the working girl, the changing role of the teen-ager from a family financial asset to a costly burden—all these promote marriage at an early age. In the United States, in 1965, more girls were married at eighteen than at any other age.

Teen-age marriages are particularly prone to failure. Numerous studies repeatedly emphasize the high divorce and poor adjustment rates of teen-age unions. One investigator found "that the proportion of remarried women among those who first married below the age of 18 years was about three times as high as that for women who first married between the ages of 22 to 24 years." [70] Particularly hazardous are marriages between the very young. The divorce rates of marriages between people sixteen or younger is 400 percent higher than for marriages in which husbands were from twenty to twenty-six years old and wives twenty-two to twenty-four. [71] In addition, "teen-age marriages forced by pregnancy are the most unstable of all." [72]

How old should one be before getting married? Some students of marriage recommend twenty-nine for the man and twenty-four for the woman. Others suggest twenty-five and twenty-two. Setting the same age for everyone is pointless. Emotional stability and maturity are better indices of marital success than chronological age. One good way of deferring a possibly premature marriage while at the

---

[70] Paul C. Glick, "Stability of Marriage in Relation to Age at Marriage," in Robert F. Winch et al., eds., *Selected Studies in Marriage and the Family*, rev. ed. (New York, 1962), p. 624.

[71] Thomas P. Monahan, "Does Age of Marriage Matter in Divorce?" *Social Forces*, Vol. 32, No. 10 (October 1953), p. 86.

[72] Judson T. Landis, "Danger Signals in Courtship," p. 43.

same time learning more about a potential partner is a reasonably long engagement. How long should the engagement period be? A year should tell the couple enough. "The best insurance policy against divorce in our society is a thorough engagement."[73] As Chaucer wrote:

> *It is no childes pley*
> *To take a wyf with-oute avysement.*[74]

Seek, then, advisement for marriage.

[73] Ersel Earl LeMasters, *Modern Courtship and Marriage* (New York, 1957), p. 168.
[74] Geoffrey Chaucer, *The Merchant's Tale,* lines 1530-31.

marriage: 8 "the craft so long to lerne"

Next, when they had got them huts and skins and fire and woman was appropriately mated to one man, and the laws of wedlock became known and they saw offspring born of them, then first mankind begun to soften. For the fire saw to it that their shivering bodies were less able to endure cold under the canopy of heaven and Venus sapped their strength and children easily broke their parents' proud spirit by coaxing. Then also neighbors began eagerly to join in a league of friendship amongst themselves to do no hurt and suffer no violence, and asked protection for their children and womankind, signifying by voice and gesture, with stammering tongue, that it was right for all to pity the weak. Nevertheless concord could not altogether be established, but a good part, nay the most part, kept the covenant in good faith or else the race of mankind would even then have been completely destroyed, nor would birth and begetting have availed to prolong their posterity.[1]

So did the Roman poet Lucretius (96?-55? B.C.) tell about the beginnings of the family of man. Families banded together and established protective societal rules. Those breaking the rules imperiled the group and were punished. Sex and love, and marriage too, were essentially controlled by the group. In that sense, man's deepest intimacy was public business. So it is today. Although marriage has ancient origins, it remains as rich and complex an adventure as life itself. And just as six centuries ago the poet Chaucer described life as "the craft so long to lerne," so is marriage a craft no more quickly learned.

No known human society allows promiscuity—sexual life without rules—to be its governing way of life. In every society, marriage and

---

[1]Lucretius, *On the Nature of Things,* quoted in Felding H. Garrison, *Contributions to the History of Medicine* (New York, 1966), p. 25.

the family exist. All societies, moreover, have chosen marriage as the arrangement for having children. And "in every known human society, there is a prohibition against incest."[2] These pervasive behavior patterns prevent social convulsions that would be inimical to child-rearing. Without such restrictions, the group would die, the victim of its own rulelessness. "It is marriage which is the basic social instrument of man's survival . . . for survival there must be an accommodation between the sexes . . . enduring enough to provide protection, care, and reasonable security for the offspring."[3]

Marriage serves man's needs to resolve loneliness and to perpetuate his kind. And society pressures him to resolve these needs through marriage. In relatively recent years, however, new dimensions of marriage have developed. Have they weakened the married state?

Today, the date of the marriage does not await the completion of either education or military service. Never before have so many students and soldiers married. And they share with all recently married people a new awareness of sexual relationships. No longer, for example, are woman's sexual needs incidental. Rapid social change, moreover, has added threats to the stability of marriage. The mobility of the family and the emancipation of the woman are but two of the factors contributing to fresh perspectives of marriage. What are some of the aspects of marriage so characteristic of these times?

war and marriage

War is the youth's premature introduction to age. On the battlefield he is old enough to die. Escaping death, it is there that he leaves his youth. Nobody ever returned young from a war. This the young today share with the young of yesterday. And both young men and women today ask an old question: how can we cope with a separating war?

During the First World War, British posters urged young women to jilt men who failed to volunteer for military service. How effective

[2]Bernard Berelson and Gary A. Steiner, *Human Behavior* (New York, 1964), pp. 313-16. Let it not be assumed, however, that the avoidance of mating with relatives (the "incest taboo" in humans) is limited to the culturally learned and determined influences of human beings. Behavioral mechanisms for the avoidance of inbreeding seem to have evolved in many creatures lower in the evolutionary scale, such as the white-throated sparrow and a species of moth. A similar mechanism, moreover, exists in certain inbred strains of mice that have been studied. Among these particular mice, "incest" depended on a fascinating variable in their rearing. "Females which stayed with their fathers until the day before testing preferred to associate and mate more with unfamiliar males. The females which had been reared with their fathers, however, only until weaning did not show any preference." Part of the testing procedure involved allowing a female mouse in induced estrus (see page 265, footnote 20) to choose between two males with previously confirmed abilities to perform sexually. (Joseph Yanai and Gerald E. McClearn, "Assortive Mating in Mice and the Incest Taboo," *Nature*, Vol. 238, No. 5362 [August 4, 1972], p. 282.)
[3]William M. Kephart, *The Family, Society, and the Individual* (Boston, 1961), p. 64.

this method of obtaining soldiers was is unknown. Today, draft boards seem to do well enough. But even a little more than a generation ago there were no seemingly permanent draft boards. In the public mind, war and peace were curiously separated from each other. When war came, it was but a temporary tragedy to be gotten over with. It was peacetime that lasted long enough for planning. Afer a war was over, the arena of conflict was returned to politicians. Except for a few nostalgic songs such as "It's a Long Way to Tipperary" or "Lili Marlene," the war was fought to be forgotten.

This attitude is long past. Yet there is still no true promise of peace. To prevent one biggest war, modern man seems destined to agonize over smaller wars. The draft board is the culminating sickness of the times. How can young people deal with the anxiety it creates? How can they fit the draft board in their need to love and to marry?

The draft board may inadvertently help decide the date of a wedding. But it should never decide whether a marriage will take place. The decision to marry should not await the decision of a draft board. The suitability of the couple, the adequacy of the courtship— such factors, not "better times in which to get married," should determine the course of action. Some people spend their lives preparing for hurdles they never meet. When, at long last, they are forced to meet life's obstacles, they are alone. Impending military service is not a signal to ignore caution. There are many valid reasons to defer marriage. However, military service is not necessarily one of them.

In this, most parents will need help. Fathers and mothers remember the fragile marriages during the Second World War and the Korean "police action." Sometimes they may use the man's military service as an excuse because they oppose the marriage itself. However, parents can be remarkably sympathetic and helpful and should be consulted.

Whether the young wife should follow her enlisted husband to his post will depend on circumstances. If at all possible, the wife should live with or near her husband. On or around military bases, living costs are high. Housing may be inadequate. Transportation may be a trial. Overcrowding is usual. Competition for jobs is great. Recreational facilities are often poor. Social contacts may be limited. Yet the problems are not comparable to those that may occur with prolonged separation. If a baby is expected, the young wife may well choose to live with her parents temporarily. Those who go into marriage secure in their love and willing to work at making their marriage a success will find even the hardships on or near a military post an enrichment. The insecure will not usually find security in a marriage, no matter where they live.

Nonetheless, there are those for whom war means long separation.

Are intimacy, love, closeness—the meanings of marriage—transmissible over great distances of time and space? In one study[4] of Iowa couples separated during the Second World War, these factors were found to ease the pain of separation:

1. Frequent, even daily, letters were exchanged detailing daily doings and hopes. These letters were more than mere reiterations of love. The sender communicated. The receiver shared.

2. Snapshots of each other, family, and friends were frequently exchanged.

3. Gifts were exchanged often between the couple and their families.

4. Special occasions, such as anniversaries and birthdays, were celebrated by cablegram and long-distance telephone.

Should a married woman date while her husband is away on military duty? No. Jealousy and gossip would result. Eventually, moreover, the jealousy could become justified; the gossip, true. If an engaged couple has agreed on it beforehand, the girl may date randomly while her fiancé is away on military duty. Such random dating may test an inadequate courtship. This is fair. Few engaged servicemen refrain from dating.

For some, war hastens marriage. A hasty marriage is a risky one. "Married in haste, we may repent at leisure," wrote William Congreve. Those considering hasty service marriages will do well to examine their motives. Some young women panic, fearful that all eligible men will be gone. Others desire "to have his baby so he will have something to remember while he's gone." Such immaturity resulted in numerous Second World War marriages. Many failed.

Service marriages are more successful if time has been taken for courtship and if the marriage takes place at least several months before or after the induction. A new marriage, combined with boot camp, demands too much adjustment in too little time.

Even the trial of unkind separation can be turned to some advantage. Seasoned by a major mark of maturity—the deferment of gratification—the bonds between the partners are deepened. So it is with many campus marriages. Again, gratification is deferred. But in the very planning together for a mutual future, there are opportunities for sharing. Of course, there are problems to be considered and solved. What are some of them?

the campus marriage

At the turn of this century the average boy left school at fourteen. Not until twelve years later, not until he had settled into his life work

---

[4] Reuben Hill, *Families Under Stress,* cited in E. E. Le Masters, *Modern Courtship and Marriage* (New York, 1957), p. 218.

and had saved a tidy sum, did he chance marriage. The dictum of Benjamin Franklin, "First thrive, then wive," was the order of that day. Furthermore, in 1890 only 63.1 percent of the population of this country ever married. In this country today more than 80 percent of all people over eighteen are married. The average man now marries at about twenty-three rather than twenty-six. In 1967 one-half of the men in the United States who married did so between twenty and twenty-six (one-quarter by twenty, and three-quarters by twenty-six). About one-half of all women who married did so between nineteen and twenty-three (one-quarter are married by nineteen, and three-quarters by twenty-three).[5] In the United States the average age of first marriage is the lowest of any advanced country in the world. So permanent a commitment by the college students in this group poses singular problems.

It was not until the Second World War was over that married students were first seen in appreciable numbers on the nation's college campuses. Thousands of veterans used their benefits to obtain an education. Today's graying professors remember them well. They were not college boys. They were older, tougher men. Some were filled with a speechless anger. Most were intensely purposeful. They had no time to fool around. They had been through a war and knew something about time. Many were married. Their wives worked. There was always pregnancy to think about. It was, for most vets, a difficult time. It was, for their wives, a time for marking time. Veterans were used to waiting. Their wives quickly learned.

One of the chief concerns of married students is money. A nation-wide survey showed that parents pay for 61 percent of students' expenses.[6] Marriage changes that picture. Some married students want to make it on their own. Often parents are reluctant to help because of a sincere belief that such a prolonged dependency might harm the marriage. Others are more abrupt: "If you're old enough to get married, you're old enough to support yourself." Many parents do help. Nevertheless, married students receive much less parental cash than do single students. Some married students are aided by the GI Bill. Most work. Not uncommonly the wife supports her student husband. Whatever the plan, it is beset with risks. That the vast majority of campus marriages succeed speaks well for the maturity of those who venture into them.

It is the campus wife's education that is at greatest risk. Marriage may dilute her motivation; the purchase of an economics text cannot compare with her first investment in a Picasso reproduction for the bedroom wall. No philosophy professor will gain her attention as a whimpering baby will. Yet, occasionally, an educationally mixed

[5] Clark E. Vincent, "Sex and the Young Married," *Medical Aspects of Human Sexuality,* Vol. 3, No. 3 (March 1969), p. 13.
[6] Robert O. Blood, *Marriage* (New York, 1964), p. 163.

marriage may result, and her sacrifice multiplies. Her husband becomes involved in the world of the slide rule or the stethoscope or Byzantine art. Her world may become a matter of warming a typewriter or yesterday's stew. Or she may seek contentment in recipes and afternoon television shows. (There is no evening television. He has to study.) A conversation gap occurs and widens. In a class in Russian literature, the student husband hears a quote: "If you are afraid of loneliness, do not marry."[7] But he is already married. He studies guiltily. She is lonely too. "If it hadn't been for you . . ." they both think. The bubble of love bursts, and mutual blame takes over.

Moreover, the married student is pressed for time. He may need to devote every evening of the week to study. Restlessly, his wife remembers the ruthless exclusion of the married from campus activity. She seeks to be busy. She may read or do mechanical things or perhaps go to the movies alone. She worries about their inadequate sexual relationship, a surprisingly common problem among married college students.[8] To maintain her aspect of the mutual vision of an educational investment, she will need to draw from the deepest wellsprings of her maturity. For the wife, handling spare time may become an issue. Her youth does not help the situation. Conflicts over leisure time are a major cause of marriage failure among college students. Campus marriages now occur at an earlier age than they used to. The college student must bring security into a student marriage. To count on finding security within marriage is a mistake.

Pregnancy may also complicate the student marriage. It ends the wife's immediate plan for a college education. Often it concludes her husband's schooling. Some college fathers successfully lead a tripartite life. Their time is divided between job, school, and family. In one study it was found that "only 52 percent of the graduate-student fathers were going to school full-time compared to 79 percent of the childless graduate students."[9]

Grades may be a problem. Some studies do indicate that married-student grades are equal to, or even better than, those of single students. However, marriage can hardly be recommended as a means of improving grades. There is a significant lack of data regarding the number of married students who drop out of school because of poor grades. The relationship between the married student's age and grades needs further study. Sometimes grades, as such, create dissension. The wife who consistently does better than her husband may find herself in the same position as the unmarried coed who feels it necessary "to play dumb" with her dates. The young, nonbreadwinning husband, his masculine role further diminished,

[7]*The Personal Papers of Anton Chekhov,* introduction by Matthew Josephson (New York, 1948), p. 75.
[8]James A. Peterson, *Education for Marriage,* 2nd ed. (New York, 1964), p. 216.
[9]Robert O. Blood, *Marriage,* p. 166.

may add resentment to regret. It requires a tactful wife to weather the storm. With the developing idea of equality of the sexes, this is less of a problem. For those who do not yet accept this concept, it can be a major concern.

Premarital planning helps. Realism must temper romanticism. What must be accomplished? What resources will be needed? From whom will help come? What about pregnancy? For those who wish to marry while in college, at least these questions should first be objectively answered.

And so it is apparent that student marriages demand much from the young couple. By far the greatest majority do have what it takes.

So far in this chapter two circumstances of marriage that must be dealt with early have been considered. Indeed, they are best discussed and planned for before the marriage takes place. The next problem is rarely considered, even expected. So insidiously does it develop that neither partner clearly sees it as a threat to their future. Too, for some it hardly exists. Others accept it. Still others resent it. It is the problem of monotony in marriage.

marital monotony

Love never dies of starvation, but often of indigestion.[10]

In the pattern of everyday married life, there is much that is honored by time. Custom and ceremony, no matter how subtle, add to the richness of the marital fabric. But mere repetition makes for a drab cloth. Individuality and custom can, however, be compatible. Indeed, customs provide an opportunity for sharing individuality. Her custom may be as simple as a best tablecloth for dinner. But unless he occasionally brings a bunch of flowers to decorate the table too, the time will come when neither sees the tablecloth. What is left? Monotony.

Many people find some marriage monotony a comfort, not a problem. They see it as a mark of their certainty about each other. Whether one can count on the other is a valid test of courtship. In marriage it is part of the loving. Life cannot be perpetual excitement. There is surely some truth in this reasoning.

Others refuse to even recognize tedium as a possible part of marriage. They hark back to the "good old days," when people (meaning women) had no time for nonsense like boredom. "In the past," they say, "women knew their place; they never thought about being bored, and they never got a divorce either." Just how far back the good old days go for such philosophers is never clear. That Grandpa was a kindly soul, in whose beneficent light Grandma was

[10]Ninon De L'Enclos, "L'Esprit des Autres," line 3.

ever content, may be true. Maybe. For those, however, who forever seek improvement only from the distant past, a code of sixteenth-century Russian family practices, called *The Domostroy* (Domestic Ordinance), will be enlightening. It was prepared by Pope Sylvester in the reign of the first tsar of Russia, that monstrous murderer Ivan IV (1530-84), called "the Terrible." This is an excerpt:

> *If she does not obey . . . then the husband should punish his wife and fill her with fear, and punish her with love.*

Gentleness, however, is urged.

> *The husband should not hit her eyes or ears nor beat her with his fists or feet under the heart . . . whoever beats her that way . . . causes much trouble; blindness, deafness, broken hands and feet . . . But to beat carefully, with a whip, is sensible . . . healthy . . . In case of grave offense, pull off her shirt and whip politely . . . saying "Don't be angry."* [11]

Before a young man married in those days in Russia, the father-in-law presented the groom with a whip. It was a symbol of authority. Often it was hung over the bridal bed.

Such bizarre brutality diminished with time, but the wife's essential situation in society did not improve. In the early nineteenth century, *The Ladies' Book* quoted the following advice of a minister to a bride: "Your duty is submission . . . Your husband is, by the Laws of God and of man, your superior; do not ever give him cause to remind you of it." [12] So wifely self-expression continued to be discouraged and her total obedience to be expected. But the role of woman changed (not surprisingly, Russian women were among the leaders of this revolution). The shackling notion of feminine obedience was discarded. Millions of women in this country found work outside the home. (Some of their singular problems are discussed on pages 210-12.) But a great number of those who remain at home are bored. This is not to say that the working woman is never oppressed by monotony. Nor is homemaking a tedious occupation for most women. But many a stay-at-home woman certainly finds little opportunity to relieve the monotony of housekeeping. Sheer boredom then erodes her marriage. And her husband, tired and perhaps also bored with his work, joins her in an unrelieved tedium.

Many marriages, then, die on the vine. Husband and wife simply stop noticing each other. True, the arithmetic of living—the baby's allergy, the leaking roof, the plugged sink—does not add up to ro-

---

[11] Elaine Elnett, *Historical Origin and Social Development of Family Life in Russia,* cited in Austin L. Porterfield, *Marriage and Family Living as Self–Other Fulfillment* (Philadelphia, 1962), p. 39.
[12] Cited in Vance Packard, *The Sexual Wilderness* (New York, 1967), p. 244.

mance. But to keep a marriage alive takes work and planning. The couple must make time to do things together both at home and away from the home and office. Daily opportunities to share thoughts and feelings must be created. Privacy is not always easy to achieve. But no home needs to be the private preserve of a small child. Often a good babysitter helps. Timing is also crucial. A woman, exhausted by a toddler, may find it hard to end the day by concentrating on her husband's office difficulties. In turn, he may be too weary, at the moment, to be concerned about the television repairman. And so, at times, silence is the wisest and most appreciated course.

In a marriage marred by boredom, a word of appreciation is usually long overdue. Sincere praise for accomplishment is a need of both marital partners. There is the story of the unhappy man who ran around with other women, not because his wife did not understand him, but because she understood him only too well. To her, knowing him meant undermining him. The woman who cannot regard her husband without foil in hand, ready to pierce his ego, will destroy her marriage. Marriage is not a competition. One does not gain by the other's loss. Between the married, "oneupmanship" is a dangerous game. There is no victim in a good marriage. Moreover, the husband who does not accentuate his marriage with expressed appreciation may reap (and deserve) a bitter harvest.

"It was a lot of little things," then, explains many a happy marriage as well as many a divorce. The difference is that the happily married couple, having worked at it, knows what happened to them. They know why it was that the customs and ceremonies of their marriage never lost freshness and meaning.

PREVENTING SEXUAL APATHY IN MARRIAGE

Boredom in marriage includes boredom with its sexual aspects. "The trouble in America," one woman says tartly, "is that most men and women can't communicate on a mattress." But that is not where most of the trouble begins. If men and women cannot communicate on a mattress, they usually cannot communicate off a mattress either.

"Better to sit up all night than to go to bed with a dragon." [13] This was written three centuries ago by Jeremy Taylor, an English bishop. It is just as applicable today. Many modern wives and husbands regard their marital beds with a sinking sense of despair. They may well have heeded the advice of William Penn (also written three centuries ago): "Never Marry but for love, but see that thou lovs't what is lovely."[14] But what once seemed lovely has become ugly. Now anything—even the late late television movie—is better than bed. Hoping that her husband will fall asleep, a wife may spend an hour

[13] Jeremy Taylor, *Holy Living.*
[14] William Penn, *Some Fruits of Solitude,* No. 79 (1693).

or more in the bathroom. Or, to escape, the husband will stare, half unseeing, at a 1944 war film being shown on the television. The joy of sexual expression is gone. What can be done?

agreeable surroundings for sexual expression

Does the bedroom suit the personalities of both occupants? Or is a masculine or a feminine haven cunningly designed to make one of the marital partners feel as an intruder? Is it attractive and clean? Can the lighting be dimmed to be subtly revealing? Are there twin beds? For many a marital partner the distance between twin beds is a long mile. Separate beds may prolong marital quarrels. To be near, to touch, to fall asleep in one another's arms, to awaken from a nightmare by the side of another's comforting presence, to awaken and share the first moments of mornings in loving—these do more than encourage sexual intercourse. They add meaning to some marriages. George Bernard Shaw described marriage as combining the maximum of temptation with the maximum of opportunity; the double bed does no less. "O for the deep, deep peace of the double bed after the hurly-burly of the chaise-longue!" [15] said Shaw's actress friend, Mrs. Patrick Campbell, doubtless a trifle wearily. Abyssinian husbands and wives "share not only the same bed, but the same night-shirt, each being entitled to one sleeve." [16] This is true togetherness.

There are, however, couples who find the togetherness of a double bed a trial. One of the pair may be a thrashing, mumbling "active sleeper." A sleepless night does not help one to be affectionate in the morning.

How about the bedroom lighting system? Men are more stimulated by visual stimuli than are women.[17] Some men and women prefer to have sexual intercourse in a lighted room.[18] However, the tendency of some women to cover their bodies and conceal their sexual responses may have an erotic effect on men. It is his revelation of both her nakedness and the throes of her sexual excitement that stimulates him. Many people learn to enjoy the subtleties of the visual aspects of sexual expression.

Personal appearance is also important. The wife will hardly be enticed by a husband who wears dirty and ragged pajamas, and who is unshaven. Nor will the husband be sexually stimulated by a woman who wears a coffee-stained nightgown. Sexual responses are total, and attention must be given to the cleanliness of the total body. Careful bathing, making sure that there is no disagreeable odor about

[15] Lawrence Wright, *Warm and Snug* (London, 1962).
[16] Ibid., p. 202.
[17] Alfred C. Kinsey, Wardell B. Pomeroy, Clyde E. Martin, and Paul H. Gebhard, *Sexual Behavior in the Human Female* (Philadelphia, 1953), p. 662.
[18] Ibid., p. 664.

the genital and anal areas, the mouth and armpits, is essential. The wife need not always wear a black nightgown and perfume. They are particularly good when they remind the couple of a former satisfying sexual encounter. Some people, however, prefer only the clean smell of a washed body. Very few do not seem to object to pungent body odor; fewer still are sexually excited by it.[19]

The effect of odor on human sexual desire has yet to be understood. When man's ancestors finally stood upright, they stopped sniffing the ground and started losing their acuity of smell. The human male is much less sexually sensitive to odors of the opposite sex than is the male of other species, such as the dog.[20]

about sexual mechanics

The bedroom is not the only place where the marital couple might enjoy sexual intercourse. Routine kills the essential spontaneity of sexual expression. The couple that guides their sexual life by rule of thumb will often succeed only in being all thumbs. Sexuality is "a human function to enjoy, not an awesome task to be mastered." [21] The attempted mechanization of human sexuality, like the attempted computerization of the personality, should be resisted.

This is not to say that knowledge of sexual technique dehumanizes sexual expression. The reverse is often true. However, when technique is stressed at the expense of a warm, loving relationship, it may indeed be mechanical rather than human. Jacques Barzun wrote that "to remain alive in mind and body a democracy must compare as well as count." [22] By this he meant that no democracy could survive without appreciating the value of each human being. So must it be between lovers. Sexual technique is a supplement (albeit an impor-

[19] A rare sexual aberration is characterized by an undue interest in body excrement; such obsessive individuals may be sexually stimulated by consuming urine and feces. But such behavior is far removed from the ordinary sexual experience.

[20] In some circumstances odor may have an effect on the function of the human female's reproductive organs. It was recently reported that roommates and close friends in a dormitory tended to develop menstrual cycles that were synchronized, that is, their menstrual cycles tended to occur within a few days of one another. (Martha K. McClintock, "Menstrual Synchrony and Suppression," *Nature*, Vol. 229, No. 5282 [January 22, 1971], pp. 244-45.) This did not happen between groups of women throughout the dormitory who did not spend time together. One possible explanation of the trend toward menstrual synchrony between the women is that there is a subtle influence between them. Experiments with female mice have shown that the mere presence of a male mouse promptly produces *estrus* (the cycle of physiological changes in female mammals that prepares the generative organs for the fertile period). This so-called Whitten effect is produced by odor; these odors are chemical messengers that travel through the air and are called *pheromones*. If the male mouse causing the estrus effect is removed from the cage within a day or two after copulation and a strange male mouse is substituted, pregnancy is blocked. (Robert A. Schneider, "The Sense of Smell and Human Sexuality," *Medical Aspects of Human Sexuality*, Vol. 5, No. 5 [May 1971], p. 160, citing A. S. Parkes and N. M. Bruce, "Olfactory Stimuli in Mammalian Reproduction," *Science*, Vol. 134 [1961], p. 1049.) It has been suggested that in the human female pheromone interaction may suppress estrus, which then occurs on week-end dates with males. However, this does not explain why menstrual synchrony existed only among close friends living together and not among women in the dormitory who dated as a group.

[21] Dennis Brisset, "A Human Function to Enjoy—Not an Awesome Task to be Mastered," *Sexual Behavior*, Vol. 1, No. 9 (December 1971), p. 80.

[22] *Men and Affairs*, compiled and edited by Colin Bingham (New York, 1967), p. 218.

tant one) to their appreciation of one another's value as a human being. In this way, sexual technique becomes part of the art of loving.

Masters and Johnson have deplored the prevalent assumptions by both sexes that the male can instinctively "discern exactly what a woman wants sexually, and when she wants it" and that "sexual expertise is the man's responsibility."[23] "In truth," they write, "no woman can know what type of sexual approach she will respond to at any given opportunity until faced with absence of a particularly desired stimulative factor. How can a woman possibly expect any man to anticipate her sexual pleasure, when she cannot accomplish this feat with consistency herself?"[24]

They emphasize their rejection of the mechanical approach to human sexuality: "Spontaneous sexual expression which answers the demand to be sexually needed and gives freedom for comparable male and female interaction, is universally the most stimulating of circumstances."[25] Stressing the importance to the couple of developing communication, they continue:

Of course, individual preferences will rapidly become known and will repetitively produce the desired pleasure and stimulation. However, to record mentally these preferences and execute them by the numbers, either partner for the other, is to change the freedom of natural interaction back to one of stereotyped performance. The fact is that sex removed from the positive influence of the total personality can become boring, unstimulating, and possibly immaterial.[26]

The happy marital partners spontaneously find variety in their sexual life. Their very search can stimulate them. They will discard rules as to time and place and technique. They may find added pleasure by using a new innovation—the water bed (a piece of hospital furniture recommended a century ago that is used today for the prevention of bedsores with bed-ridden patients).[27] It has been suggested that "the pelvic action of a man is well suited for use on a water bed."[28] If they tire of the bedroom, a couple may find that the floor by the fireplace, the back seat of their car on a lonely road, or a long-forgotten hotel room, help renew their old excitement with one another. For diversity of place and position, Elsa Lanchester expressed enthusiasm about the chaise longue:

[23] William H. Masters and Virginia E. Johnson, *Human Sexual Inadequacy* (Boston, 1970), p. 87.
[24] Ibid.
[25] Ibid.
[26] Ibid.
[27] Richard F. Jones and G. C. Burniston, "The Water Bed in a Spinal Injury Unit," *The Medical Journal of Australia,* Vol. 2, No. 24 (December 11, 1971), pp. 1215-21.
[28] "Sex Does Not Belong to the Physician," *Modern Medicine,* Vol. 39, No. 24 (November 29, 1971), pp. 57-58.

There are so many ways
On this very longue chaise.[29]

There are couples who go through the maneuvers of sexual intercourse every Saturday night at about eleven o'clock. To avoid boredom they would do well to try Tuesday morning, or Wednesday afternoon, or any other time that they feel the desire and can find privacy. But privacy is essential. Rearrangement of the furniture can often avoid the desparate warning "the children will hear!" They should not. The sounds of sexual intercourse, as well as the sights, may frighten a small child. The mother's ecstatic moan means only one thing to the listening child: she is being hurt. Such a memory can last a long time—long enough to impede future sexual expression.

mechanical devices for sexual stimulation

It is not uncommon for some people to use mechanical devices to attain the rhythmic sexual stimulation necessary to attain orgasm. Various ways of mechanical sexual stimulation are used. Electric vibrators sold for skin massage are the most effective; they are certainly capable of imparting a considerable physical stimulus. Some persons studied by Masters and Johnson used them. Their application to the sensitive parts of the genital area may provide an exciting variation of sexual expression for some men and women. In some instances, the husband may use a vibrator to satisfy a wife who has difficulty having an orgasm; or he may help her enjoy multiple orgasms, particularly if he is growing tired; or he may provide her with an orgasm in this manner if he is physically incapable of doing so.

In carefully selected situations, these devices do have limited therapeutic use. There is some opinion that their indiscriminate use should be avoided. For some individuals a mechanical device may be threatening, thereby suppressing an erotic response. Moreover, dependence on it may "create indifference towards the physically less exciting stimulus of coitus." [30] Mechanical devices may be dangerous. "Battery-operated facial vibrators . . . may cause lacerations." [31] The woman who is unacquainted with or is unable to localize her anatomic sexual structures is at particular risk when using vibrators or other mechanical devices such as a douche nozzle. This is because of possible trauma to the vulva, vagina, perineum, urethra, and anus. There may be secondary infection or the development of a dermatitis.

[29] Lawrence Wright, *Warm and Snug*, p. 316.
[30] David R. Mace, "Mechanical Devices in Sexual Stimulation," *Medical Aspects of Human Sexuality*, Vol. 4, No. 12 (December 1970), pp. 69, 71.
[31] Albert Altchek, "Masturbation with Mechanical Devices," *Medical Aspects of Human Sexuality*, Vol. 6, No. 1 (January 1972), p. 177.

what is "normal"?

As long as nobody is hurt, as long as the husband and wife enjoy their sexual expressions, there are no "perversions." In his *Answer to Some Elegant Verses Sent by a Friend,* Byron wrote:

> *When love's delerium haunts the glowing mind*
> *Limping decorum lingers far behind.*

There need be no limits to mutually enjoyable love play between man and wife. The activities preferred by one couple may be astonishing to another, but each couple should be free to make and enjoy its own ways of loving. One couple may use a vibrator. Another may want to make love in front of a mirror. Still another may use provocative language during love play. It all remains a private matter between two people who need to give and to take and to express intimacies.

masturbation while married

Not uncommonly, a married person masturbates when he or she is alone. Usually, it may be considered an ordinary means of sexual expression. When a husband or wife are temporarily separated, masturbation may help to avoid a complicating extramarital affair. However, solitary and compulsively frequent masturbation by a married person may be a symptom of an underlying conflict that has to be resolved. It should be emphasized, however, that this need not always be the case.

A married person may masturbate rather than risk the embarrassment of rejection. Or masturbation may be an expression of hostility. In this way, the husband or wife denies the need for the partner. Thus, masturbation may indicate an inability to relate to the opposite sex.

> *One physician discussed a patient whose weight fluctuated widely at rather frequent intervals. She eventually told him that all periods of marked weight reduction were accompanied by compulsive masturbation to orgasm many times daily. Periodically she would become flooded with feelings of guilt and self-contempt and discontinue the masturbation, but invariably she substituted overeating and rapidly became obese again. This cycle occurred many times over about 15 years of marriage.*[32]

[32] A variety of reasons have been given to explain why some wives overeat. Some researchers suggest that the women desire to make themselves so unattractive that their husbands will avoid sexual intercourse with them. Others believe it sometimes is due to husbands who encourage their wives to eat, thereby creating a sort of fleshy chastity belt. According to two investigators at the Medical Research Institute of Chicago's Michael Reese Hospital and Medical

*Armed with this knowledge, her physician directed his attention
to the anxiety and its causes rather than to the physical manifestations.*[33]

who can help the ailing marriage?

Of course, sexual problems are not usually isolated as the only
difficulties in an ailing marriage. Too often they are merely a manifestation of a variety of other tensions. Masters and Johnson have
created a renaissance of scientific interest in sexual problems.
Several, but not enough, professional people have already completed
training at their institute. It can only be hoped that the training
program will expand through their trainees. With or without sexual
problems as a primary symptom complex, where can those with
marital difficulties seek help?

Family, friends, and relatives often must act as willing (or un-
willing) family counselors. Doubtless, they are the ones most frequently asked for advice. Not enough are reluctant to give it. Some,
however, are mindful that "marriage resembles a pair of shears, so
joined that they cannot be separated; often moving in opposite
directions, yet always punishing anyone who comes between
them." [34] They are faced with the twin handicaps of involvement and
lack of training—two serious shortcomings in an often explosive
situation. In considering the intimate, interrelated complexity of the
three elements of the ailing situation—the husband, the wife, and their
marriage—one appreciates more clearly the need for professional
objectivity and experience.

The family physician or gynecologist often acts as a marriage
counselor. Particularly if the problem is physical, he is in an invalu-
able position to promptly discover its source and to give practical
advice. The average physician is profoundly aware of the emotional
needs of patients. He may feel that the services of a professional
counselor are indicated.

The specialist marriage counselors have organized the highly
professional American Association of Marriage Counselors, composed
of sociologists, psychologists, lawyers, physicians, and clergymen.
These counselors have both training and experience in a field requiring sensitivity and wisdom. Unfortunately, there are not enough

---

Center, neither notion need be true. They found that of fifteen overweight wives that were
questioned, a higher number (thirteen) wanted intercourse more often than did wives who were
not overweight. There was no difference between the husbands of the two groups. The investigators concluded that for the overweight women they studied, food did not replace sexual intercourse. Both food and sexual intercourse were desired for the same reason: "to satisfy needs of
affection that were not fulfilled when they were children." ("Why Wives Overeat," *Science News*,
Vol. 102, No. 6 [August 5, 1972], p. 89.)

[33] James L. Mathis, "Masturbation After Marriage," *Medical Aspects of Human Sexuality*, Vol.
5, No. 3 (March 1971), p. 199.

[34] Sydney Smith, "Lady Holland's Memoir," Vol. I, Chapter 10.

of them. The more accessible Family Service Association of America is comprised of local Family Service agencies, which are found in most cities. Staffed by social caseworkers, these agencies charge fees based on ability to pay. Many such marriage counselors hope to explore the marital dilemma with both parties. Frequently, however, the tension between the two precludes this.

A basic first step is the acceptance by both partners that they need help. Sometimes "talking out" a problem, in the presence of an attentive third party, opens a road to its solution. Often, the marriage counselor can guide a degree of interaction between marital partners that is a revelation to both of them. Many married people simply do not talk enough to each other. As the years go by, they tend to confide less and less in each other. Some couples do not talk—they quarrel. Fear and pride and the sheer habit of quarreling have shipwrecked many a marriage.

Should the marriage counselor discover a deep emotional base to the marital problem, he may urge the couple to seek the help of a psychiatrist. One person may have been taught that sex is dirty. Another may have had an acrimonious mother who taught her daughter only of the baseness of men. Still another may be afraid of giving or taking love. "She can't give. I can't take." This tragic dialogue has been expressed in many ways to more than one therapist.

A marriage cannot be put on and taken off like a coat. It must be mended and refitted. But it can wear well.

It can last a lifetime.

senior citizen sexuality

> *Do you set down your name in the scroll of youth, that are written down old with all the characters of age? Have you not a moist eye? A dry hand? A yellow cheek? A white beard? A decreasing leg? An increasing belly? Is not your voice broken? Your wind short? Your chin double? Your wit single? And every part about you blasted with antiquity? And will you yet call yourself young? Fie, fie, fie, Sir John!*[35]

Thus is age described by the Chief Justice in Shakespeare's *Second Part of King Henry the Fourth*. It is not a pretty picture. Perhaps the greatest pain of the aged is in thinking that this is youth's view of them. To lose desirability without losing desire is a cruel blow for most people. In this youth-oriented society the aged shuffle by, unnoticed, untouched, and thus they are often cruelly deprived of two basic human needs—to be noticed and to be touched. The old

[35] William Shakespeare, *The Second Part of King Henry the Fourth*, I.ii. 201-09.

man who ventures to pat the head of a child may be regarded with suspicion, even with hidden horror. In this respect the elderly woman has the advantage; it is considered quite natural for her to cuddle and pet children. Aged males comprise less than 10 percent of adult child molesters.[36] Yet fear of the "dirty old man" runs deep in this society. Not many old people can satisfy their needs as did Mahatma Gandhi. Throughout his life he had castigated himself (and some of those who were close to him) for what he considered his ungovernable lust. In his old age he still felt sexual needs, but he found a way to forgive them in himself.

As communal riots raged between Hindus and Mohammedans and foreshadowed a partition of India and an end to Gandhi's vision of the unified state, the seventy-seven-year-old Mahatma became subject to violent, trembling disorders. To quiet these inner tremors he took to being cradled by middle-aged women, though the standard rumor—by no means disproven—has it as young women. The purpose was supposedly medicinal; the warmth of the bodies comforted him. Gandhi's friends, disquieted over the fact that these women were sometimes naked, protested to the Mahatma. These protestations, however, were of no avail. Rather than quit this practice of being held by naked women, Gandhi publicly proclaimed that it provided him with a good test of his own ability to suppress arousal.[37]

THE SEXUALITY OF THE AGING MALE

about the aging Aristotle's philosophy

A wonderful legend about Aristotle will serve well to introduce the subject of the aging male's sexuality. The conquerer Alexander the Great, the legend goes, was himself conquered by an Indian girl of great beauty named Phyllis. So enchanted was he by her that he neglected his duties. But Phyllis was part of a plot to destroy the Macedonian ruler. She was a "poison maiden." This was a common strategy in ancient Persia. At intervals over a prolonged period of time, these women were fed small doses of snake poison. In this way they built up a resistence to it. It was incorrectly believed that they could then transmit the poison to a victim by kissing or by sexual intercourse. They reasoned that the lover, unconditioned to the poison, would thus be killed. The old philosopher Aristotle uncovered

---

[36] H. L. Kozol, M. I. Cohen, and R. F. Garofolo, "The Criminally Dangerous Sex Offender," *New England Journal of Medicine,* Vol. 275 [1966], p. 79, cited in Frederick E. Whiskin, "The Geriatric Sex Offender," *Medical Aspects of Human Sexuality,* Vol. 4, No. 4 (April 1970), p. 126.
[37] Stanley J. Pacion, "Gandhi's Struggle with Sexuality," *Medical Aspects of Human Sexuality,* Vol. 5, No. 1 (January 1971), p. 89.

the plot. He warned Alexander to cease his attentions toward Phyllis. Alexander heard and obeyed. He refused Phyllis and slept with her no more.

Phyllis was furious with the great philosopher for his interference. Using her womanly wiles she set out to even the score. It was not long before Aristotle was at her feet. So smitten was he that he agreed to do anything she asked. The courtesan enticed the philosopher into her bedroom. She then ordered him to get down on all fours. The befuddled philosopher obeyed. Phyllis put a bridle in his mouth and a saddle on his back, mounted him, and then had the greatest thinker of the age ride her around the room on his back like a donkey as she whipped him. But her planned humiliation of Aristotle was not yet complete. She had concealed Alexander behind a curtain. The young conqueror stepped out from the hiding place and demanded that Aristotle explain his inconsistency.

The aged philosopher rose to his feet and dusted himself off. (First, he doubtless rid himself of the bridle and saddle.) This is what he said: "If a woman can make such a fool of a man of my age and wisdom, is she not even more dangerous for those who are younger and less wise? To my precept I have added an example, and you may profit from both."

the aging male's active sexual expression

There is some correlation between strong sexual feelings in youth and continued sexual interest in old age.[38] Despite the taboos in this culture against sexual expression among the aged, such sexual expression exists and, happily, to a considerable extent. "There are only two basic needs for regularity of sexual expression in 70–80-year-old women. These necessities are a reasonably good state of general health and an interesting and interested partner."[39] The same is true of the aging male.[40] The sexual excitement of the older male may not result in as much testicular elevation, scrotal sac congestion, or testicular engorgement as does sexual excitement in the younger male. However, these facts need not inhibit him. For the male older than fifty years of age, the ability to have an erection is usually not lost. What may be lost is his confidence to have and to maintain an erection. An understanding of the normal physiological changes that accompany aging is essential for a continuously gratifying sexual life. The speed of attaining an erection may be slower. The young man attains an erection three to five seconds following stimulation. The

[38] G. Newman and G. R. Nichols, "Sexual Activities and Attitudes in Older Persons," *Journal of the American Medical Association,* Vol. 173 (1960), pp. 33–35, cited in Eric Pfeiffer, "Geriatric Sex Behavior," *Medical Aspects of Human Sexuality,* Vol. 3, No. 7 (July 1969), p. 23.
[39] William H. Masters and Virginia E. Johnson, *Human Sexual Inadequacy,* p. 350.
[40] Ibid., p. 326.

older man requires two to three times as long, or even minutes. The rigidity of the erection may also be noticeably less as may be the volume of the ejaculate and the force of the ejaculation.[41]

The young man experiences ejaculation in two stages. First, the two- to four-second state of *ejaculatory inevitability,* in which the male can no longer control the ejaculation. Then, the second stage of *orgasmic expulsion.* In the older man the entire ejaculatory process may occur as a single stage. The duration of ejaculatory inevitability may be diminished to one or two seconds, or it may be lost altogether. Sometimes, however, it is just lengthened. Also lengthened is the *refractory period*—the period following ejaculation during which the male is unresponsive to sexual stimulation (see page 87). After ejaculating, the young man may require only minutes before he can again have an erection. Some aging men may also be able to do this; most, however, require hours. Following ejaculation, the aging man usually loses an erection much more rapidly than the young man.

The innate drive to have an ejaculation with each coital connection—*the ejaculatory demand*—also diminishes with age. This occurs between the ages of fifty and seventy years. At the age of sixty, for example, the man may find that an ejaculation with each second or third coital connection is entirely satisfying. He may be able to have an ejaculation more often, but he does not have to do so to be sexually satiated. *"This factor of reduced ejaculatory demand for the aging male is the entire basis for effective prolongation of sexual functioning in the aging population."*[42] Here the woman can help both her aging sexual partner and herself. Believing that his ejaculation is her sexual duty, she may try to force him to have an ejaculation with each coital connection. This is a mistake. She must leave the determination of the frequency of ejaculation to her partner. The man, thus relieved of any threat, is then able to have and share an erection with her. In this way, the aging couple may enjoy sexual functioning well into their eighties.[43]

Thus, the aging male's sexual expression is a compromise. For the enjoyment of having and maintaining an erection he exchanges a proportion of his ejaculations. This compromise brings a dividend: the older man generally has better control of the ejaculatory process than does a man in the twenty- to forty-year-old age group. So functional changes in the aging male do not detract from the pleasure of orgasmic experience.

[41] In young men, the ejaculated fluid is under enough pressure so that it may travel a distance of twelve to twenty-four inches beyond the external opening of the penis. Masters and Johnson have found that in older men this expulsive force may be diminished to between three to twelve inches. (William H. Masters and Virginia E. Johnson, *Human Sexual Inadequacy,* p. 320.)
[42] William H. Masters and Virginia E. Johnson, *Human Sexual Inadequacy,* p. 323.
[43] Ibid., pp. 322-25.

THE SEXUALITY OF THE AGING FEMALE

The aging female's sexual response may also be slowed with advancing years. This does not mean that she cannot enjoy active sexual expression. In the older woman the vaginal mucous lining thins and sometimes becomes too fragile for comfortable sexual intercourse. There is, moreover, some delay in the speed of vaginal lubrication, and the amount of lubricating material may be diminished. There may also be a reduced potential for vaginal expansion. The orgasmic phase of the woman's sexual response may be shortened. More distressing may be the loss of the regularity of uterine contractions during the orgasmic phase; the regular contractions may be replaced by uterine spasm, which can cause pain during orgasm. Most, if not all, of these changes are easily reversible by appropriate hormonal replacement therapy. Like the male, the aging female should enjoy a prolonged sexual life.

Nor are the later years a time to discontinue sexual experimentation. Indeed, the reverse is true. During the husband's middle and later years it may take more than a cerebral stimulus to initiate and maintain his erection. The husband's anxiety about his performance is easily transmitted to his wife. The knowing and understanding wife can help her husband (and herself) by massaging and manipulating his penis. And there are other ways to achieve full sexual satisfaction than direct genital contact that may be considered. "Proficiency in these (oral, manual and digital manipulations) not only provides powerful sources of sexual arousal, but also leads to distracting of attention from the sufferer's genital problem through focusing on pleasures being bestowed by the partner. The primary sexual difficulty is overcome without further formal treatment when a couple learns to accept that sexual satisfaction does not necessarily depend on coitus."[44]

FREQUENCY OF SEXUAL INTERCOURSE
AMONG OLDER PEOPLE

To what extent do older people engage in sexual intercourse? Kinsey's data revealed that by seventy years of age approximately 73 percent of white males remain sexually potent.[45] In their study, the oldest sexually active person was an eighty-eight-year-old man married to a ninety-year-old woman. The Kinsey investigators noted little evidence of a diminished sexual capacity among aging women. Indeed, unlike many younger women who reported less interest in sexual intercourse than did their husbands, a considerable number of older women expressed a greater desire for sexual intercourse than did

[44] J. Wolpe and A. A. Lazarus, *Behavior Therapy Techniques* (London, 1966), pp. 105–06.
[45] Alfred C. Kinsey, Wardell B. Pomeroy, and Clyde E. Martin, *Sexual Behavior in the Human Male* (Philadelphia, 1948), p. 237.

their husbands.[46] Another study (1960) concerned 250 people ranging in age from sixty to ninety-three years.[47] One hundred forty-nine were still married. When both partners were reasonably healthy sexual activity continued into the seventh, eighth, and ninth decades of life. Still another report (1961) indicated that 75 percent of the men (average age seventy-one years) in a group continued to experience sexual activity.[48] The gap between desire and activity is often considerable. In research carried out at the Duke University Center for the Study of Aging and Human Development it was found that in both men and women sexual desire outstrips activity. Women experience diminished desire and activity at a younger age than do men. It was found that

> *while about 2 out of 3 men in their early sixties are still sexually active, only 1 in 5 is still active in his eighties, though these older men still have desires. Thus there seems to be a growing discrepancy between the number of men who are still sexually interested and the number still sexually active. Nevertheless, there does not seem to be any single age beyond which all men have stopped having sexual intercourse. The story is a good deal different for women. When women arrive at their sixties the proportion who are no longer interested and who are no longer sexually active is already a good deal larger than for the men.[49]*

> *Women reported overwhelmingly (86%) that they had stopped having sexual intercourse because their husbands had either died, become ill, lost interest, or lost potency. Even when death of the husband was eliminated as a reason for stopping, the large majority of women still blamed their husbands, and the men also tended to blame themselves. Thus there was good general agreement that it was the husband who was usually responsible for the termination of sexual activity within the marriage of two aged people.[50]*

One of the most striking findings of the Duke study was that "some 13% to 15% of aged persons, when followed over a period of years, actually showed rising patterns of sexual interest and activity."[51]

[46] Ibid., pp. 235-37, and Alfred C. Kinsey et al., *Sexual Behavior in the Human Female*, pp. 353-54.
[47] G. Newman and C. R. Nichols, "Sexual Activities and Attitudes in Older Persons," p. 33, cited in Jack Weinberg, "Sexuality in Later Life," *Medical Aspects of Human Sexuality*, Vol. 5, No. 4 (April 1971), p. 223.
[48] J. T. Freeman, "Sexual Capacities in the Aging Male," *Geriatrics*, Vol. 16 (1961), p. 37, cited in Jack Weinberg, "Sexuality in Later Life," p. 223.
[49] Eric Pfeiffer, "Geriatric Sex Behavior," p. 26.
[50] Ibid., p. 28, citing E. Pfeiffer, A. Verwoerdt, and H. S. Wang, "Sexual Behavior in Aged Men and Women, I. Observations on 254 Community Volunteers," *Archives of General Psychiatry*, Vol. 19 (1968), pp. 753-58.
[51] Ibid., citing E. Pfeiffer, A. Verwoerdt, and H. S. Wang, "Sexual Behavior in Aged Men and Women, I. Observations on 254 Community Volunteers," pp. 753-58, and A. Verwoerdt, E. Pfeiffer, and H. S. Wang, "Sexual Behavior in Senescence, II. Patterns of Sexual Activity and Interest," *Geriatrics*, Vol. 24 (1969), pp. 137-54.

Such data should certainly lay to rest any misconceptions concerning older persons' impotence or disinterest in sexual intercourse. The work of Masters and Johnson emphasizes the need for active sexual expression among aged people. In their *Human Sexual Response,* Masters and Johnson reported their studies of sixty-one menopausal and postmenopausal women ranging in age from forty to seventy-eight years. Despite the above-noted diminished physiological sexual response in the older woman (see page 000), all were able to reach orgasm. Of the thirty-nine elderly males in the study, the oldest was eighty-nine. "The mere fact," wrote the researchers, "that full penile erection could be obtained and an ejaculation produced by an 89-year-old man during episodes of active cooperation as a study subject is considered worthy of report."[52] But all the elderly men actively cooperated in the program. True, these men experienced varying degrees of diminished sexual vigor. But by no means does this indicate decreased enjoyment of coitus. Significantly, moreover, many aging men and women suffering from sexual inadequacies respond well to treatment. Also men and women who have set aside sexual expression for physical or social reasons can often be successfully restimulated. And so not every part of either the aging man or woman is as "blasted with antiquity" as Shakespeare supposed. Growing and irrefutable evidence plainly supports the heartening contention stated by Masters and Johnson that "there is every reason to believe that maintained regularity of sexual expression coupled with adequate physical well-being and healthy mental orientation to the aging process will combine to provide a sexually stimulating climate within a marriage. This climate will, in turn, improve sexual tension and provide a capacity for sexual performance that frequently may extend to and beyond the 80-year level."[53]

epilogue

Then Almitra spoke again and said, And what of Marriage, master?
And he answered saying:
You were born together, and together you shall be forevermore.
You shall be together when the white wings of death scatter your days.
Ay, you shall be together even in the silent memory of God.
But let there be spaces in your togetherness,
And let the winds of the heavens dance between you.

[52]William H. Masters and Virginia E. Johnson, *Human Sexual Response* (Boston, 1966), p. 181.
[53]Ibid., p. 270.

Love one another, but make not a bond of love:
Let it rather be a moving sea between the shores of your souls.
Fill each other's cup but drink not from one cup.
Give one another of your bread but eat not from the same loaf.
Sing and dance together and be joyous, but let each one of you be alone,
Even as the strings of a lute are alone though they quiver with the same music.

Give your hearts but not into each other's keeping.
For only the hand of Life can contain your hearts.
And stand together yet not too near together:
For the pillars of the temple stand apart,
And the oak tree and the cypress grow not in each other's shadow.[54]

[54] Kahlil Gibran, *The Prophet* (New York, 1923), pp. 16-17.

correcting problems of sexual expression

9

Masters and Johnson's study of human sexual inadequacy

Physiology is the science dealing with the functions of the living organism and its parts. The initial work of Masters and Johnson was largely physiological. In their study of the physiology of the female sexual response, for example, they observed 382 women in their laboratory during more than ten thousand cycles of sexual response. There is a basic wisdom to this approach. Inadequate sexual response is an all too common human problem. One can hardly expect to effectively treat disturbances of sexual function without an accurate and complete understanding of the function itself. The results of their research were published in the now famous *Human Sexual Response*. The book is based on knowledge gained from studies of sexual anatomy and physiology begun in 1954 and reported in 1966. Although *Human Sexual Response* is a classic addition to the scientific literature, like all such contributions it will have to be expanded as more research information is gathered.

In 1959 Masters and Johnson began their treatment program for a variety of sexual dysfunctions. In 1970 the methods and results of their treatments were published in their book *Human Sexual Inadequacy*. Included in the evaluation of the results of the treatment program were the findings of a five-year follow-up study of their treated patients. Such a delayed appraisal of the effects of treatment surely increases the significance of the data.

In the development of their various treatments for sexual inadequacies, Masters and Johnson were guided by certain basic concepts. First, they emphasized that sexual activity is a form of communication and personal interaction. Their second concept (a corollary of the first) was the principle that it was the sick marital relationship, and not only the sick individual, that required treatment. Here Masters and Johnson parted company with tradition. Previous failures by some therapists to understand that there is no such person as an uninvolved partner in a marital relationship, or, when that was understood, the lack of practical effort to treat the relationship itself may well explain some of the failures of more traditional approaches.

A third concept resulted in another treatment innovation. Masters and Johnson believe that no man can fully comprehend a woman's sexual response; no woman can fully comprehend a man's sexual response. This realization has resulted in their development of the *dual-sex treatment team.* Composed of a man and a woman, the treatment team deals with the sexual inadequacies consequent to the ailing marital relationship. This approach now seems obvious and logical. Yet in the past it was not generally taken. Single therapists, usually men, saw patients alone. The patients' marital partners were not included in the therapeutic process. Again the results were only too often disappointing.

The fourth concept was the necessity of taking careful histories of all patients as well as paying meticulous attention to a complete physical and laboratory examination. A patient's history might reveal, for example, that she was taking an oral contraceptive. This could cause her inadequate sexual response. In such a case, the cure could be the simple discontinuance of the pill. In another case, a physical and laboratory examination might reveal a diabetic husband. This, rather than a psychological problem in the marital relationship, could cause his impotence. Purely physical factors are but a small percentage of the total causes of sexual inadequacy. But if these factors are not first eliminated therapy might be based on mistaken diagnoses and may even magnify problems rather than alleviate them.

The fifth concept involved the use of partner surrogates (substitutes) in the treatment of single male patients. During the two-week treatment period these women assumed the role of the male patient's sexual partner. After intensive screening of thirty-one women volunteers by both investigators, thirteen were finally selected. Although attractiveness played a part in determining the selection, it was by no means the deciding factor. "Of far greater importance is the partner surrogate's ability to identify with the male, her ability to evaluate the situation, and to handle the experience with grace and dignity . . . Her psychological support and compassionate involvement with the male's problem contributes immeasurably to success of the treatment."[1] Surrogate partners ranged in age from the early twenties to the early forties. All but one were used no more frequently than approximately once a year. The one exception was a physician; she was particularly helpful in establishing treatment techniques.

[1]"An Interview with Masters and Johnson on 'Human Sexual Inadequacy,'" *Medical Aspects of Human Sexuality,* Vol. 4, No. 7 (July 1970), p. 29.

Partner surrogates were not provided for female patients. Masters and Johnson consider this culture not yet ready to accept such a procedure.

CRITICS OF MASTERS AND JOHNSON

The treatment procedures for sexual inadequacy practiced by Masters and Johnson are not without their critics. Nor are all their critics ill-informed traditionalists. The distinguished psychiatrist Rollo May has said that "they put the emphasis on orgasm when it should be on love. They help some couples, and I congratulate them for that, but their total impact on society is to send us further down the road of misunderstanding ourselves and our need to love one another."[2] In a recent review of *Human Sexual Inadequacy* in the *Journal of the American Medical Association,* psychiatrist Natalie Shainess wrote:

> The ideas within this book can be summed up quite briefly: marital units (not couples, please!) are advised to "pleasure" (touch) each other—a leaf taken from sensitivity and encounter groups—but to delay actual coitus until given permission by the therapists; wives are taught to squeeze the penis to prevent ejaculation; husbands are taught to use metal dilators on wives who have vaginismus. In short, each is placed in the power of the other, depending on the condition. This reviewer cannot resist asking: can faulty and inadequate sex truly be corrected in this joyless way, and ignoring the psychological forces at work?
>
> Tucked away neatly in the chapter on primary impotence comes an astonishing innovation: a section on "replacement partners" and "partner surrogates." A case is made for these women surrogates (provided for single men by the authors): they are described as "fully sexually responsive, confident, understanding and compassionate." Apparently, a superbreed. Why are they not busy with their own confident, fully responsive men?[3]

A brief review of some of the material presented in *Human Sexual Inadequacy* is included in this chapter. It is doubtless too early to judge the total societal effect of Masters and Johnson's work. However, both May and Shainess do emphasize a valid concern held by other investigators. The sheer objectivity of the approach to sexuality by Masters and Johnson might indeed lead some to unthinkingly

---

[2]Paul Wilkes, "Sex and the Married Couple," *The Atlantic Monthly,* Vol. 226 (December 1970), p. 92.
[3]Natalie Shainess, review of *Human Sexual Inadequacy, Journal of the American Medical Association,* Vol. 213, No. 12 (September 21, 1970), p. 2084.

consider sexual expression as a mechanical event. The danger would certainly seem greatest with those who have not considered sexuality as an expression of the whole personality. Masters and Johnson can hardly be said to make this error. Masters has defined sexuality as "a dimension of the personality and sex as a specific physical activity." [4] Recently, the authoritative journal *Medical Aspects of Human Sexuality* devoted a considerable portion of one issue to a careful and generally appreciative description of the Masters and Johnson technique. In an introductory statement the editors emphasized that *"the following descriptions constitute the physical procedures utilized in treatment of sexual dysfunctions. It is to be emphasized that the techniques are of little or no value without supportive psychotherapy for the marital relationship, for the* relationship *and the interaction of the couple are the primary focus of Masters' and Johnson's therapeutic program."* [5] It is with this same caution that the Masters and Johnson material is presented in this chapter.

Masters and Johnson classify and treat sexual inadequacy

EARLY PATIENT DAYS

To become patients at the Reproductive Biology Research Foundation in St. Louis, the marital couple must be referred by a physician, psychologist, social worker, or clergyman. It is common for couples who are members of these professions to refer themselves. Certain aspects of the therapy program are common to all patient-couples no matter what their sexual dysfunction. All take rooms at a St. Louis hotel. The staff provides each couple with a program of the available recreation and entertainment in the surrounding area. This relaxed "vacation" approach is geared according to patient tastes and is an important part of the treatment program. All patients are scheduled to be seen seven days a week for two weeks. Depending to some extent on the ability to pay, the cost at this writing is $2500 per couple.

During the first four days the program is very much the same for all couples. An initial fifteen-minute interview establishes the basic rules of the program. For example, no overt sexual activity may take place until permitted by the therapists. All sessions are recorded to minimize the possibility of a loss of confidential information that might occur with the need for transcription by a third person. A

[4] Mary Harrington Hall, "A Conversation with Masters and Johnson," *Psychology Today,* Vol. 3, No. 2 (July 1969), p. 52 (see also page 84).
[5] "Highlights of Masters and Johnson Therapy Techniques," *Medical Aspects of Human Sexuality,* Vol. 4, No. 7 (July 1970), p. 36.

complete history of both individuals usually takes a full day. It is designed to reveal the development of past personality and sexual problems that contribute to the present pattern of sexual disability. Both individuals also undergo a thorough medical examination, designed to ferret out those physical ailments that interfere with proper sexual functioning.

The patients and therapists meet at a series of round-table conferences. At the first meeting, the therapists discuss their initial findings with the couple. So begins an education program about sexuality. It is an integral and continuing part of the therapy. Long held misapprehensions and myths about sexuality are aired. Problems revealed by the history of each patient are explored. Sometimes one member of the marital pair wishes a secret fact kept from the other. This desire is generally respected, although there are occasions in which the sharing of such information is necessary for the resolution of a sexual problem. Permission to discuss the secret is usually obtained in a private interview between one of the therapists and the patient.

If the first round-table conference is successful the couple is given their homework. This consists of "sensate focus exercises" to be carried out in the privacy of their hotel room. The exercises are simple, but they have profound meaning. Lying naked, the pair stroke and feel one another. The breasts and genitals are not touched. At this stage coitus is not to take place. This pleasing of one another is free from any demand by either member of the pair. Neither is required to perform. People who have been married for many years may, at first, be clumsily self-conscious with their partners. Sometimes it seems very funny to them. This is good. Humor and sexual expression are old companions, and they get along well with one another. After a few such sessions, most couples look forward to these experiences. They may come to have a poetic quality. It is as if Robert Browning's lines had truly come to pass:

> *Your soft hand is a woman of itself,*
> *And mine the man's bared breast she curls inside.*[6]

Following the fourth day increased sexual expression is permitted. The breasts and genitals are now touched and stroked. The communicating wife or husband guides the hands of the partner. They tell one another what is most pleasurable. They share information about the areas of greater pleasure, the speed of stroking, the degree of pressure desired. In the clinic the round-table discussions are continued. The various aspects of the developing sexual experience are discussed. The couple, moreover, receives information on the next procedure.

[6]Robert Browning, "Andrea del Sarto," lines 21-22.

During the pleasuring exercises, an old problem arose that led Masters and Johnson into a new area of research. Dry or rough hands interfered with the pleasure of some couples. A variety of well-advertised lotions had been tried by them. Because they were sticky or too cooling, or otherwise unpleasant, an effort was made to develop a more agreeable lotion. Thus it was finally possible to offer each couple the choice of a variety of lotions that were variously scented, or an unscented lotion could be chosen. An odor can have a profoundly stimulating effect on the sexual emotions (see page 265). Moreover, the use of a lotion helped some couples to overcome their revulsion of vaginal secretions or seminal fluid. A number of couples (eighteen of one hundred) refused the use of a moisturizing lotion. They considered it immature and undignified. As it turned out, the treatment failure rate was extremely high among those couples. The number of couples involved was too small for final conclusions. However, the rejection of the lotion as a medium of giving and taking sexual pleasure seemed to be an astonishingly good indicator of a future inability to overcome the sexual inadequacy.

On the fifth day the therapy is directed to the specific problem affecting the partners. Some of these problems will now be considered.

INADEQUATE SEXUAL RESPONSE IN WOMEN

definition of terms

Frigidity is used as a general term to indicate inadequate sexual response in women. The word has been used to describe anything from the woman's total revulsion by sex, to the result of her severe pain during intercourse, to her mild indifference, to her sexual enjoyment without orgasm, to her sexual pleasure with occasional orgasm. It has such a wide spectrum of meanings that Masters and Johnson reject its use as a diagnostic word.[7] "They feel that the maximum meaning of the word should indicate no more than a prevailing inability or subconscious refusal to respond sexually to effective stimulation."[8] In this book, the word *frigidity* will be avoided and the term *inadequate sexual response* will be used instead.

[7]Like most labels, the word *frigid* can do harm. Its application to a woman may increase her anxiety and decrease her self-esteem. One can hardly expect to help her to sexual adequacy in this way. In addition, more than one young male has countered a girl's rejection with the epithet *frigid!* Interestingly, one student of the subject points to a significant misuse of the word *frigid:* "When the norms forbade all extramarital sex relations, a girl or woman could easily refuse male requests. When the norms are permissive, she has nothing to hide behind. If she does not wish to engage in sex relations—and most teenage girls probably do not—she is left in an exploitable position. If in the past she had to say no to safeguard her self-respect, she must now say yes for the same reason—to avoid the dreaded epithet *frigid.*" (Jessie Bernard, "The Fourth Revolution," *Journal of Social Issues,* Vol. 22, No. 2 (1966), pp. 76–87.)

[8]Philip Polatin, "The Frigid Woman," *Medical Aspects of Human Sexuality,* Vol. 4, No. 8 (August 1970), p. 12.

Inadequate sexual response in women may be due to a wide variety of physical or emotional factors. Occasionally both physical and emotional factors may be involved. Three aspects of female inadequate sexual response have been studied by Masters and Johnson: *dyspareunia* (painful coitus), *orgasmic dysfunction,* and *vaginismus* (painful spasm of the vagina). (Dyspareunia also occurs in the male.)[9]

female dyspareunia

Painful sexual intercourse may result from physical causes or from insufficient lubrication of the vagina (see page 85) due to psychological problems.

Physical causes   Therapists at the Masters and Johnson clinic may discover causes of female dyspareunia as a result of the physical examination. An intact membrane or its ragged, bruised remnants may be the cause of pain at the vaginal opening. Clitoral pain may result from an irritating collection of smegma.[10] Moreover, dyspareunia may occur when precoital play or masturbation has irritated the clitoris beyond any sense of pleasure (see pages 56-57).

Vaginal infections may be another factor causing painful coitus. The normal acidity within the vagina keeps harmful bacteria at bay. During menstruation, the vaginal environment becomes alkaline, and bacteria are more able to thrive. This explains the greater incidence of infection during the menstrual period. The physician is able to treat the causes of greatly diminished vaginal acidity. The vagina often becomes infected as a result of anal intercourse. This is particularly likely when anal intercourse is a form of foreplay. Contaminated by rectal microbes, the penis transfers them to the vagina. When anal intercourse is practiced, the male should ejaculate in the rectum, not in the vagina. "There should never be penetration of both rectal and vaginal orifices during any single coital episode."[11] And, after anal intercourse, penile cleanliness is mandatory. Other vaginal infections that may produce dyspareunia include those caused by trichonomads, and fungi such as monilia (see pages 72-73).

The vagina may also become irritated by inserted chemicals. Among these may be contraceptive creams, jellies, suppositories, and

[9]The work of Masters and Johnson is emphasized in these discussions. Instances in which this is not the case are indicated. For example, the descriptions of the causes of some sexual dysfunctions may include the opinions of other investigators. An outline summary highlighting the *physical* procedures of the Masters and Johnson therapy techniques was published in *Medical Aspects of Human Sexuality,* Vol. 55, No. 7 (July 1970), pp. 36-37. Both it and the book *Human Sexual Inadequacy* (Boston, 1970) were used for most of the consideration of the therapy that is in this text.

[10]The matter secreted by any of the sebaceous glands is composed in great part of fat. Specifically, the sebaceous matter that collects around the clitoris and labia minora, or between the glans penis and the foreskin.

[11]William H. Masters and Virginia E. Johnson, *Human Sexual Inadequacy,* (Boston, 1970), p. 271.

foams. The rubber of the diaphragm or the condom may also cause vaginal sensitivity reactions. A singularly common cause of female dyspareunia is based on the mistaken belief that douching is necessary after coitus in order to insure cleanliness. It is not. In considering douches, and, indeed, the whole subject of the woman's genital hygiene, it is well to remember that nature long ago provided woman with a vaginal environment that is essential to her well-being. Frequent douching, even with plain water, can be harmful because it will interfere with the survival of beneficial microbes that are necessary to protect the vagina from outside infection. It is true that soap and detergent solutions kill spermatozoa. Nevertheless, the chemicals they contain often irritate the vaginal mucosa and the vulva. Indeed, chemical douches are a common cause of vaginal sensitivity reactions. Plain water also immobilizes spermatozoa. However, as soon as ejaculation occurs, spermatozoa enter the cervical canal. Therefore, no vaginal douch is a contraceptive, because the douch liquid does not get into the small cervical canal that leads from the opening of the cervix to the uterus. A vaginal douche under increased pressure should never be used; such a hazardous procedure can force infection upward and into the pelvic organs.

If desired for personal hygiene, and not for contraceptive purposes, the vulva may be cleansed after coitus with plain tepid water. An extremely light soapy solution, although needless, may be used. However, care should be taken that the soapy solution does not enter the vagina; the soaping should, moreover, be followed by careful rinsing. A woman should no more think of putting a soapy solution into the vagina than she would consider putting one into her eye. Some women insist on douching. Plain water is enough. Highly advertised "feminine hygiene" preparations may smell better, but they may also be harmful. There is no confirmed evidence that a douche will prevent major venereal diseases, trichomonas vaginalis, or monilial infection (see pages 60–73).

It is advisable for the male to wash his genitals with soapy water every day, whether or not he has had coitus. This is done for hygienic reasons; such washing is particularly helpful to the uncircumcised male. Many physicians recommend that the male wash his genitalia after sexual intercourse. This is a good procedure for desirable personal hygiene; supportable evidence that it prevents venereal infection remains unconfirmed.[12]

[12] Aquiles J. Sobrero, "Genital Hygiene," *Medical Aspects of Human Sexuality*, Vol. 6, No. 9 (September 1972), pp. 161, 165.

It is the healthy acid reaction of the vagina that keeps yeast, fungi, and bacteria from overgrowing. Regrettably the menstrual blood is alkaline. For this reason, a menstruating woman does lower her barrier against infection every month. Most women handle this functional paradox without problems. For some, however, even a prolonged menstrual flow may result in vaginal infection. This needs treatment. Part of the therapy might be an acid douche. It should never be used unless specifically advised by a physician. (Robert N. Rutherford, extracted from *Audio-Digest Family Practice*, Vol. 19, No. 17, in the Audio Digest's subscription series of tape recorded programs. Cited in "Combating Alkalinity in Vaginitis," *California Medicine*, Vol. 116, No. 5 [May

It has been suggested that part of the physician's treatment of recurrent vaginal infections might include the advice to, at least temporarily, discontinue the wearing of form-fitting clothing, such as panty hose and panty girdles. Worn by an estimated 76 to 80 percent of U.S. women, they are thought to promote vaginal infections because they produce the warmer temperatures in which organisms flourish.[13]

Older women (past the age of fifty) often complain of dyspareunia. When this is due to the thinning of the vaginal mucous membrane, it quickly responds to adequate therapy.

Psychological causes   Psychological problems can cause insufficient vaginal lubrication, which results in dyspareunia. This chain of events parallels the male's inability to have an erection. Insufficient lubrication may be due to fear, hostility, conflict,[14] or combinations of any of these three. The woman may be afraid of pregnancy (legitimate or illegitimate) or the pains of childbirth. She may fear men, venereal disease, or genital injury (his or hers). She may be haunted by the fearful memory of overly restrictive or denigrating parents. All these, and more, may block her sexual responsiveness. And just as these fears may inhibit penile tumescence and erection in the male, they may block the venous engorgement about the vagina that is necessary for vaginal lubrication.

As a companion of fear, hostility may be a major component of the psychological problem. Some women fear yielding to men because they are resentful of their dependence on them for sexual pleasure. Others fear the abandonment of a sexual experience; they resist revealing the depth of their orgasmic emotion for fear of becoming vulnerable. Sometimes the hostile woman withholds from her husband her complete submission to sexual pleasure, in this way diminishing his pleasure and punishing him. She is not unlike a country invaded by a hated army. The invader receives as little pleasure as possible, and he is hurt where he is most vulnerable—in his ego.

Such fears and hostilities may be rooted in long established and unresolved conflicts. A Lesbian orientation (see page 304, footnote 20), an unresolved Oedipus complex (see pages 11–13), an attachment to a domineering mother—these may be among the conflicts that

---

1972], p. 24.) It should, moreover, be emphasized that sexual activity is not a major cause of urinary infection. True, since the opening of the urethra is separated from the vaginal orifice by a very small distance (see Figure 2-4, page 40), urethral infection during coitus can conceivably (although uncommonly) occur. Some women seem more susceptible to this than others. Some physicians advise certain of their patients to urinate after intercourse and, moreover, to drink a glass of water to encourage another voiding of urine during the night. ("The Female Infection: Watch It," *Medical World*, Vol. 13, No. 29 [August 4, 1972], pp. 20–23, 29, 33–35.)

[13] *M.D., Medical Newsmagazine*, Vol. 16, No. 9 (September 1972), p. 87.

[14] Terence F. McGuire and Richard M. Steinhilber, "Frigidity, the Primary Female Sexual Dysfunction," *Medical Aspects of Human Sexuality*, Vol. 4, No. 10 (October 1970), pp. 108–23.

contribute to a woman's inadequate sexual response. Another conflict may be due to an untruth that the woman learned as a child; she may have been taught that she can take without giving. But it is only by giving that she can receive most fully.

Fear, hostility, conflict—these three may cripple the sexual life of the husband as well as the wife. This is yet another reason for the importance of approaching the problems of inadequate sexual response via the marital unit—the husband and the wife. In some cases of female dyspareunia, relief may be provided through psychotherapy. Therapy is least likely to succeed in those cases in which the marital relationship is poor beyond reasonable chances of repair, or in marriages that have only a socioeconomic basis, or, finally, when the woman's orientation is toward homosexual behavior.

female orgasmic dysfunction

Until quite recently, the woman's sexual potency was primarily defined by her ability to accept her husband's penis on demand. If she did reach the attention of a physician it was because her husband was hampered by an imperforate hymen or (as occurs very rarely) by the absence of a vagina. As late as the nineteenth century, the London physician William Acton wrote "that most women happily for them [or as in a later edition, "happily for society"] are not much troubled with sexual feeling of any kind."[15]

Today, happily for both society and its men and women, this misconception is being corrected. In their treatment of nonorgasmic women, Masters and Johnson consider it of paramount importance to educate the husband about his wife's sexuality. To a considerable degree the success of their efforts is dependent on his acceptance of this responsibility. It is of more than parenthetical interest that many so-called cases of female orgasmic dysfunction are really due to the male's premature ejaculation.

Treatment of female orgasmic dysfunction   During the conferences with Masters and Johnson, or their associated therapists, the history of the couple's past sexual experiences and sexually tinged memories are carefully explored. Those factors that sexually stimulate or depress the woman are also discussed. During premarital dating many young couples try to neck their way out of their conflicts. For a while it may work. But in a continuing relationship like marriage problems are not so easily ignored. No woman can enjoy her sexual life if the rest of her life is a nightmare. She cannot be deeply hurt at 9:00 P.M. and deeply loving at 10:00 P.M. Angry reminders of wifely duties accomplish nothing except, at times, indifferent sub-

[15] Melva Weber, "Sexual Inadequacy: How Masters and Johnson Treat It," *Medical World News,* Vol. 11, No. 18 (May 1, 1970), p. 47.

mission, which is worse than nothing. Only a secure wife, sure of being loved, finds joy in sex.

The couple must also learn that, just as the male cannot will an erection, neither can the female will her sexual excitement or orgasmic release. During the treatment of female orgasmic dysfunction the wife is encouraged to seek and share sexually stimulating experiences with her husband. After sensate focus exercises have proved effective, the couple may engage in genital play. For this Masters and Johnson recommend a particular position. The husband is seated or is reclining slightly. The wife is between his legs with her back resting against his chest. In this way the husband has full access to his wife's body. By guiding his hand or squeezing his legs, the wife can direct her husband's caresses. His gentleness and his willingness to consider her wishes, combined with his consideration and the warmth of his feeling toward her, are important factors in the success of the treatment of the woman's orgasmic dysfunction. In the above described position the wife's back is protected, and her sense of security is enhanced. And her self-conscious role as a spectator of her own sexual response is diminished.

In his genital play the husband is cautioned not to approach the clitoris directly. The extreme sensitivity of this organ often makes direct stimulation an irritating, even a painful, experience for the woman. Varied and random hand-finger stimulation of the breasts, abdomen, thighs, and labia can be intermingled with stroking the less sexually sensitive areas previously stimulated during the sensate focus exercises. The husband's fingers may maneuver lubricating fluid from the vaginal outlet to the clitoral area. Throughout the experience the couple is under no pressure; they know that they are making a beginning and that the experience will be repeated soon.

Success in manual excitation may be followed by nondemanding coitus. The female-superior position is used. The husband lies still on his back. On top of him, the wife's slow, controlled pelvic thrusting makes her more aware of the pleasures of penile containment. As vaginal sensation develops, the husband may thrust, but nondemandingly. His pace should be guided by the wife. Periodically the coital position and activity should be interrupted with an episode of love play. Should the husband ejaculate, as indeed he might, the experience can be enjoyed as such. Soon there will be an opportunity to try again, to make further progress. When the wife has begun to appreciate the sensate pleasure of the penis in her vagina, the couple may have sexual intercourse in a lateral (side face-to-face) position. In the lateral position recommended by Masters and Johnson, the husband lies on his back with his legs slightly spread. The wife lies on her right side and stomach to his left with her legs more or less straddling his right leg. Thus the wife's right thigh is the only weight that must be supported. Since neither is supporting the other's

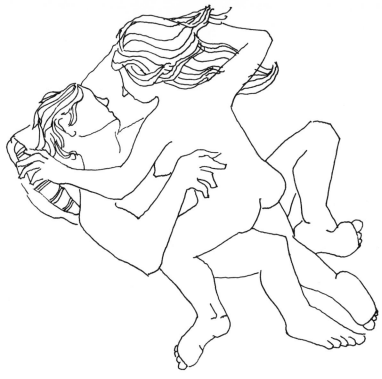

9-1 Masters and Johnson's lateral position

total weight, pelvic movement is easy for both. Both husband and wife will find a pillow under their heads an added comfort; a pillow under the wife's right side may also be supportive.

vaginismus

Vaginismus is a spasm of the vagina that results in a constriction of the vaginal outlet. The spasm is involuntary; it is in no way under the control of the woman who experiences it. It is brought about by "imagined, anticipated, or real attempts at vaginal penetration. Thus, vaginismus is a classic example of a psychosomatic illness."[16] Vaginismus is easily diagnosed by the examining physician. While the patient is on the examining table, any suggestion that the physician is about to insert an examining finger into the vagina causes

---

[16] William H. Masters and Virginia E. Johnson, *Human Sexual Inadequacy,* p. 250. The term *psychosomatic* is from the Greek *psychikos,* mind + *soma,* body. Psychosomatic disorders originate in the mind and are manifested as physical symptoms. Emotional stimuli are referred by the brain to body organs, resulting in effects ranging from goose flesh to vaginismus. The ancients were well aware of psychosomatic influences. "Diseases of the mind impair the powers of the body," wrote Ovid. Nor did the seventeenth-century Englishman John Donne contradict Ovid when he wrote that "the body makes the minde."

the woman "to escape the examiner's approach by withdrawing to the head of the table." [17] To avoid examination she may raise her legs and draw her knees together. Her apprehensive distress is thus immediately apparent. Gentle insertion of the examining physician's finger into the vagina soon confirms vaginismus. Since penile penetration is impossible or, at best, extremely difficult, vaginismus is commonly the cause of unconsummated marriages and marriages in which coitus is very infrequent. Understandably, the husband may be severely affected by his wife's disability. Male sexual inadequacies, such as impotence, are not uncommonly associated with vaginismus. This emphasizes the importance of a diagnostic and treatment approach involving both members of the marital couple. Among the causes of vaginismus is repressive sex education from which the child learns that sex is dirty and sinful. The psychic trauma of rape or a painful initial coital experience may also result in vaginismus. A previous homosexual orientation may be another cause.

Treatment of vaginismus   Masters and Johnson have had considerable success with a procedure that first involves a thorough exploration of the misconceptions about sexuality that may contribute to the wife's tension.[18] Both husband and wife may profit from this discussion. They gain an initial idea of the physical nature of vaginismus from anatomical charts illustrating the involuntary constriction that occurs in the outer third of the vaginal barrel. They are then given a practical demonstration. With the woman properly placed on the examining table and draped, the physician inserts a rubber-gloved finger into the constricted vagina. With a rubber-gloved finger the wife then feels her own vaginismus. She is then examined by her husband.

When the couple fully understand the nature of the problem they can try to solve it together. In the privacy of their bedroom the husband gently inserts lubricated, graduated sizes of metal dilators into his wife's vagina. To avoid discomfort he does this under his wife's direction. The wife retains a dilator of a comfortable size in her vagina. Increasingly larger dilators are used during succeeding treatments. When penile insertion is attempted, it may be preceded by the insertion of a dilator. "Usually a major degree of involuntary spasm can be eliminated in a matter of 3 to 5 days, presuming daily renewal of dilating procedures." [19]

Of the use of the dilator in treating vaginismus it was written more than twenty years ago that "it will not cure phobias, it will not make a disliked husband attractive, but it will make coitus physically painless, and when no deep-seated prejudices exist, responsiveness

[17] William H. Masters and Virginia E. Johnson, *Human Sexual Inadequacy,* p. 251.
[18] Ibid., pp. 262–65.
[19] Ibid., p. 263.

may develop." [20] This serves to emphasize the importance of the Masters and Johnson round-table conferences and their educational techniques. However, some women, as well as their husbands, may require prolonged psychiatric help. Relief of the problem of vaginismus makes both members of the couple more responsive to such help, if needed. Of twenty-nine women reported treated for vaginismus by Masters and Johnson, all recovered from the disorder: sixteen were orgasmic for the first time in their lives during their two-week stay at the Foundation; six who had been orgasmic before the onset of vaginismus experienced a return of orgasmic ability; four became orgasmic during the follow-up period; three remained nonorgasmic although they were relieved of vaginismus.[21]

INADEQUATE SEXUAL RESPONSE IN MEN

male dyspareunia

Only the most common of the considerable number of causes of male dyspareunia will be presented here. These are generally physical in nature. Poor personal hygiene may lead to an infection beneath the foreskin. The resultant inflammation may be painful even without the stimulation of sexual intercourse. Old scars within the urethra from a subsided gonorrheal infection (see Table 2-2, page 63) may cause a stricture of the urethral passage, which may result not only in painful coitus but, indeed, may interfere with the passage of the urine through the penis. Many, but by no means all, strictures are due to untreated gonorrhea. Early and adequate treatment of gonorrheal infection is the best preventative of gonorrheal strictures. A third cause of male dyspareunia is phimosis (Greek *phimosis,* muzzling, closure). Men with phimosis have an unusually long prepuce (foreskin) that is so tight that it cannot be drawn back from over the glans penis. As with many other penile problems, the condition may be painful even when the man is not attempting sexual intercourse. Phimosis can become quite complicated if it is not treated. Fibrous tissue may grow between the prepuce and the glans. These fibrous adhesions make the prepuce even less retractable. Smegma (see page 284, footnote 10) collects and may cause infection, inflammation, and even ulceration, all of which may be very painful. Fortunately, these disagreeable and inhibiting circumstances are easily

---

[20] R. T. Frank, "Dyspareunia: A Problem for the General Practitioner," *Journal of the American Medical Association,* Vol. 136 (1948), p. 361

[21] William H. Masters and Virginia E. Johnson, *Human Sexual Inadequacy,* p. 264.

The use of tampons during menstruation is believed to have reduced the incidence of vaginismus among young women. Familiarity with the anatomy, and the frequent introduction of tampons into the vaginal opening seem to minimize the reflexive protective action that leads to vaginismus. By using tampons, young women become aware that neither a physician's examination nor a first coitus is necessarily painful. (John C. Weed, "Tampons," *Medical Aspects of Human Sexuality,* Vol. 6, No. 4 [April 1972], p. 10.)

rectified—usually by circumcision and administration of medication to relieve the infection.

Still another cause of male dyspareunia may be found within the environment of the vagina. Not uncommonly contraceptive chemicals and douche preparations may cause allergic manifestations of sensitive penile tissue. Masters and Johnson report the case of a man who, despite numerous changes in sexual partners, found "glans constraint in the vaginal environment intolerable. There was a constant blistering and peeling of the superficial tissues of the glans' surface . . . This individual simply could not tolerate the natural pH levels of the vagina." [22] He was, therefore, advised to wear a condom during intercourse. Occasionally, a vaginal infection that is not due to gonorrhea may, as the consequence of a coital connection, result in enough inflammation of the penis to cause pain. A chronic infection of the prostate may also be responsible for male dyspareunia.

impotence

"It is the heaviest stone that Melancholy can throw at a man, to tell him he is at the end of his nature." So did the seventeenth-century English physician and writer Sir Thomas Browne describe the despair of impotence. It is a disability that has tormented men throughout the ages, and men have always sought ways of releasing themselves from its torment (see pages 346–48). Men who suffer from primary impotence have either never had an erection or have been unable to maintain an erection long enough to have sexual intercourse. Those who suffer from secondary impotence were once sexually capable but have lost the ability to have an erection and maintain it long enough to enjoy coitus.

The causes of impotence   Primary impotence usually is the result of a deep-seated psychological problem. A boy may grow up to be impotent if he is denigrated, or taught that sex is sinful and dirty, or is overwhelmingly impressed by his mother that her sex is preferable to his. Masters and Johnson have reported relatively little success in the treatment of primary impotence. Nevertheless, their results have improved as they have gained experience with their methods.

A wide range of causes are responsible for secondary impotence. Biological-physical causes include disease, injury, and impotency-inducing medication.[23] Among the psychosocial factors are rigidity during childhood training, an affiliation with an orthodox religious

[22] Ibid., p. 290. The glans penis is the head of the organ (see Figure 2-1, page 34). pH is a symbol for the degree of alkalinity or acidity in a solution.

[23] A Canadian study suggests that some cases of impotence may be due to obstructed blood flow to the penis. The technique for measuring penile blood pressure involved the use of a small blood pressure cuff placed at the base of the penis; while the cuff was slowly deflated, an instrument was used that could detect the earliest appearance of oxygenated blood. Both old and young men

group with highly restrictive sexual mores, and an orientation toward homosexual behavior. By holding out little or no hope for the cure of impotence some physicians inadvertently deepen the problem for their patients. But the major cause of secondary impotence in the Masters and Johnson population is premature ejaculation (see pages 294-96). Such impotence may take years to develop. The drinking of too much alcohol is the second major cause of secondary impotence. Impotence from this cause may occur suddenly (see pages 340-41). Sometimes excessive alcohol consumption can lead to a single episode of impotence. In most cases this is no cause for undue concern. However, to be convivial or to build up his courage a man may consistently drink a small amount of alcohol before engaging in sexual intercourse. If this becomes habitual, he may increase his intake. Soon he experiences an episode of impotence. Building up an anxiety about the next performance may result in still another failure. He may try to drown his fear of failure in more alcohol. Soon fear of failure to have an erection haunts the afflicted man. Like an angry bystander he observes himself with anxiety. No longer does an erection occur as naturally to him as does breathing. He watches to see if he will perform, and he cannot. He curses his flaccid penis, hoping that by his very frustration he can will it erect. But no man can will an erection. If he seeks treatment, this is one of the first facts that he has to learn.

The treatment of impotence   One nonmedical advisor promised a cure for impotence through regular church attendance for one year. This failed. But many men who suffer from impotence can be helped by therapy. Besides accepting the fact that he cannot will an erection, the patient has to learn how his own mounting anxieties aggravate his problem. True communication between the members of the marital unit may have ceased to exist. In the Masters and Johnson population the middle-aged men (average age fifty-three) and their wives had suffered the problem for more than two years. Communication between the marital partners must be restored. Taboos must be

---

who are not impotent have a penile blood pressure equal to or higher than the mean blood pressure that is taken in the usual way with a cuff on the arm. The study revealed that twenty-one impotent nondiabetic men had a penile pressure definitely lower than the mean of that taken from the arm. The highest penile blood pressure that was observed in this study was with a potent eighty-seven year old. (Peter Gaskell, "The Importance of Penile Blood Pressure in Cases of Impotence," *Canadian Medical Association Journal*, Vol. 105, No. 10 [November 20, 1971], pp. 1047-51.

Still another approach to the problem of impotence has been a study of the nocturnal erection. While asleep during the night, males often have such erections. Young men may have four or more. These may last half-an-hour or longer. Most of these erections occur during the period of rapid eye movements (REM) or dream sleep. Nocturnal emissions also occur during the REM period. It is postulated that REM sleep is a necessary part of brain function. Possibly the sensory input from the erect penis may play a part in the development and maintenance of association areas in the cerebral cortex that are sex related. (Ismet Karacan, Carolyn Hursch, Robert L. Williams, and John I. Thornby, "Some Characteristics of Nocturnal Penile Tumescence in Young Adults," *Archives of General Psychiatry*, Vol. 26, No. 4 [April 1972], p. 351.)

eliminated. The strains of having to perform sexually, of being on trial, of increasing anxiety, have to be alleviated.

During the first days of therapy no coital connection is attempted, even if erection occurs. Through the sensate focus exercises, the man and wife rediscover one another. Their attention is directed at one another and not at their performance. This can be a uniquely binding experience. No demands are made. No coital performance is expected, just gentle tenderness.

On successive days, the couple progress to manipulative pelvic play leading to erection. Even then coitus is delayed. The manipulation continues until the erection is lost, then resumed until it recurs. Slowly the man learns that he is able to achieve and maintain an erection. Nondemanding coitus may be begun with the wife astride the husband. Without concentrating on satisfying the wife or on forcing the ejaculation, the couple hopefully learn to interact with one another in a sexual way.

premature ejaculation

With this condition, the male loses much of his erection as soon as he ejaculates. He is thus unable to continue intravaginal intercourse. Should the ejaculation occur before his partner is sexually satisfied, it may be considered premature. A variety of reasons may account for premature ejaculation. By no means are all of them unusual. The time between his sexual contacts may have been too long. Or he may have enjoyed too prolonged a period of foreplay. An occasional premature ejaculation should not concern either partner. When it becomes a chronic part of the sexual pattern serious problems arise.

Many men in this culture regard the ability to satisfy their sexual partner as one measure of masculinity. The persistent failure to do so causes the man to lose confidence in his masculinity. Even a few failures may make him feel that he is on trial. This makes him anxious, and his mounting anxiety causes him to ejaculate prematurely—often even before his penis enters the vagina. At first his wife may be patient with him. Hopefully, she avoids stimulating him before intromission. When this fails, she may resort to self-pity. "You're just using me," she may tell him bitterly. Now their sexual experience is out of its context of love. It is no longer an expression of understanding mutuality. It is surrounded by embarrassment, anxiety, failure—even hate.

Masters and Johnson consider premature ejaculation a problem if the male cannot control his ejaculation during vaginal containment long enough to satisfy his partner for at least 50 percent of their coital exposures. Of all the male dysfunctions, they find premature ejaculation the easiest to cure. They are convinced that the problem could be brought under complete control in this country within ten years with the help of enough trained physicians.

What can be done for premature ejaculation?   Early in the discussion of the treatment of this dysfunction, the couple is honestly assured that it can be controlled. Only five of the reported eighty-six men afflicted with premature ejaculation who were treated by Masters and Johnson failed to bring their problem under control. To the man and woman so long frustrated by failure this news is indeed heartening. It is emphasized that the physical procedures practiced in the treatment of premature ejaculation are only part of the therapeutic program. The psychological complexities of the marital relationship are also carefully explored.

The couple begins, as do all patients, with the sensate focus exercises. When the therapists allow it, the couple proceeds to genital play. As in the treatment of female orgasmic dysfunction, the therapists recommend a particular position for this. The wife sits with her legs apart, her back resting against pillows at the head of the bed. The husband lies on his back with his pelvis between her legs, his legs over hers. To encourage erection the wife stimulates her husband's penis with her hand. When the husband feels he is about to ejaculate, he tells his wife. Masters and Johnson found that the time during which the husband can no longer control his ejaculation occurs two to four seconds before emission. This is the period of ejaculatory inevitability—the point at which the man can no longer control the ejaculation.[24] In order to delay the period of ejaculatory inevitability, the wife then employs what is called the "squeeze technique" by firmly squeezing the tip of the penis with her thumb and first two fingers. Firm pressure is applied by the wife for three to four seconds. Immediately the husband loses his urge to ejaculate. The wife's role is essential. The man cannot successfully use the squeeze technique by himself. To teach the squeeze technique, Masters and Johnson employ a manikin for demonstration and practice. The wife may alternately stimulate the penis and employ the squeeze technique four or five times during the couple's first session. The husband thus learns to maintain an erection for many minutes without orgasm and ejaculation.

During succeeding sessions, the husband and wife learn to apply the squeeze technique during coitus. The female-superior position is used at first. In order to accustom her husband to having his penis in her vagina without ejaculating, the wife at first remains motionless. Should the husband feel that he is about to have an orgasm, he warns his wife in time for her to apply the squeeze technique. If necessary the husband thrusts to maintain an erection. As the husband learns ejaculatory control the lateral coital position described above (see Figure 9-1 and pages 288–89) is tried. At no time should either partner be made to feel that he or she is on trial or that a particular position

[24] There are two stages in the man's orgasmic experience: the period of ejaculatory inevitability; the period of orgasmic expulsion. Once started, the male goes through both stages without voluntary control (see page 273).

entails a demand for successful sexual performance. The couple continues to use the squeeze technique for six months to a year. After that time it may be used as needed.

ejaculatory incompetence

The man with ejaculatory incompetence usually has no difficulty in having an erection. However, he cannot ejaculate in the vagina. It is "the clinical opposite of premature ejaculation . . . separate from impotence." [25] Fortunately, this disability is rare. A severely restrictive upbringing, a fear of causing pregnancy, or a shocking emotional upset may be among the causes of ejaculatory incompetence. Sometimes a single traumatic event may cause the problem. It has been noted that wives of husbands with this condition may feel rejected. Despite this, they may frequently experience multiple orgasms.

In the treatment for this condition the wife is advised to manually manipulate the penis until ejaculation occurs. The couple engages in a mutual search for what is stimulating for the man. Gradually the husband will associate ejaculation with a coital experience with his wife. When the man's orgasm seems imminent intromission of the penis into the vagina is finally effected. The female thrusts in an attempt to encourage intravaginal ejaculation. If this fails, manual manipulation of the penis by the wife is repeated. Penile irritation may be minimized by the use of moisturizing lotions.

[25] William H. Masters and Virginia E. Johnson, *Human Sexual Inadequacy,* p. 126.

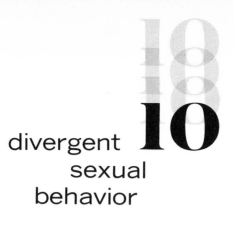

divergent 10
sexual
behavior

*I am a man: nothing human
is alien to me*[1]

homosexual behavior

*She who superintended the wedding comes and clips the hair
of the bride close around her head, dresses her up in man's
clothes, and leaves her upon a mattress in the dark; afterwards
comes the bridegroom, in his everyday clothes, sober and composed, as having supped at the common table, and, entering
privately into the room where the bride lies, unties her virgin
zone, and takes her to himself; and, after staying sometime
together, he returns composedly to his own apartment, to sleep
as usual with the other young men.*[2]

In this way the Greek biographer Plutarch (46?-120?) described the
wedding night of a Spartan girl who had been dressed as a boy. The
groom had enjoyed a succession of male lovers since his twelfth year.
Moreover, he had been taught that he owed love to neither his wife
nor his child. The bridegroom dared not tarry long with his bride
lest he incur the jealous wrath of his male lovers in the barracks.
So casual was the marital relationship that the wife often bore a child
without ever seeing her impregnator in the daylight. Any children
born of these unions were the property of the state. Male homosexual
orientation was a cultural cornerstone of Spartan life. Its purpose
was to preserve and perpetuate the state, as it was reasoned that
love between young men increased their sense of allegiance to one

---

[1] Terence, *Heauton Timoroumenos* (*The Self-Tormentor*), line 77.
[2] Plutarch, quoted in Stanley E. Pacion, "Sparta: An Experiment in State-Fostered Homosexuality,"
Medical Aspects of Human Sexuality, Vol. 4, No. 8 (August 1970), p. 31.

another and, therefore, to the state. Marriage to a female was expected but, again, only to provide warriors for Sparta.

The Greeks considered everyone to be bisexual ("double-sexed"). Hence they worshiped the god Hermaphroditus who possessed both male genitalia and female breasts. But the origins of mythology about sexuality are even more ancient. From his earliest beginnings, man wondered how to explain the existence of two sexes and developed stories like this one told in Plato's *Symposium:* Once there were three sexes—male, female, and male-female. Zeus sliced each of them through the middle. Ever since, the two halves have sought to rejoin one another in love. "Then all men who are a cutting of the old common sex which was called manwoman are fond of women . . . The women who are a cutting of the ancient women do not care much about men, but are more attracted to women . . . But those which are a cutting of the male pursue the male."[3] Such a myth conveniently explains both heterosexual and homosexual behavior. Both forms of sexual expression exist in all societies. In some societies homosexual behavior is approved, even promoted, although Western culture has rejected it as a way of life. Modern knowledge of homosexual behavior is far from complete. There is still much to be clarified, nor have all the myths been discarded.

THE HAZARDS OF LABELING

"There are some persons," wrote Kinsey and his co-workers,

> *whose sexual reactions and socio-sexual activities are directed only toward individuals of their own sex. There are others whose psychosexual reactions and socio-sexual activities are directed, throughout their lives, only toward individuals of the opposite sex. These are the extreme patterns which are labeled homosexuality and heterosexuality. There remain, however, among both females and males, a considerable number of persons who include both homosexual and heterosexual responses and/or activities in their histories. Sometimes their homosexual and heterosexual responses and contacts occur at different periods in their lives; sometimes they occur coincidentally.*[4]

About male homosexual behavior they wrote further: "Males do not represent two discrete populations, heterosexual and homosexual. The world is not to be divided into sheep and goats . . . nature rarely deals with discrete categories. Only the human mind invents cate-

[3] Plato, *Symposium,* in *Great Dialogues of Plato,* translated into English by W. H. D. Rouse (New York, 1956), p. 87.
[4] Alfred C. Kinsey, Wardell B. Pomeroy, Clyde E. Martin, and Paul H. Gebhard, *Sexual Behavior in the Human Female* (Philadelphia, 1953), p. 468.

gories and tries to force facts into separated pigeon-holes."[5] Homosexual behavior is not an all-or-none condition, and in evaluating it
considerations of time, place, and degree are especially important.
However, the Kinsey report was apparently aimed at indicating the
essential frequency of homosexual behavior.[6] The question of whether
exclusive or preferential homosexual behavior is a disease is still
being debated. In some of the summary graphs of the Kinsey report
the term *heterosexual* is used to denote individuals who experienced
few or no episodes of homosexual behavior throughout their lives.
By the Kinsey criterion, moreover, anyone who has had even one
childhood experience of homosexual behavior may be termed a
homosexual.[7] Thus the report states that "the actual incidence of the
homosexual is at least 37 to 50 percent."[8] However, fantasies, dreams,
and the transient homosexual behavior of adolescents can hardly be
a basis on which to label people "homosexuals." Nor are infrequent,
isolated, or situational episodes of homosexual behavior indicative
of a true homosexual orientation. The Kinsey report fails to distinguish between homosexual behavior that is a preferential or generally
exclusive pattern in which the individual actively seeks sexual gratification with a member of the same sex, and the vast number of
relatively insignificant episodes of homosexual behavior occurring
among a large proportion of the population. Such labeling of human
behavior can be both misleading and harmful.

MISCONCEPTIONS ABOUT HOMOSEXUAL BEHAVIOR

It is apparent, then, that no single series of events or factors can
explain homosexual behavior. Several causative factors operating in
the individual environment over a prolonged period of time are
usually responsible. As will be seen, heredity has not been proved
to be directly related to homosexual behavior. Furthermore, it is a
mistake to associate body type or mannerisms or occupation with
homosexual behavior. A brawny football player may actively and
exclusively prefer a homosexual behavior pattern; a graceful male
ballet dancer may just as likely prefer a heterosexual pattern. Only
a small percentage of people whose behavior is homosexual (fewer
than one in twenty men and probably the same number of women)
can be identified by such attributes as mannerisms or dress.[9] There
is a widespread belief that people whose behavior is homosexual are
unusually creative, based on the observation that some professions

---

[5] Alfred C. Kinsey, Wardell B. Pomeroy, and Clyde E. Martin, *Sexual Behavior in the Human Male*
(Philadelphia, 1948), p. 639.
[6] Ibid., cited in Warren J. Gadpaille, "Homosexual Experience in Adolescence," *Medical Aspects
of Human Sexuality*, Vol. 2, No. 10 (October 1968), p. 30.
[7] Alfred C. Kinsey et al., *Sexual Behavior in the Human Male*, pp. 474, 658.
[8] Ibid., p. 626.
[9] Warren A. Ketterer, "Homosexuality and Venereal Disease," *Medical Aspects of Human Sexuality*,
Vol. 5, No. 3 (March 1971), p. 119.

demanding unusual creative ability seem to attract a large proportion of people who engage in homosexual behavior. However, this is most likely due to the tolerance shown by most of the members of these particular professions toward people whose homosexual behavior is overt. It has been noted that many men whose behavior is homosexual are involved in the designing of women's clothes. A psychological explanation has been offered for this fact (which may well be more apparent than real): "Idealization of the thin female form is the homosexual's expression of admiration for this body configuration. Without question, however, it is rather a boyish figure that he finds beautiful. On the other hand, many of the male homosexuals may be taking unconscious revenge on females, with whom they feel competitive, by obliterating the secondary sexual characteristics which are the female symbols of sexual allure."[10] How well all the aspects of this interesting theory would fit those men who participated in the design of the miniskirt and the bikini would certainly stimulate some interesting discussion.

THE EXTENT OF HOMOSEXUAL BEHAVIOR
AND HOW IT IS EXPRESSED

How many individuals participate in homosexual behavior? Possibly millions. Kinsey estimated that the behavior of 4 percent of the adult white males in this country was exclusively homosexual after the onset of adolescence. Thirty-seven percent was estimated to have had at least some overt homosexual experience to the point of orgasm between adolescence and old age.[11] This last figure must be considered in a new light. The present director of the Institute for Sex Research, founded by Kinsey, recently revealed that this estimate is now considered to be high. Since he had ready access to prisoners, Kinsey used them for many of his interviews. He thought that their experience was typical of the lower socioeconomic group. Such is not the case.[12] Indeed, recent revelations of rape of new prisoners by long-term prisoners have shocked the nation.

Among the more common methods of erotic stimulation used by men are fellatio (the penis is taken into the mouth and licked), mutual masturbation, anal intercourse, interfemoral (between the thighs) intercourse, and rubbing of bodies.

The available data on the incidence of homosexual behavior among females is, at best, open to question. Female homosexual behavior seems to be treated with studious indifference. Unlike the male who is often hounded by the police, the female whose behavior

[10] Harold Greenwald, "Fashion Models and Sex," *Medical Aspects of Human Sexuality,* Vol. 4, No. 6 (June 1970), p. 87
[11] Alfred C. Kinsey et al., *Sexual Behavior in the Human Male,* pp. 650–51.
[12] "In the News," *Medical Aspects of Human Sexuality,* Vol. 3, No. 7 (July 1969), p. 104.

is homosexual is rarely arrested. In this culture, deep emotional involvements between women are more acceptable than those between men. So are their expressions of such involvements. Kinsey's data revealed that female homosexual responses had occurred in about one-half as many females as males. Homosexual contacts to orgasm had occurred in about one-third as many females as males. At any age, the behavior of one-half to one-third as many females as males was primarily or entirely homosexual.[13] There is much present-day disagreement with Kinsey's estimates of female homosexual behavior. Some research suggests that the number of females participating in homosexual behavior may approximate the number of males. In addition, there is some reason to believe that more women than men are inclined to engage in both homosexual and heterosexual relationships at the same time. A study of twelve hundred women revealed that 26 percent had experienced some specific homosexual episode. However, these women were not representative of the population as a whole;[14] they were unmarried and employed, and homosexual behavior could be expected to be more common among them. A smaller study indicated that stimulation of the genitalia, particularly the clitoris, with the tongue or lips (cunnilinction) was the most common form of sexual expression used by the women. Mutual masturbation, self-masturbation, caressing of the breasts, and close rubbing of bodies were also used.[15] It should be noted that both these studies are over thirty years old. New studies are needed.

THE ROOTS OF HOMOSEXUAL BEHAVIOR

varying influences at varying times

Basically, human sexuality depends on three factors—*genetic, endocrine,* and *psychological.* All are involved in human sexuality, but the degree of their influence on human development varies at different stages of growth. Genetic combinations are established as a result of fertilization and subsequent cellular division. The cells contain the fundamental arrangement of chemical materials (DNA) necessary for the development of genital, nervous, and muscular structural patterns. Endocrine tissue has an early influence on the direction that the developing embryo will take. Its critical role in determining nervous and genital system structure has been discussed elsewhere in this book (see pages 80–82). But this early activity of the endocrine hormones is not the only instance these gland products assume

[13] Alfred C. Kinsey et al., *Sexual Behavior in the Human Female,* p. 475.
[14] Clellan S. Ford and Frank A. Beach, *Patterns of Sexual Behavior* (New York, 1951), p. 134, citing K. B. Davis, *Factors in the Sex Life of Twenty-Two Hundred Women* (New York, 1929).
[15] Ibid., p. 135, citing G. W. Henry, *Sex Variants* (New York, 1941).

A term used for the mutual friction of the genitals between women is *tribadism* (Greek *tribein,* to rub). It is a word referring to a particular sexual practice; it is not an alternative word for female homosexual behavior.

primary importance. Puberty is marked by a second surge of endocrine activity. Androgen in the male and estrogen in the female, along with other hormones, stimulate further growth and development of the sexual organs. Hormones also increase the sensitivity of the sex structure to stimulation. Still other hormones, such as those from the thyroid gland that affect vitality and strength, have an indirect influence on sexual development.

But neither the genes nor the hormones determine the human choice of the sex object. It is the cultural influences that teach heterosexual behavior. The instruction may be as subtle as a boy's haircut or as blunt as a child's jeering at a young boy's long, curly hair. So, starting at birth, environmental influences begin to supersede and augment the now visible genetic-endocrine influences on the child. Not until puberty do the endocrine glands temporarily take over again and partly supersede the psychological influence of the environment. In the late teens or early twenties, when endocrine maturity is complete, the psychological factors engendered by the environment again become paramount. To summarize: within the uterus, the genetic and endocrine factors are of import. In early childhood, the environment molds most of the sexual response. During adolescence, the endocrine glands again assume primary importance. By the late teens or early twenties, psychological influences again become supreme. Although different influences are dominant at different times, they all operate to a certain extent all of the time. The see-saw effect resulting from the varying influences of genetic, endocrine, and psychological factors at different stages of human development can hardly be expected to guarantee one single form of sexual behavior. Considering the complexity of these relationships, it is not surprising that there is so much homosexual behavior. It is surprising that there is so little.[16]

[16] The endocrine glands are ductless. From the many chemicals in the blood of the arteries, they manufacture hormones, which are released into the veins in perfectly accurate doses to govern a wide variety of body processes. The pituitary gland, the testes, and the ovaries are endocrine glands (see page 30).

The complexity of sexual behavior is well illustrated by a recent animal experiment. Male rats were exposed to prenatal (before birth) or postnatal (after birth) stress, or to both. Prenatal stress was induced by enclosing pregnant mothers in restraining glass tubes across which distressing lights were directed. Postnatal stress was caused by placing male pups on a plastic ice cube tray mounted on a vibrating metal rack. Among the prenatally stressed animals there was a marked reduction of male copulatory (coital) behavior and a high rate of female coital behavior. This did not occur with postnatally stressed pups. The combination of prenatal and postnatal stress did not enhance the effect caused by prenatal stress alone. Why did not the sexual behavior of male rats subjected to postnatal stress become feminized? For the first ten days after birth, rats pass through a period during which they do not respond to stress. What accounts for the feminizing and demasculinizing effect on the sexual behavior of the male rats that were subjected to stress before they were born? Mention has already been made of several male hormones, the androgens, and particularly of the potent male hormone testosterone, produced in the testes (see page 35). Also producing small amounts of testosterone, but a larger amount of another weaker male hormone *androstenedione,* are the outer portions of the adrenal glands, one of which is situated on top of each kidney. Stress, it appears, causes an increase in the weak adrenal androgen androstenedione from the adrenal glands of either or both the stressed mother or the unborn rat, and a simultaneous decrease in the potent androgen testosterone from the fetal testes. (Ingebord L. Ward, "Prenatal Stress Feminizes and Demasculinizes the Behavior of Males," *Science,* Vol. 175, No. 4017 [January 7, 1972], pp. 82–85.)

preadolescent sexual behavior

Earlier in the book it was pointed out that before the onset of puberty, when surges of hormonal activity intensify the sexual drive, there is much curiosity and, indeed, sexual play among both boys and girls (see pages 9-10). Both may masturbate and be capable of orgasm. Both are exceedingly curious not only about their own genitalia but also about the sexual organs of others of the same sex as well as those of the opposite sex. A very few may even accomplish coitus. Occasionally small groups of children, usually of the same sex, participate in prepubescent sexual play. Unless they are treated with senseless harshness by adults, they experience no particular anxiety as a result of this passing behavior.

early adolescent needs: homosexual-like behavior

The increased sexual drive that occurs at puberty can be an overwhelming experience. The anxious young person is often entirely unsure of his relationship to the opposite sex. Understandably, he or she may retreat to more familiar ground—to members of the same sex. Many young people pass through a period of intense interest in the same sex before proceeding to a heterosexual adjustment. They share tremendous secrets and derive needed comfort in the knowledge that they all have problems. The variety of sexual expression during this ordinarily transient period may be considerable. Group exhibition and masturbation as well as mutual masturbation may occur among boys. Anal or interfemoral (between the thighs) intercourse and oral-genital stimulation are certainly less frequent, but they do take place. Girls who go through this stage may experience hand-holding, kissing, breast fondling, genital petting, and mutual masturbation. During the early adolescent period of a relatively small number of these young people, there may be some oral-genital stimulation. However, "this is not a clinically significant homosexuality and should not be so labeled. At this age homosexual behavior should be viewed as a temporary defense against the fear associated with the move towards full heterosexual relationships." [17]

To summarize:

> One therefore finds early adolescents involved in various forms of normal, mutual "homosexual" exploration, including comparing of sexual knowledge, sex talk, and some sex acts. Overt homosexual explorative acts (including mutual masturbation) may also occur and be essentially normal. These acts

[17] Group for the Advancement of Psychiatry, Committee on Adolescence, *Normal Adolescence* (New York, 1968), p. 77, cited in Warren J. Gadpaille, "Homosexual Experience in Adolescence," p. 33.

are no more indicative that such a child will become a homo-
sexual than the sexual exploration at age four means that he
(or she) will become sexually promiscuous as an adult. However,
the reactions of adults to these acts can have catastrophic
results, engendering a sense of guilt which may lead to lasting
personality disturbances.[18]

early clues

The period of prepubescent and adolescent homosexual behavior
among those people with whom it occurs varies in length, and the
criteria that indicate a later homosexual orientation are not well
established. Age alone is not a dependable criterion. A great number
of variables are involved, including such environmental factors as
interaction among family members, the nature of the homosexual
behavior, the frequency of its occurrence, and the evidences of sexual
identity.

Most young people develop a heterosexual dating pattern by the
time they are sixteen or seventeen years of age. "Continued homosexual behavior into the late teens in normal environmental circumstances, particularly if repetitive or habitual, is more likely to be an
enduring predilection." [19] This does not mean that this is always the
case. A recent study conducted by the Research Committee on
Female Homosexuality established by the Society of Medical Psychoanalysts of New York City suggests the beginning ages of adult
female homosexual behavior. Part of the data gathered by this committee was from 157 corresponding members of the Daughters of
Bilitis.[20] The correspondence revealed that "while the lesbian experiences of the Daughters of Bilitis group ranged from age 6 through
44, the largest had their first homosexual encounter between 16 and
20, with a mean age of 19 to 20. Again, this is considerably later than
one finds among male homosexuals, the majority of whom have their
first homosexual episode before their 14th birthday." [21]

Another possible clue to a future homosexual orientation may be
found in the kind of homosexual behavior in which the adolescent
engages. The more ordinary forms of adolescent homosexual behavior
are mutual masturbation and group masturbation. It is possible (but
by no means certain) that the adolescent's experience with the less
common types of adolescent homosexual expression, such as anal

[18] Marshall Shearer, "Homosexuality and the Pediatrician," *Clinical Pediatrics,* Vol. 5, No. 8 (August
1966), p. 515.
[19] Warren J. Gadpaille, "Homosexual Experience in Adolescence," p. 33.
[20] The Daughters of Bilitis is a women's group seeking to promote the integration into society
of individuals whose behavior is homosexual. The name of the organization is derived from *The
Song of Bilitis* by Pierre Louÿs. In this work, Bilitis, whose behavior had been heterosexual, turned
to Sappho, became her disciple, and adopted homosexual behavior. Sappho was a Greek poetess
of the sixth century B.C. who lived on the Greek island of Lesbos. Hence the term *Lesbian* for
the female whose behavior is homosexual.
[21] Harvey E. Kaye, "Lesbian Relationships," *Sexual Behavior,* Vol. 1, No. 1 (April 1971), p. 83.

intercourse and oral-genital stimulation, might indicate future homosexual behavior. The "love phenomenon"—the adolescent experience of being "in love" with a partner of the same sex—might also have some significance as to later behavior. However, many adults who actively choose a homosexual behavior pattern do not remember such a "love" experience during adolescence. Moreover, it is common for the searching adolescent to literally worship an adult who is younger than the parent.

Some psychiatrists have found, through their research and clinical experience, that much homosexual behavior may be detected as early as childhood and early adolescence. One psychiatrist considers signs of future Lesbian behavior to be found in such tendencies as seeking physical fights; disliking dolls; playing with guns; preferring boys' games and disliking girls' games such as "house"; seeing themselves as "tomboys"; having strong "crushes" on women, particularly during puberty; and being particularly competitive with their mothers.[22] Still another psychoanalyst, however, warns that

tomboy behavior does not in itself presage a homosexual outcome, though many lesbians consider themselves to be tomboys during childhood. A vigorous, spirited, athletic girl need not be boyish. The tomboy is one who is having a conflict about her femininity. She may be reacting to maternal preference of a boy, to a father or mother who treats her like a boy, or to her own envy and admiration of what it is boys do. With the strong upsurge of sexuality as adolescence approaches, a feminine identification may assert itself and then the tomboyishness will dissipate.[23]

Irving Bieber considers the following to be some of the possible characteristics of the boy whose tendency toward adult homosexual behavior can be identified during preadolescence: an obsessive fear of physical injury and an avoidance of fights with other children; isolation from peer groups (this child is a "lone wolf"); avoidance of competitive games and the rough-and-tumble activity of other boys; a preference for playing with girls or boys like himself; and an overly pronounced attachment to the mother.[24]

[22] Ibid., p. 84.

[23] Tony Bieber, "The Lesbian Patient," *Medical Aspects of Human Sexuality,* Vol. 3, No. 1 (January 1969), p. 10.

[24] Irving Bieber, "Advising the Homosexual," *Medical Aspects of Human Sexuality,* Vol. 2, No. 3 (March 1968), pp. 34–35.

A study of sixty young men (sixteen to twenty-two years old) who had experienced at least one orgasm with other men whose behavior was homosexual, revealed that they had certain experiences in common before saying to themselves, "I am a homosexual." These were: early behavior of a homosexual nature (sex play) before or after puberty; the active seeking out of men whose behavior was homosexual; and participating ("coming out") in the "gay world." "This period was, for many, one of extreme emotional turmoil. Of sixty subjects, twenty-nine (48%) had visited a psychiatrist and nineteen (31%) had made what they considered to be a significant suicide attempt." (Thomas Roesler and Robert W. Deisher, "Youthful Male Homosexuality: Homosexual

It should be emphasized that none of the behavioral clues listed in the above paragraphs is, by itself, an absolute indicator of an eventual orientation to an active preference for homosexual behavior. It may be a clue. When several appear to define the behavior pattern of an individual and seem a cause for concern, the advice of a trained psychologist should be promptly sought. Delay is inadvisable, for it neither dispels parental concern nor hastens childhood change.

possible parental factors in homosexual behavior

One recent study of New York adolescent girls whose behavior pattern is homosexual identified a disruptive and unstable family background (and not only an unresolved Oedipus complex, see pages 11-13) as a major contributing factor in their homosexual behavior. In these cases a wide variety of emotionally traumatic experiences led to a deep sense of insecurity that was at least minimally relieved by a woman. This led to the seeking of female relationships.[25] British studies support this view: "Children reared in families which are incomplete, disturbed by distortions in personal relationships, or whose sexual attitudes are markedly clouded by repression or ignorance appear to be particularly vulnerable . . . It is particularly important to stress that these homosexual feelings do not inevitably imply homosexuality." [26]

It should be emphasized that parental attitudes are by no means the only (and sometimes not the major) factor in the development of a homosexual behavior pattern. Some studies reveal that men whose behavior is homosexual may have had reasonably good relationships with their parents. The son of a close-binding and intimate mother and a dominated, detached father often develops a homosexual behavior pattern, but just as often he develops a heterosexual pattern. This is not to deny the profound effect of parental attitudes on children. However, it must be pointed out that a simple cause-and-effect relationship between parental behavior and a homosexual orientation in their children has not been established.

It is just as tenable to assume that the father of a prehomosexual son becomes detached or hostile because he does not understand his son, is disappointed in him, as it is to assume that the son becomes homosexual because of his father's rejection . . . Similarly, it is as reasonable to assume that a mother becomes intimate and close-binding with her potentially homo-

Experience and the Process of Developing Homosexual Identity in Males Aged Sixteen to Twenty-two Years," *Journal of the American Medical Association*, Vol. 219, No. 8 [February 21, 1972], p. 1018.)

[25] "Research with Adolescents Sheds New Light on Early Lesbianism" *Science News*, Vol. 96, No. 3 (July 19, 1969), p. 45.

[26] "Female Homosexuality," *British Medical Journal*, Vol. 1, No. 5640 (February 8, 1969), p. 331.

sexual son because of the kind of person he is, as to assume he becomes homosexual because she is too binding and intimate with him.[27]

Nevertheless, there are many cases of homosexual behavior that would certainly seem to be strongly associated with parental actions. With his son, a father is harsh, unforgiving, punitive. With his daughter, he is gentle and understanding. Will not the son then contemplate the advantages of being a girl? An overbearing, domineering mother constantly ridicules the father, who is but a shadow in the home. How can the son then perceive the advantages of manhood? So may it have been with the female whose behavior is homosexual. Possibly the girl's mother gave her reason to fear womanhood. Or the mother may compete with the daughter. She defeminizes her by repeatedly telling her that she is gawky and unladylike. The father may be too submissive to help his denigrated daughter. Or, uneasy about the girl's budding sexuality, he is only too glad to avoid her. More commonly, however, he subtly seduces his daughter. He ruthlessly criticizes both her male and female friends. Feeling guilt because of his interest in the girl's body, he forbids her every expression of femininity—playing with dolls, using cosmetics, shopping for pretty dresses. "This image of a close-binding overly intimate father [is] a counterpart to the close-binding, intimate mother found in studies of male homosexuality."[28]

The wise parent avoids such pitfalls and helps the child to establish a rewarding sexuality by discussing his or her problems calmly and intelligently. As the child gains the knowledge that homosexual feelings are commonly a part of growing up, the fears will dissipate. The parent can also show appreciation of the child's budding heterosexual interests.

homosexual behavior: partly a biochemical basis?

The profound effect of the male hormone androgen on the developing embryonic brain has been discussed elsewhere in this book (see pages 80-82). The period of this hormonal activity is so critical that any deviation from it might help to explain some divergent sexual behavior. The German neurologist and psychiatrist Baron Richard von Krafft-Ebing suggested in 1892 that an imbalanced body chemistry might be involved in the determination of homosexual behavior patterns. An endocrinologist has produced preliminary evidence that male homosexual behavior is possibly associated with an imbalance between two chemicals that are related to the male sex hormone

[27] Ray B. Evans, "Parental Relations and Homosexuality," *Medical Aspects of Human Sexuality,* Vol. 5, No. 4 (April 1971), p. 176.
[28] Harvey E. Kaye, "Lesbian Relationships," p. 83.

testosterone. When testosterone is broken down in the male's body, two chemicals, *androsterone* and *etiocholanolone,* are produced in the urine. Studies have shown that in men whose behavior is heterosexual the amount of androsterone in the urine is greater than the amount of etiocholanolone. Preliminary research suggests that in those who practice homosexual behavior the ratio is reversed.[29] The researchers emphasize that there is no cause-and-effect relationship between the urine's chemical content and homosexual behavior.

British research on a possible chemical factor contributing to homosexual behavior was stimulated by the discovery that severely painful menstruation (dysmenorrhea) was often related to a low output of urinary estrogens.[30] Dysmenorrhea had previously been attributed only to emotional stress. This discovery led to a further finding: impotence (see pages 292-94) was not necessarily and always a manifestation of only psychological problems; a certain proportion of impotent men had low levels of testosterone in their urine. Further research revealed a low level of urinary testosterone in two men whose behavior was exclusively homosexual.[31]

In 1971, a group of U.S. researchers reported a significant reduction of blood serum testosterone and spermatozoa counts in a group of thirty males whose behavior was homosexual. In addition, there was a significant correlation between the degree of the biochemical defect and low spermatozoa count and the rated degree of homosexual behavior.[32] Further work with the same men revealed sig-

[29] M. Sydney Margolese, "Homosexuality: A New Endocrine Correlate," *Hormones and Behavior,* Vol. 1 (1970), pp. 151-55, and "The Homosexual: Is It Chemistry?" *Medical World News,* Vol. 12, No. 16 (April 23, 1971), pp. 4-5.

[30] John A. Loraine, "Hormones and Homosexuality," *New Scientist,* Vol. 53, No. 781 (February 3, 1972), pp. 270-71. It is, however, questionable that a testosterone deficit in the urine is a principal cause of impotence. Testosterone levels are increased by sexual activity; thus a low urinary testosterone level may be the result rather than the cause of impotence. Also, the administration of testosterone to men whose testosterone excretion is low has not cured their impotence. (Thomas G. Benedek, "Aphrodisiacs: Fact and Fable," *Medical Aspects of Human Sexuality,* Vol. 5, No. 12 [December 1971], p. 58.)

[31] John A. Loraine, A. A. A. Ismail, D. A. Adamopoulos, and G. A. Dove, "Endocrine Function in Male and Female Homosexuals," *British Medical Journal,* Vol. 4, No. 5732 (November 14, 1970), pp. 381-442.

"But though our outward man perish, yet the inward man is renewed day by day" (II Corinthians 4:16). So does the Bible take note of the inherent rhythmicity of humankind. But there is rhythm in all things and beings, and they are bound by their rhythms into a universal whole. The majestic division of a single cell in mitosis is in harmony with and rivals the movements of the heavenly bodies. The basic timing mechanisms—the inner biological clocks—may lie in the chemical configuration of the cell's DNA. And those inner biological clocks, set millenia ago during the course of evolution, are in concert with the outer cosmic clocks.

There are the obvious rhythms of a beating heart, of walking, sleeping, breathing, loving. There are the more subtle harmonies within the body between such functions as the daily rise and fall of temperature and hormone release. There is a rhythm both to ease and disease. A highly unusual but enigmatic example of sexual rhythmicity is cited by the case of a young man "who underwent cyclic alternations between feeling and acting male or female. He would be male for three or four days and then female for three or four days, in extremely regular alternation. Observation of patients with attacks of homosexual feelings every four weeks has also led to the suggestion that there must be oscillations in the output of sex hormones or oscillations in the susceptibility of target organs." (Gay Gaer Luce, *Biological Rhythms in Human and Animal Physiology* [Washington, D.C., 1970], p. 114, citing H. A. Reimann, *Periodic Disease* [Oxford, England, 1963].)

[32] Robert C. Kolodny, William H. Masters, Julie Hendryx, and Gelson Toro, "Plasma Testosterone

nificantly higher than usual levels of gonadotropins (see page 127). Luteinizing hormone levels (LH, see page 31) were significantly higher in men whose behavior was almost exclusively or exclusively homosexual than in men whose orientation was heterosexual. Four of thirteen of the men with low blood plasma-testosterone levels had raised LH and FSH levels. A lack of spermatozoa was demonstrated in their semen. This indicates dysfunction of the testes. The other nine men with low testosterone levels were shown to also have low levels of LH in their blood plasmas. They would appear to be experiencing a hypothalamic disturbance. In men whose behavior was exclusively homosexual, blood plasma levels of prolactin were somewhat higher than in men whose orientation was not homosexual. The relationships between FSH, LH, spermatogenesis, and testosterone have been described elsewhere in this book (see page 32). Suffice it to say here that some of the men in this study certainly presented correlations that deviated from those of men whose behavior is ordinarily heterosexual. It must be emphasized that these results must be viewed with caution. However, they do suggest that

> *endocrine dysfunction must be considered in association with homosexuality. Available data do not allow a conclusion to be drawn relating endocrine disturbances in homosexuality to either cause or effect. . . Endocrine dysfunction is unlikely to be found in most men with a history of homosexual involvement; whereas in men with a predominantly or exclusively homosexual behavior pattern, such dysfunction may be quite common. The approach to understanding homosexual behavior should include assessment of the interaction of biological and psychological factors.*[33]

Another study of the hormone levels excreted in the urines of only four young women whose behavior was homosexual also suggest a hormonal imbalance. Readings of the urinary level of the male hormone testosterone were higher and of the female hormone estrone were lower than in women whose behavior was heterosexual.

---

and Semen Analysis in Male Homosexuals," *The New England Journal of Medicine,* Vol. 285, No. 21 (November 18, 1971), pp. 1170-74. A letter written by Jack Baker was received by the editor of the journal that published this article criticizing the "patent bias" of the authors against homosexual behavior. In answer, the senior author (Kolodny) wrote that "we view homosexual behavior as a normal form of sexual functioning." A second letter written by Herbert Barry, Jr. and Herbert Barry III, also questioned the results, pointing out that testosterone levels ordinarily fall during the day and are replenished during sleep, and that, moreover, heavy alcohol consumption is known to adversely affect the testes and male sexual activity. However, the habits of the homosexually oriented men who were studied were such as to invalidate these as factors of importance. ("Homosexuality and Testosterone," *The New England Journal of Medicine,* Vol. 286, No. 7 [February 7, 1962], pp. 380-81.)

[33] Robert C. Kolodny, William H. Masters, Laurence S. Jacobs, Gelson Toro, and William H. Daughaday, "Plasma Gonadotropins and Prolactin in Male Homosexuals," *Lancet,* Vol. 2, No. 7766 (July 1, 1972), p. 20.

"Such abnormalities could stem from the impingement of psychological factors on hypothalamic centers (or) a hormonal imbalance occurring during periods of life at which the direction of future sexual behavior is determined could play a role."[34]

These findings raise more questions than they answer. Is the hormonal imbalance found in the majority of individuals whose behavior is homosexual? Is it the result or the cause of a homosexual orientation? Does this hormonal imbalance occur at those periods of life during which the direction of future sexual behavior is determined? Today, the answers to these and other questions are being actively sought. It seems quite possible that endocrine factors are among the many that are involved in homosexual behavior.

WHAT IS HOMOSEXUAL BEHAVIOR?

By the mid-1930s, Sigmund Freud was known as the greatest living physician of the human mind. His name had become a household word, and a bewildered mother had written him imploring his help. Freud's answer is now part of psychiatric literature. "Homosexuality," he wrote her, "is assuredly no advantage, but it is nothing to be ashamed of, no vice, no degradation, it cannot be classified as an illness."[35] However, this statement raised as many questions as it answered. Is homosexual behavior a disease? If so, it should be treated. Or is homosexual behavior a different way of sexual expression, a mere departure from the average? A large number of professionals today disagree with Freud.[36] Many of them consider homosexual behavior a disease that requires prolonged, albeit expensive, psychiatric therapy. However, the scientifically based opposition to their view is formidable and merits serious consideration.

the dilemma: is homosexual behavior a disease?

The differences among professionals concerning the need for therapy for those whose behavior is homosexual are based on whether they consider this form of sexual expression as diseased behavior. One group claims that the sickness and misbehavior that can be associated with homosexual behavior is due to society's cruel appraisal. "Educate society," they say, "then the sickness and maladjustment will be lessened." Members of the opposing group declare that this approach is unrealistic, and assert that a practical adjustment to existing cultural mores is essential for emotional health. In this country,

---

[34] John A. Loraine, D. A. Adamopoulos, K. E. Kirkham, A. A. A. Ismail, and G. O. Dove, "Patterns of Hormone Excretion in Male and Female Homosexuals," *Nature*, Vol. 234, No. 5331 (December 31, 1971), p. 553.

[35] Ernst L. Freud, ed., *Letters of Sigmund Freud* (New York, 1960), p. 423.

[36] Freud did consider homosexual behavior "a variation of the sexual function, produced by a certain arrest of sexual development." (Ibid.)

they continue, it is impractical to expect society to soon accept homosexual behavior. Moreover, they point out that since heterosexual orientation is begun at an early age, homosexual behavior unavoidably generates conflict, depression, self-denigration, and guilt. Individuals suffering from these problems fill the offices of psychotherapists. (Of course, not all are suffering only the consequences of homosexual behavior.)

The opposition answers that these psychotherapists treat only those homosexually oriented individuals who seek therapy. Millions of individuals whose behavior is homosexual do not wish to change their sexual orientation. They point to ample data to show that people whose behavior is homosexual are no more emotionally maladjusted than are people whose behavior is heterosexual. The work of Evelyn Hooker is often cited to support this view. She argues that "apart from the specific difference in sexual orientation, many of the homosexuals she had studied reveal, on psychological testing, no 'demonstrable pathology' that would differentiate them in any way from a group of relatively normal heterosexuals."[37] Additional evidence for this opinion is not difficult to find. Another study group reported that "there was little difference demonstrated in the prevalence of psychopathology[38] between a group of 89 male homosexuals and a control group of 35 unmarried men . . . Despite the slight increase in disability and the changes in their lives, the homosexual men functioned well."[39] Moreover, a study involving almost seventeen hundred males whose behavior was homosexual revealed that the men older than forty-five years were no more lonely or unhappy than those who were younger. They worried less about exposure of their behavior (possibly because their parents were no longer living), accepted themselves more, and felt less inadequate. Many of these changes are characteristic not only of aging men with a homosexual orientation but also of aging men whose behavior is heterosexual.[40] Some years ago the aging male with a homosexual orientation was depicted in this way: "In Greenwich Village gay boys laughingly pass around cards which read: Nobody loves you when you're old and gay."[41] The young often underestimate the ability of the old to adjust.

However, the professionals who consider homosexual behavior a disease to be treated emphasize the need for integration of sexuality

[37] Judd Marmor, ed., *Sexual Inversion: The Multiple Roots of Homosexuality* (New York, 1965), pp. 15, 16.

[38] The word *psychopathology* is from the Greek *psycho*, mind + *pathos*, disease + *logus*, word, reason (the science or study of). *Psychopathology*, then, means the study of emotional disorders or disease.

[39] Marcel T. Saghir, Eli Robins, Bonnie Walbran, and Kathye A. Gentry, "Homosexuality: III. Psychiatric Disorders and Disability in the Male Homosexual," *The American Journal of Psychiatry*, Vol. 126, No. 8 (February 1970), p. 63.

[40] Martin S. Weinberg, "The Aging Male Homosexual," *Medical Aspects of Human Sexuality*, Vol. 3, No. 12 (December 1969), pp. 66-67, 71-72.

[41] Ibid., p. 66, citing Jesse Stearn, *The Sixth Man* (New York, 1961).

into the total life style. A dynamic adjustment to living today, they state, is hardly compatible with a deep-seated terror of women, fleeting and meaningless sexual involvements, depression, inadequacy, and pathetic passivity. "Sexual relations with a person of the same sex," one psychiatrist recently stated, "represent a deviation or a short-circuiting of a very definite biological intention."[42] For individuals who constantly participate in homosexual behavior, the family—mother, father, sisters and brothers, wife and children—is usually not a significant component of their lives. Often "they are people who have failed to find something meaningful in themselves or in their lives, and pursue one sex act after another trying to make up for the deficit. And after the tenth sex act in a night they are as empty inside as when they started."[43] These professionals consider married men whose behavior is bisexual also in need of psychiatric treatment. Experience has shown that without therapy they tend to develop exclusively homosexual behavior.[44] Some psychiatrists consider homosexual behavior a symptom rather than a disease itself. Domination by a brother, for example, may so diminish the male's sense of adequacy that, as a compensation, his sexual orientation changes.[45] In such cases, psychiatric intervention may reorient the man to heterosexual behavior.

Pressures from societal condemnation   The alienation so characteristic of many men whose behavior is homosexual surely indicates emotional distress. "What is striking about male homosexual alliances, in contrast to both heterosexual and female homosexual alliances, is their fragility, their tendency to be transitory, and the all-pervading promiscuity that characterizes them."[46] Why is this?

The individual who first feels a homosexual orientation has learned no words to express his emotions. At first he thinks himself entirely alone. Often guilt-ridden, he tries desperately to control his feelings. It takes years for the person with a homosexual orientation to "come out"—to identify himself as a person who has this feeling and to participate in sexual expression with others who are like him. "On the average there [is] a six year interval between the time of first sexual feelings toward persons of the same sex and the decision that one [is] a homosexual."[47] He may meet others like himself in a convenient environment—jails, boys' dormitories, mental institu-

---

[42]Lawrence J. Hatterer, "Debate: Can Homosexuals Change with Psychotherapy?" *Sexual Behavior,* Vol. 1, No. 4 (July 1971), p. 45.

[43]Ibid.

[44]Irving Bieber, "The Married Male Homosexual," *Medical Aspects of Human Sexuality,* Vol. 3, No. 5 (May 1969), pp. 76, 81-82, 84.

[45]Lawrence J. Hatterer, "Debate: Can Homosexuals Change with Psychotherapy?" p. 44.

[46]Martin Hoffman, "Homosexual," *Psychology Today,* Vol. 3, No. 2 (July 1969), pp. 43, 70.

[47]Barry M. Dank, "Coming Out in the Gay World," *Psychiatry: Journal for the Study of Interpersonal Processes,* Vol. 34, No. 2 (May 1971), p. 182.

tions, the military, public restrooms (known as "T-rooms"), and the YMCA. Undoubtedly the most popular meeting place is the "gay bar."[48]

Not all men with this sexual orientation frequent these places in order to make sexual contacts. Some men and women share a homosexually oriented life with one individual for many years. Sometimes "'near communities' have developed, especially in residential areas of the city with heavy concentrations of homosexuals. These areas are described by homosexuals as 'the swish Alps' or 'boys' town.' In these sections, apartment houses on particular streets may be owned by, or rented exclusively to, homosexuals."[49] Nor are people with this orientation persecuted in every country. In France homosexual behavior (between consenting adults) has not been a crime since the *Code Napoleon* was promulgated in 1810. More recently, most of the other European states have made the same ruling.

Some professionals feel that the promiscuity of the man whose behavior is homosexual is due to his being labeled sick and criminal. For many men this "disease concept" combined with societal condemnation is a double shock. The societal reaction to homosexual behavior doubtless arose from the efforts of the early Hebrews and Christians to perpetuate and protect the family and the group. Many people cannot endure prolonged societal condemnation without coming to condemn themselves. Although not universal among people whose behavior is homosexual, self-condemnation and guilt are common among them.

The individual who engages in predominantly homosexual behavior points to the writings of Plato and other ancients,[50] as well as to the disagreement among many professionals concerning the medical status of the homosexual orientation. As has been said above, commonly in this society the individual whose behavior is actively homosexual (particularly the male) frequently forsakes the comfortable warmth of family and friends for a life of casual contact. He may have to endure public contempt and ostracism. And for the male (very rarely for the female) it may be a life of frequent conflict with the law.

Whether the homosexually oriented person is sick or merely different, his treatment as a criminal and a social outcast when he

[48] Ibid., pp. 183-84.
[49] Evelyn Hooker, "Male Homosexuals and Their Worlds," in Judd Marmor, ed., *Sexual Inversion: The Multiple Roots of Homosexuality*, p. 93.
[50] The early Romans were tolerant of homosexual behavior but considered it unworthy of a Roman. Julius Caesar, who apparently was bisexual, was known variously as "The Bald Adulterer" or "The Bald Lecher," while the historian Cato referred to him as "every woman's man and every man's woman." The Roman poet Ovid was intolerant of homosexual behavior. "Let youths," he wrote in *Heroides*, "got up like women, keep away!" (IV, line 73). In his *Metamorphoses* (IX, lines 731-33), he is just as explicit: "No bird of air, nothing that breathes, endures female to mate with female." If by "mate," Ovid meant only a sexual relationship, he was wrong. Homosexual behavior among animals is not uncommon, and in some human societies it is an acceptable form of sexual expression.

is not predatory and does not bother children is unwarranted. Harassment only creates or increases much of his emotional distress. There is some evidence that there is growing understanding and tolerance of this form of sexual behavior.

the hope: treatment for those who want it

Several studies have been designed to prove that homosexual behavior can be changed through psychiatric treatment. Moreover, it is claimed that many (although not all) of those who seek treatment want to develop a heterosexual behavior pattern. Both men and women have successfully changed their homosexual orientation. One study, extending over eighteen years, included 710 patients drawn from both clinics and private practice. Including partially and fully heterosexual adjustments, the reported "change rate" was about 45 percent.[51]

A recent survey suggested that among many women who are homosexually oriented there is a basic attraction for members of the opposite sex. In this study twenty-four women whose behavior was homosexual were compared with twenty-four nonhomosexually oriented women. Both groups of women were in psychoanalysis. Heterosexual dreams were not significantly fewer in the homosexually oriented group, nor was the desire for pregnancy less prevalent. Even before any psychoanalytic therapy, a majority of these women (53 percent) had experienced heterosexual activity. Indeed, 75 percent overtly sought social contact with men whose behavior was primarily heterosexual. With adequate treatment, the probability of a change to heterosexuality among the homosexually oriented women was considered to be about 50 percent.[52] Another professional notes that

> *most lesbians are bisexual. Some will have had heterosexual experiences before their homosexual debut, some move back and forth pendulum style, from heterosexual to homosexual, affairs . . . Interest in heterosexuality is never completely abandoned by homosexuals of either sex—if not consciously, then on a subconscious level. The dreams of even confirmed homosexuals continue to reveal conflicts about their sexual direction. Since women need not concern themselves with problems of potency and erection on purely functional grounds, it is easier for them than for male homosexuals to satisfy heterosexual curiosity and yearnings. However, a firmly established heterosexual adaptation is rarely, if ever achieved without psychiatric intervention.*

[51] Lawrence J. Hatterer, *Changing Homosexuality in the Male: Treatment for Men Troubled with Homosexuality* (New York, 1970), p. 492.
[52] H. E. Kaye et al., "Homosexuality in Women," *Archives of General Psychiatry*, Vol. 17, No. 5 (November 1967), pp. 626-34.

Today lesbianism is a treatable condition. About 50 percent who undertake psychotherapy, and stay with it, shift to heterosexuality, although the younger the patient the more favorable the outlook.[53]

In 1953 still another psychiatrist began a study of 106 men whose behavior was homosexual. All were receiving psychoanalytic treatment. They were compared with 100 men who were also undergoing treatment but whose behavior was heterosexual. "One-third of the homosexuals who entered psychoanalytic treatment became heterosexual."[54] Follow-up studies were obtained on the majority of these patients.

A study of 123 women whose behavior was homosexual revealed that one in four wished her orientation to be heterosexual.[55] Although the desire to become heterosexually oriented is not always characteristic of those whose behavior is exclusively homosexual, modern therapy offers hope for those who want it. Long-term psychotherapy has been helpful. Homosexual behavior "is eminently curable—as curable as any other chronic psychologic disorder. Of the people presenting for therapy—and these are the only ones who can be counted legitimately—. . . more than one-third correct their homosexual orientation."[56]

Two newer attempts to treat homosexual behavior   Group therapy has recently been reported to be effective in helping to reorient some individuals to heterosexual behavior. In a group, individual rationalizations are broken down, and support by others "in the same boat" is given. "I make it clear," writes one psychiatrist about a group, "that to me there is no such thing as 'a homosexual'; that I regard them as individuals who, in their developmental period, acquired many patterns of maladaptation, of which homosexuality is the one that they regard as the most serious and disturbing . . . As emphasis is placed on their other neurotic traits, they soon give up the idea that a homosexual orientation is as normal as it is to be left handed." Interestingly, "about one-third of those persisting in treatment reach an effective heterosexual adjustment."[57]

In West Germany an astonishing treatment for homosexual behavior has recently been tried. Somewhat radical, the treatment is still in the experimental stage and is certainly too new to be routinely

[53] Tony Bieber, "The Lesbian Patient," p. 12.
[54] Irving Bieber, "Advising the Homosexual," p. 38.
[55] F. E. Kenyon in *Journal of Neurology, Neurosurgery, and Psychiatry*, Vol. 31, No. 5 (October 1968), p. 487, and in *British Journal of Psychiatry*, Vol. 114, No. 11 (November 1968), p. 1337, cited in "Female Homosexuality," p. 330.
[56] Daniel Cappon, "Understanding Homosexuality," *Postgraduate Medicine*, Vol. 42, No. 4 (October 1967), p. A-131.
[57] Samuel B. Hadden, "Group Therapy for Homosexuals," *Medical Aspects of Human Sexuality*, Vol. 5, No. 1 (January 1971), pp. 120, 126.

employed in this country. By means of a series of tiny electrical brain-burns, a neurologist at the University of Göttingen has knocked out part of the so-called sexual switchboard of the brain. Seven of eleven men so treated were transformed from a homosexual to a heterosexual orientation.[58] Further results of this treatment are still to come.

transvestite behavior

"Connie isn't bossy, she isn't demanding, she doesn't fly into jealous rages. She exists only for me, and she knows I'm her lord and master. I like it that way."[59]

This is how one man deals with his fear of women. Connie is his ideal. But she is not a nonthreatening woman. She is he: the man speaking is a male transvestite, and "Connie" is his female role. Such a man derives his sexual satisfaction by dressing in the clothing of a woman. There are also female transvestites.[60] This behavior is a form of fetishism—the worship of an inanimate object as the symbol of a loved person.

But the transvestite secures more than erotic satisfaction from his fetishism. It also provides him with a fantasy social life. The transvestite has heterosexual needs, and since he himself is both the male and the female he is in a position of complete control. He gives himself a girl's name that he likes, like Connie. No gift, whether it be high-heeled shoes or lacy nightgowns, is ever rejected. Connie is never sullen, never demanding, never nagging. When his day's work is done he does not come home to an unhappy wife who may whittle away at his already diminished masculinity. Perhaps shaving before applying cosmetics, he changes into woman's clothes. He becomes the woman who gives him not only sexual pleasure but social status too. Connie continues:

[58] *Medical World News*, Vol. 11, No. 39 (September 25, 1970), pp. 20–21.

[59] H. Taylor Buckner, "The Transvestic Career Path," *Psychiatry: Journal for the Study of Interpersonal Processes*, Vol. 33, No. 3 (August 1970), p. 385, citing Larry Maddock, *Sex Life of a Transvestite* (Hollywood, Calif., 1964), p. 120.

[60] A strong suggestion of transvestism is frequent in the plays of Shakespeare. Although Falstaff is dressed as a woman in *The Merry Wives of Windsor*, examples of female transvestism are more apparent than those of male transvestism. Playing the role of a male lawyer in *The Merchant of Venice*, the woman Portia is dressed as a man. In *Twelfth Night*, Viola disguises herself as her dead brother. Julia dresses as Sebastian in *Two Gentlemen of Verona*. (Matthew Besdine, "Shakespeare: The Homosexual Element in the Life of a Genius," *Medical Aspects of Human Sexuality*, Vol. 5, No. 2 [February 1971], p. 177.) In Shakespeare's day, moreover, the role of a girl was usually played by a boy. So it was, in those times, with Rosalind who is disguised as the young countryman Ganymede in *As You Like It*. What is it about Rosalind that has so long fascinated men? Is it her beauty alone? "Here is Professor Wilson Knight's intuition: 'A boy actor playing a girl disguised as a boy pretending to be a girl . . . Rosalind-Ganymede rings all the changes on love'." (Wilson Knight, *The Golden Labyrinth*, cited in H. F. Rubenstein and J. C. Trewin, eds., *The Drama Bedside Book* [London, 1966], p. 147.)

Keeping her lovely is a full-time job. It literally takes several hours a day—but when I look into the mirror and see what we have made, it's worth every bit of hard work and discomfort involved. When we walk down the street, our feet flying in their tight patent leather pumps because Connie's skirts are so narrow at the knees, our heels clicking in precise feminine rhythm, it's a great feeling to know that heads are turning. The women look, and they envy Connie her wardrobe; the men look and they envy whoever she belongs to, and maybe they think she doesn't belong to anybody, but they're wrong. She belongs to me. I'm the man whose hands run over her body, the man who touches her where only a lover is allowed to touch.[61]

The sexual problems of the transvestite are basically psychological and probably began in a childhood environment that discouraged masculine expression. At an early age (between five and fourteen years) he may have associated some item of feminine clothing with sexual gratification, often by masturbating with it. Later, perhaps as a young adult, he may have doubted his adequacy as a male. Perhaps his own standards of maleness were too high, or the masculine roles with which he was involved were too strenuous for him, or he failed in some masculine sport. Then, if homosexual opportunities were not open to him, he developed a fantasy life. He became his own woman, his own ever pleasing wife. His real marriage may not be as satisfying as his imaginary marriage. "For some of the reasons that happily married couples do not get divorced, transvestites do not give up transvestism." [62]

Two-thirds of male transvestites marry. Transvestite behavior can continue well into later life. Although overt sexual activities may diminish or cease entirely, cross-dressing has been observed to persist in a number of persons between the ages of sixty and eighty-three years.[63] Transvestites rarely disturb the law.

Many masculine demands on Western man are diminishing (see pages 355-56). This, plus the increasing tolerance of homosexual behavior, may preclude an increased rate of a transvestite orientation. Psychiatric treatment aimed at this sexual deviation is generally unrewarding. Newer psychotherapeutic efforts seem to recognize the need to closely analyze the social gratifications of transvestism.

Aversive therapy using electric shocks has been successful in treating transvestism. One behavior therapist reported a patient who

[61]H. Taylor Buckner, "The Transvestic Career Path," p. 385, citing Larry Maddock, *Sex Life of a Transvestite,* pp. 120-21.
[62]H. Taylor Buckner, "The Transvestic Career Path," p. 386.
[63]Walter C. Alvarez, "The Need for Expression of Femininity in Man," *Modern Medicine,* Vol. 39, No. 3 (February 8, 1971), p. 83.

was unable to have sexual intercourse with his wife unless he first dressed up as a woman, and he frequently went out on the streets at night dressed in this fashion and wearing a wig. This symptom had become especially uncomfortable to the patient because he feared that his young son, as he grew up, would learn about it. The treatment prescribed was extremely simple. Electrodes were fastened into the woman's clothing that the patient habitually wore; he was encouraged to dress up but warned that at some point he would receive a painful shock or hear a buzzer and that the shock or buzzer would then be repeated at irregular intervals until he had removed the clothing. Each session of therapy included five starts at dressing followed by the shock or buzzer, with a one-minute rest period between each trial. After 400 trials, the treatment was considered ended.[64]

transsexual behavior

In 1746 in Somersetshire, England, Mary Hamilton was tried for the crime of polygamy. Assuming a series of aliases, she had married fourteen women. As *The Newgate Calendar* reported it, a learned, if bewildered, quorum of justices

"In full-blown dignity of wigs,
Mounted on blocks, thus cogitated

That he, she, the prisoner at the bar, is an uncommon notorious cheat; and we, the Court, do sentence her or him, whichever he or she may be, to be imprisoned six months, and, during that time, to be whipped in the towns of Taunton, Glastonbury, Wells, and Shipton-Mallet, and to find security for good behaviour as long as they, the learned justices aforesaid, shall or may, in their wisdom and judgment, require"; and Mary, the monopolizer of her own sex, was imprisoned and whipped accordingly, in the severity of the winter of the year of 1746.[65]

One cannot be certain about what type of divergent behavior Mary Hamilton exhibited. The Newgate report mentions nothing about her feelings in the matter. But Mary Hamilton could very well have been a transsexual. Transsexual behavior is related to both homosexual and transvestite behavior. This divergence was recently

---

[64]C. B. Blakemore et al., "The Application of Faradic Aversion Conditioning in a Case of Transvestism," cited in Jerome Kagan and Ernest Havemann, *Psychology: An Introduction* (New York, 1968), pp. 443-44.
[65]"The Woman Who Married Fourteen Wives," from *The Newgate Calendar,* in Alexander Klein, ed., *Grand Deception: The World's Most Spectacular and Successful Hoaxes, Impostures, Ruses, and Frauds* (London), p. 70.

demonstrated by a seventeen-year-old who was admitted to a hospital in the East for attempted suicide. A feminine creature, the young patient wore an attractive gown and an alluring hairdo. Not until the patient stubbornly refused to shower for three days was the truth discovered. He had normal-sized male genitalia.

> *As far back as he could remember, he had the feeling of a girl trapped in the wrong body of a boy, with the feeling that his apparent original sex was wrong. Although fully aware of the reality of his biological-physical sexual organs, he felt cross-sexed—that is, a member of the opposite sex. In addition, he never obtained sexual pleasure from his own male sex organs. He never had erections or ejaculations.*[66]

This patient wanted nothing more than the removal of his penis and the acquisition of female sexual organs. His inability to achieve this sex-change depressed him so much that he attempted the suicide that led to his hospitalization.

Men whose behavior is homosexual, transvestite, or transsexual may all cross-dress. But the first two experience penile pleasure. Only the male transsexual hates his penis and derives no sexual pleasure from it. The effeminate man whose behavior is homosexual enjoys the sexual interests of other men. The male transvestite may have a heterosexual or, rarely, a homosexual behavior pattern, or both, but he usually considers himself a male. The male transsexual cross-dresses in order to become a female, and he seeks men who are interested in his acquired femininity, not in his male genitalia. The male transsexual rejects intercourse with a female, considering it homosexual behavior and repulsive. He often seeks and sometimes obtains a sex-change by operation as did Christine (George) Jorgensen.

How does transsexual behavior develop? There are various theories, but most indicate that this pattern originates in childhood. Before the birth of the child the parents begin hoping for a boy or girl. When the child is born most parents forget their past wishes and adjust to the gender of the child happily enough. Some do not. Parental attitudes combined with cultural influences may produce in the impressionable child a desire to be of the opposite gender. A disruptive family life may also be involved. If, for example, the mother dominates an ineffectual father, the son may not be able to relate to his father. Desperately, he may wish to be more like his mother, to be powerful enough to protect himself. In time, this desire may be transformed into a wish to be the same strong gender as his mother. But his genitalia, a repellent deformity, are a cruel reminder of his

[66] Louis R. Hott, "Transsexuality," *Medical Aspects of Human Sexuality,* Vol. 4, No. 9 (September 1970), p. 162.

inherent weakness. Finally they become the hated symbols of his imprisonment in the wrong body.

Another theory attempts to explain transsexual behavior as the result of a nervous-endocrine imbalance. This possibility is not only borne out by results of recent laboratory experiments (see page 302, footnote 16) but is also suggested by the fact that signs of possible future transsexual behavior may appear at a remarkably young age. Efforts at cross-dressing have been reported in a child less than two years old.[67] It will be remembered that all human embryos have a hypothalamic center in the brain that is basically female (see page 81). For the development of a male, the embryonic hypothalamus must be masculinized by androgen originating in the fetal testes. Should this not occur, the hypothalamic center in the brain remains female. It is theorized that in the development of the male transsexual there occurs an inadequate change in the brain from female to male, although male genitalia do develop.[68]

TREATMENT OF TRANSSEXUAL BEHAVIOR

Most experts now believe that after childhood psychotherapy is useless in treating transsexual behavior. Some therapists disagree, however, and suggest that some people choose transsexual behavior in order to have a position in society that is less stressful.[69] There are a few reports that treatment with hormones helps reverse the transsexual orientation.

Although there is no proven biological or physical basis to transsexual behavior, surgical sex-change may at least alleviate some psychological problems. For males, the operation involves the removal of the penis and the testes. Treatment with female hormones (estrogens, see page 42) effects some fat redistribution and breast enlargement. Sometimes an artificial vagina is surgically constructed. If before coitus a lubricating material is inserted into the artificial vagina, coitus may then be quite satisfactory. Male transsexuals also seek to have facial hair removed by electrolysis. Cosmetics, hair-styling and highly feminine dress complete a convincing picture. For female transsexuals the surgical procedures involve the removal of the uterus and both breasts as well as the closing of the vagina. An artificial penis may be constructed from a skin graft, although it cannot be used for sexual intercourse. Sometimes clever surgery can make it possible for the transsexual to urinate through the penis in a standing position—a capacity usually desired. For cosmetic purposes artificial testicles can be inserted into the labia majora (see page 57).

---

[67] Lawrence E. Newman, "Transsexualism: A Disorder of Sexual Identity," *Medical Insight,* Vol. 2, No. 1 (November 1970), p. 29.

[68] "Gender Identity: The Desire to Be Different," *Nature,* Vol. 223, No. 5205 (August 2, 1969), pp. 448–49.

[69] Ibid., p. 448. The male does, indeed, suffer from more stress-related diseases.

Male hormones (androgens, see page 35, footnote 3) cause an increase in body weight and muscularity. The voice deepens—a change highly prized by the transformed transsexual.

How successful are these procedures? One report states that "a good result, measured by improved psychological and social adjustment . . . is ten times as likely as a bad result." [70] Another physician is not as enthusiastic; in a review of twenty-nine men and six women patients, he found that the surgery brought a good appearance in only one-third of the men; results with the women were much more satisfactory. [71] For the male or female whose orientation is heterosexual, such genital mutilation would be devastating. For the male or female whose orientation is transsexual it is avidly sought. However, genital surgery is usually not performed until the transsexual has successfully lived as a member of the opposite sex for one year. [72] Nor are hormones used until the patient has had at least three to six months experience as a member of the opposite sex. [73]

Since 1953, about one thousand operations have been performed in various parts of the world. Marriage, orgasm, and community acceptance have all been reported. In the United States there are now six gender clinics to help the transsexual, but in only one are sex-change operations performed. These clinics are infinitely preferable to the charlatans who prey on those often distressed individuals, further robbing them of their sexual security.

the significance of the child's cross-dressing

The occurrence of cross-dressing in the child requires the parents to exhibit great sensitivity and tact in their response. Parents who jump to hasty conclusions can irreparably harm a child. The young boy who cross-dresses once or twice in a playful way is by no means a potential transvestite. The child usually forsakes such behavior after a few experiments. Nor does the cross-dressing appear to be in any way associated with sexual excitement. Whether it is significant will depend, in part, on the intensity of the child's need to repeat the activity. Also significant are the length of time the cross-dressing has been occurring and the degree of frustration shown by the child if he is interrupted. In the Gender Identity Clinic at the University of California at Los Angeles a considerable number of very feminine

[70] I. Pauly, "The Current Status of the Change of Sex Operation," *Journal of Nervous and Mental Disease,* Vol. 147 (1968), pp. 460-71, and H. Benjamin, *The Transsexual Phenomenon* (New York, 1966), both cited in Lawrence E. Newman, "Transsexualism: A Disorder of Sexual Identity," p. 29.
[71] Russell Roth, "The Brave New World of the Transsexuals," *Modern Medicine,* Vol. 40, No. 4 (February 21, 1972), p. 161.
[72] Lawrence E. Newman, "Transsexualism: A Disorder of Sexual Identity," p. 37.
[73] H. Benjamin, *The Transsexual Phenomenon,* and Lawrence E. Newman, "Transsexualism in Adolescence," *Archives of General Psychiatry,* Vol. 23 (August 1970), both cited in Lawrence E. Newman, "Transsexualism: A Disorder of Sexual Identity," p. 37.

young boys have been examined. "A persistent desire to dress up in little girl's clothing is often accompanied by a preference for girls as playmates, preference for the female role in fantasy games, and not uncommonly by the wish to grow up to become a woman." [74] The child who is attached to this kind of behavior and who is otherwise also unduly feminine may, in time, not only be inclined to transvestite behavior, but may eventually be predisposed to transsexual or homosexual behavior. Such a child should receive a psychiatric evaluation, and possibly psychotherapy. The parents will surely need counseling.

other forms of sexual expression

EXHIBITIONISM

Societal acceptance of different forms of sexual behavior varies according to time, place, and degree as do the forms of behavior themselves. One man buys a suit of clothes that tastefully displays his masculine attributes. Another lurks near a playground and suddenly displays his genitals to children. Both exhibitions are sexual expressions. The differences lie in degree, and in the appropriateness of time and place. The sexual gratification the latter receives from his exaggerated behavior is a result of his exhibitionism. The sexual gratification the less obsessed, elegantly dressed man receives is a result of his good taste. The exhibitionist is unable to adjust to basic cultural rules. He needs help.

He may be suffering from a variety of emotional stresses that prompt his culturally unacceptable behavior. By exposing his genitals to unresisting children he may be trying to allay an unconquered fear of his own childhood—that he will lose his penis.[75] Male exhibitionists who are apprehended are usually married. Perhaps a restrictive childhood combined with an inadequate adult sexual life fills him with a constant sense of waning masculinity. To reaffirm his manhood he displays his genitalia.

VOYEURISM

Voyeurism, or *scoptophilia,* is a form of sexual behavior in which gratification is derived from looking at another person's genital organs. As with other forms of sexual behavior, whether it is to be considered a matter for concern or not depends on the degree of involvement in this behavior and the appropriateness of the time and

---

[74]Lawrence E. Newman, "Cross Dressing in Children," *Medical Aspects of Human Sexuality,* Vol. 5, No. 2 (February 1971), p. 219.
[75]For a discussion of the fear of castration, see pages 13–14.

place of its occurrence. A related form of behavior is *troilism,* which refers to sexual intercourse involving three persons; two are of the same sex, and the third person looks on. Sometimes two or more couples have sexual intercourse at the same time as others watch. There is considerable reason to believe that this last form of sexual expression (often referred to as group sex) is occurring with increasing frequency. The effect of group sex on the individuals involved and on society in general has yet to be reliably evaluated. Much has been made of the fact that persons in the upper socioeconomic levels participate in troilism and group sex. However, there is no reason to believe that sexual inadequacy and homosexual behavior are not commonly present in these population groups, and there may be reason to suspect that both may be common among those people who seek to participate in troilism and other group sexual expression.

is voyeurism a national problem?

There is some opinion in this country that the degree of voyeuristic sexual behavior has become detrimental to the welfare of the social group. Not without some justification, this era has been called the Age of Voyeurism. It is speculated that "we seek and look and ingest with the eye to a degree that is unparalleled in human history . . . the great increase in voyeurism is taking place at the expense of coitus and other interpersonal kinds of sex expression." Sexually explicit films and magazines "may be expected to move people in the direction of masturbating activities rather than interpersonal relations involving sex." [76] One may rightfully be concerned about a societal trend in which there is widespread substitution of sexual isolation for involvement. But there is also, in this country, an increasing tolerance of sexually specific visual materials. Some of this tolerance may be an overreaction to an overly restrictive past. At times the restrictions bordered on the ridiculous. In October 1913, for example, an art magazine was held up at the New York Post Office on the grounds that it contained reproductions of "objectionable" paintings, while at the same time the original paintings were on exhibit in the Brooklyn Museum. [77] "Man," said Mark Twain, "is the only animal capable of having a dirty mind." In March 1953, zealots in Cleveland withdrew from sale Freud's *General Introduction to Psychoanalysis* along with the classic second-century satire *The Golden Ass (Metamorphoses)* by Lucius Apuleius. [78] Even the instructive word *chaste* was once deleted from a book because it was "too suggestive." [79]

[76] Charles Winick, "The Desexualized Society," *The Humanist,* Vol. 29, No. 6 (November–December 1969) pp. 6–8.
[77] Ralph Slovenko, ed., *Sexual Behavior and the Law* (Springfield, Ill., 1965), citing *Publishers Weekly,* Vol. 84 (October 25, 1913), p. 1380.
[78] Ralph Slovenko, ed., *Sexual Behavior and the Law,* p. 818.
[79] Ibid., p. 811.

Somewhere between such nonsense and common sense the people of this nation are trying to establish a standard that represents the views of the majority. Meanwhile, trial and changes are inevitable. Unfortunately, legal interpretations are not helpful. "If a man walking past an apartment stops to watch a woman undressing before a mirror, the man is arrested as a peeper. If a woman walking past an apartment stops to watch a man undressing before a window, the man is arrested as an exhibitionist." [80]

When may voyeuristic sexual expressions become possibly harmful to the individual? This behavior pattern may indicate emotional problems in those unusual cases in which it supplants sexual intercourse as the primary source of sexual gratification. Although there is much avid opinion that voyeurism is harmful, there is, as yet, no concrete evidence that sexually stimulating visual materials have a pronounced deleterious effect on either the average adult or society in general.

THE LAW AND SODOMY

The word *sodomy* is derived from the name of an ancient city that in the Bible is judged by the Lord to be a center of sinfulness. Sodomy denotes anal intercourse, which is in many cultures a crime punishable under the law. The reasoning behind these laws arises, in part, from the biblical prohibition against any sexual act that did not serve to propagate the species. Today, however, considering the problem of overpopulation of the human species, this reasoning is no longer as valid as it once might have been. There is surely a more tolerant attitude toward anal intercourse between men whose behavior is homosexual. Moreover, many people today reject the notion that sodomy is a crime when practiced by consenting adults. For some people whose behavior is heterosexual, anal intercourse is one variety of sexual expression.

Many of today's laws designed to control sexual behavior are based on yesterday's needs or ignorance. One typical statute prohibiting sodomy reads like this: "Every person who shall carnally know or shall have sexual intercourse in any manner with any animal or bird; or shall carnally know any male or female by the anus (rectum) or with the mouth or tongue; or shall attempt intercourse with a dead body is guilty of Sodomy." [81]

This single statute prohibits under the term *sodomy* a number of forms of sexual behavior, including pederasty (anal intercourse as practiced by a man with a boy), bestiality (human sexual connection with an animal, see pages 325–27), fellatio (see page 89), cunnilinction

---

[80] Paul H. Gebhard, John H. Gagnon, Wardell B. Pomeroy, and Cornelia V. Christenson, *Sex Offenders* (New York, 1965), p. 10.

[81] Robert Viet Sherwin, "Sodomy," in Ralph Slovenko, ed., *Sexual Behavior and the Law,* p. 427.

(see page 89), and necrophilism (a morbid attraction to corpses, or sexual intercourse with a dead body).

Today, some of these forms of sexual expression are considered divergent; some are not. Necrophilism would doubtless repel almost everyone in this culture. The same is true of pederasty, although it was ordinary practice in Sparta (see page 328). In some situations bestiality has been equated with masturbation; only when it persists into adulthood can it be considered as a possible emotional problem. To think of either fellatio or cunnilinction as criminal or as a manifestation of emotional illness is totally invalid (see page 89). Clearly the above-mentioned statute is both unclear and out of date. For breaking any part of it, people are subject to punishments varying from five years to life imprisonment at hard labor. Laws such as this open the parties in a divorce case to cruel blackmail. And such laws do little to foster marital sexual security. One couple "turned themselves over to the local police station for punishment, when they discovered that their specific acts of love subjected them to sixty years to life in prison." [82] There is little question that senseless guilts are often propagated by senseless laws.

The very concepts of divergent sexual behavior change in different times. As Judd Marmor has written:

> It is necessary to put aside our culturally acquired biases to achieve an objective perspective on what constitutes "normal" and "deviant" sexual behavior. Sexual practices and mores have varied widely in the course of human history and in different cultures. Our present concept of normal and deviant behavior cannot be divorced from the value systems of contemporary society. Since value systems are always in the process of evolution and change, we must be prepared to face the possibility that some patterns of sexual behavior currently considered deviant may not always so be regarded. [83]

LESS COMMON FORMS OF SEXUAL EXPRESSION

bestiality

On September 8, 1642, the governor of Plymouth Plantation recorded the execution of seventeen-year-old Thomas Granger for "buggery" (another term for sodomy) with a mare, a cow, two goats, five sheep, two calves, and a turkey. "A very sad spectacle it was," wrote the aggrieved Governor William Bradford. "For first the mare and then the cow and the rest of the cattle were killed before his face . . . and

[82] Ibid., p. 428.

[83] Judd Marmor, "'Normal' and 'Deviant' Sexual Behavior," *Journal of the American Medical Association*, Vol. 217, No. 2 (July 12, 1971), p. 165.

then he himself was executed.[84] As a result of a similar trial, held fifty years later, a New Jersey man was sentenced to be "hanged by the neck till the body be dead, dead, dead and God have mercy on thy Soule; and that the Cowe with which thou committed the Buggery shall the same day be slaine."[85] In France another fifty years later, the offending human was hanged, but the animal (a she-ass) was spared execution when several good citizens of the town "signed a certificate stating that they had known said she-ass for four years, and that she had always shown herself to be virtuous both at home and abroad."[86] Occasionally, bestiality has been used to explain the origin of a supposedly inferior race of people. Among the Copper Eskimos, for example, intercourse between a human and a dog is believed to have resulted in white men.[87]

Sexual intercourse between humans and animals continues to this day. Since in recent decades there has been a massive migration from the farms to the cities, this has doubtless diminished the frequency of sexual contacts between human beings and animals. Kinsey and his group noted that "among boys raised on farms, about 17 percent experience orgasm as the product of animal contacts which occur sometime after the onset of adolescence."[88] However, even in the 1940s, when Kinsey conducted his study, bestiality accounted for the smallest proportion of the total sexual expression for the entire population. As was to be expected, the number of city boys who reported sexual contacts with animals was relatively few. Most of these occurred during visits to farms. Older rural males had markedly fewer sexual contacts with animals, doubtless due to the increased availability to them of the human female.[89]

As a result of observing animals during coitus, farm girls reported much less erotic arousal than did the boys. Moreover, they experienced much less sexual contact with animals. However, unlike farm boys, many farm girls were excluded from talk about sexual matters and animal breeding. Most female sexual contacts with animals occurred with house pets such as dogs and cats. Interestingly, a male dog experiencing human sexual stimulation might become so devoted to the human as to forsake the female of his own species for sexual purposes.[90]

For most of those who experience it, bestiality is a transient and relatively harmless practice. In societies in which there are an in-

[84] William Bradford, *Of Plymouth Plantation 1620–1647,* edited by Samuel Eliot Morison (New York, 1967), p. 320.
[85] Negley K. Teeters, *Hang by the Neck* . . . (Springfield, Ill., 1967), p. 111, citing Harry B. Weiss and Grace M. Weiss, *An Introduction to Crime and Punishment in Colonial New Jersey* (Trenton, N.J., 1960), p. 87.
[86] Clellan S. Ford and Frank A. Beach, *Patterns of Sexual Behavior,* pp. 151–52.
[87] Ibid., p. 155.
[88] Alfred C. Kinsey et al., *Sexual Behavior in the Human Male,* p. 671.
[89] Alfred C. Kinsey et al., *Sexual Behavior in the Human Female,* pp. 502–09.
[90] Alfred C. Kinsey et al., *Sexual Behavior in the Human Male,* p. 677.

sufficient number of women it has been equated with masturbation. The few people who continue the practice into adulthood may fear the opposite sex. Others may be expressing their hostility to the opposite sex by deliberately choosing an animal for their sexual gratification. Because the biblical prohibition against bestiality[91] has had such lasting influence on this culture some people live with deep anxiety and guilt feelings about their youthful "transgression."

sadism and masochism

Sadism refers to the sexual gratification that is derived from dominating, mistreating, or hurting one's partner, physically or otherwise. *Masochism* is its opposite; the masochist receives sexual pleasure from being cruelly treated. Each behavior pattern is named after a singularly unwholesome character. As a young man the Marquis de Sade (1740–1814) had been guilty of a few sadistic acts. In later life he was more a "pervert of the pen"[92] than an active sadist. His third-rate writings describing sadism have perpetuated a name that, in his last testament, he himself hoped would "be wiped from the memory of mankind."[93] The term *masochism* is derived from the name of an Austrian, Ritter Leopold von Sacher-Masoch (1835–95). Like de Sade, he was of noble birth and was a minor writer who depicted some of his own sexual experiences.

Neither sadism nor masochism should be confused with the usually gentle, but sometimes vigorous, slapping, pinching, or biting that may occur during ordinary sexual intercourse. For the sadistic person the inflicting of suffering is a sexual end in itself, as is the receiving of punishment for the masochist. A common, perhaps milder, example is the sadistic husband who mercilessly beats his masochistic wife while she meekly endures her punishment. Both are really enjoying one another. A most extreme degree of sadism is lust murder. As he kills, the lust murderer experiences intense sexual pleasure and, indeed, may sexually violate his dying or dead victim.

The sadist's exceedingly aggressive sexual behavior may be an expression of a loathing of sexuality. It becomes a punishment of the sexual partner for participating in an act that the sadist finds so "degrading." Among the other explanations for sadism is the need to express power because of a deep sense of inadequacy. In contrast, the masochist hates himself. This hatred may arise from a wish to hurt the mother or father that is transformed into a perverse wish to hurt the self. Of the two, sadism is more dangerous because, unlike masochism, it harms others. The overt sadist has a tendency to repeat his crimes.

[91] See, for example, Exodus 22:19 and Leviticus 18:23, 20:16.
[92] Richard Lewinsohn, *A History of Sexual Customs* (Greenwich, Conn., 1958), p. 235.
[93] Ivan Bloch, ed., *Marquis de Sade: Life and Works* (New York, 1969), p. 89.

In this country today, violence, cruelty, and sexuality have become part of the daily emotional diet of both children and adults.[94] The influence on the young psyche of sadism, as it is portrayed in, for example, comic books and television, is cause for concern.

pedophilia

Pedophilia is defined as a morbid interest in children; *pedophilia erotica* refers to sexual perversion toward children. In ancient Greece the pedophiliac was considered neither morbid nor perverted but a man of refined tastes. Today, there are a number of cultures in which the pedophiliac is regarded with mere contempt. The pedophiliac seeks children to satisfy his sexual expression because he is unable to satiate himself sexually in another way. It is of interest to note that sexual activity between mature and immature animals is common, although apparently not preferential.

In this culture pedophilia is viewed with disgust, and the convicted pedophiliac is severely punished. It has been noted earlier that societal judgments and subconscious sexual reactions (no matter how innocently instigated) do not always coincide. "Thus a grandfather bouncing his grandchild on his lap may be aghast to discover he is developing an erection."[95] Such a reaction is hardly a cause for concern; nor is it pedophilia. But it can cause a needless sense of guilt.

Pedophilia may be manifested in a number of different ways. Most commonly, the man exhibits his genitals to a female child. The more aggressive pedophiliac may force a child to submit to genital manipulation or to reciprocate the genital contact. More rarely the offender rapes a child. Pedophilia is almost entirely an activity that is limited to men. Reports of female children being molested far outnumber those involving male children. The stereotype notwithstanding, old men comprise the least numerous of the age groups involved in child molestation.

> *The old-age group is relatively the smallest one involved in child molesting; the major age groups are the middle to late thirties (about one-third), the early forties to the early fifties (about one-fourth), the twenties (about one-fourth), and the teens (about one-tenth). Exhibitionism occurs most often in men in their mid-twenties and is rarely seen in its true form after forty.*[96]

The distress of the parents of a molested child is understandable. To this is added a sense of guilt that they are not properly caring

---

[94] For a further discussion of the relationship between sexuality and violence, see pages 331-34.
[95] Paul H. Gebhard et al., *Sex Offenders,* p. 55.
[96] *Sexuality and Man,* compiled and edited by the Sex Information and Education Council of the United States (New York, 1970), p. 87.

for their child. Perhaps long forgotten fears about sexuality, so common among human beings, may come to the fore. A relatively minor event is thus magnified and distorted. If the parents panic, their high-strung reaction may be transmitted to the child. It is important that several factors be kept in mind.[97] First of all, *"for most children, in most situations, the victim situation is of short duration and of minimal effect."* [98] The trauma to the child resulting from a hysterical parental reaction to molestation may be more injurious than the molestation itself. The child should be taught the proper (and safe) way to make friends. He should not be taught to fear all strangers as possible molestors.

Whether to report the matter to the police is a difficult problem for parents. A prime consideration may be how concerned the police department is about avoiding trauma to the child. A child psychologist may be most helpful in making this decision and in handling other aspects of a difficult situation.

[97] Ibid., pp. 83–98.
[98] Ibid., p. 86.

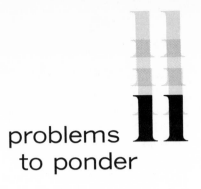

problems 11
to ponder

alienation and sexuality

Oh Father, my Father, Oh what must I do?
They're burning our streets and beating me blue.
"Listen my son, I'll tell you the truth:
Get a close haircut and spit-shine your shoes."

Oh Mother, my Mother, my confusions remove,
I long to embrace her whose hair is so smooth.
"Now listen my son, although you're confused,
Cut your hair close and shine all your shoes."

Oh Teacher, my Teacher, your life with me share.
What books ought I read? What thoughts do I dare?
"Oh Student, my Student, of dissent you beware.
Shine those dull shoes and cut short your hair."

Oh Preacher, my Preacher, does God really care?
Are all races equal? Are laws just and fair?
"Boy—here's the answer, no need to despair:
Shine those new shoes and cut short that hair." [1]

Widespread racism, war, antiquated institutions, depersonalization, pollution—these are but some of the causes of youthful alienation. And alienation profoundly influences sexual behavior.

Sociologist Melvin Seeman has written that alienated people demonstrate one or more of six attitudes toward life: (1) a sense of individual *powerlessness* in determining one's own destiny; (2) a feeling of the *meaninglessness* of one's efforts and, indeed, of one's whole life; (3) *normlessness* (cynicism), the conviction that hard work simply does not pay and success can only be achieved by cutting corners; (4) *cultural estrangement,* a separation between one's own

[1] Paul Cummins, "Advice," *The New Republic,* Vol. 157, No. 21, Issue No. 2764 (November 18, 1967), p. 26.

value system (such as artistic integrity) and societal values (such as money grabbing); (5) *self-estrangement,* the feeling that one has not been able to live up to one's own expectations and potentials; and (6) *social isolation,* one's feeling that one is rejected and unacceptable as a person.[2]

Different people experience different degrees of alienation, and they react in different ways. For example, consider two people whom Kenneth Keniston might call "postmodern youth."[3] Both were born since the end of the Second World War, both consider the older generation, its institutions and its ways, largely irrelevant to the needs of a rapidly changing society, and both are critical of the contradiction between the words and the actions of their parents. But one individual responds by turning to activism, while the other, not typical of postmodern youth, withdraws. The withdrawn person has been overcome by alienation. His sense of helplessness and meaninglessness, his separation from self and society are too much for him. The activist, however, may well go through the pains of alienation, but rather than withdrawal he seeks commitment. He may decide to work for radical change through some possibly receptive branch of the establishment, or he may become committed to the New Left. He is also more likely to be able to commit himself to a person. For him sexual expression is more than physiologic relief, it is an expression of sharing and caring. And although he may find enough cause for discouragement, depression is not his constant companion. He may experiment with drugs but will generally not abuse them chronically. He does not need drugs to escape a sense of impotence, either in his sexual life or in his other activities.

violence and sexuality

OBSESSION AGAINST VIOLENCE
REPLACES SEXUAL OBSESSION

Kenneth Keniston, in comparing Victorian sexual behavior with that of today's committed youth, has formulated a significant explanation for the reaction of many of today's youth to violence. During the Victorian era sexual expression "was not forcibly stuck into a straight-jacket, but carefully put in plaster, like the victim of an accident who must not be hurt."[4] Shakespeare's works were published in expurgated editions. For fear that men would be able to peek up their dresses, girls were warned against wearing patent

[2] Melvin Seeman, "Alienation," *Psychology Today,* Vol. 5, No. 3 (August 1971), pp. 83–84. See also Melvin Seeman, "On the Meaning of Alienation," *American Sociological Review,* Vol. 24, No. 6 (December 1969), pp. 783–91.
[3] Kenneth Keniston, *Young Radicals* (New York, 1968), p. 275.
[4] Richard Lewinsohn, *A History of Sexual Customs* (Greenwich, Conn., 1958), p. 264.

leather shoes. Women did not have *legs*. Even piano stools had limbs; in many homes they were carefully covered with ruffled crinolines. (Of course, to provide panties for piano legs was to sexualize them.) The Victorians' repression of sex was a mark of their obsession with it. It reached a height with the mid-century (1853) warning published in *Godey's Lady's Book* that "the perfect hostess will see to it that the works of male and female authors be properly separated on her bookshelves. Their proximity, unless they happen to be married, should not be tolerated."[5] Forty-three years later, England's *Electrical Journal* (1896) advertised "X-ray proof underclothing—especially made for the sensitive woman."[6]

How does Keniston compare this obsessive concern with sex with the attitude of today's committed young person?

> *In the Victorian era, what was most deeply repressed, re-jected, feared, controlled, projected onto others, or compulsively acted out was related to the issue of sex. The personal and social symptomatology of that era—the hysterical ladies who consulted Freud, the repressive moralism of middle class life, and the sor-did underlife of the "other Victorians"—can only be under-stood in the context of the Victorian era with human sexuality. The postwar generation, in contrast, is freer, more open, less guilt- and anxiety-ridden about sex. Sex obviously remains important, as befits one of the primary human drives. But in-creasing numbers of postmodern youth . . . have been able to overcome even the asceticism and puritanism of their own ado-lescences to move toward a sexuality that is less obsessional, less dissociated, less driven, more integrated with other human experiences and relationships. Inner and outer violence is re-placing sex as a prime object of fear, terror, projection, dis-placement, repression, suppression, acting out, and efforts at control . . .* The issue of violence is to this generation what the issue of sex was to the Victorian world.[7]

THE VIOLENCE OF THE BETRAYED BOY

> *You know he sat right in front of me for two years, and I'll bet I gave him an A in deportment every time . . . That little blond kid, not bristling the way many adolescents are, getting their own identity and rebelling in the process. He was absolutely cooperative. You know how teachers will talk about some*

[5] Donald Day, *The Evolution of Love* (New York, 1954), p. 392.
[6] E. Posner, "Reception of Röntgen's Discovery in Britain and U.S.A.," *British Medical Journal,* Vol. 4, No. 5731 (November 7, 1970), p. 359.
[7] Kenneth Keniston, *Young Radicals,* pp. 248, 252–53.

kids—so and so did this or that today. Well, Arthur's name was never mentioned in the teachers' lounge.[8]

That is how a former teacher of the would-be assassin of Governor George Wallace described the schoolboy Arthur Bremer.

Violence is a topic of major concern among modern students of behavior. Keniston's theory is one of several that attempts to explain the possible relationships between sexual expression, repression, and violence. Sociologist Patricia Sexton has drawn attention to a correlation between violence and the feminization of the male child in this culture.[9] Eighty-five percent of U.S. public elementary school teachers are women. In all U.S. public schools, women comprise two-thirds of the total. Although the administrators are predominantly men, schools are essentially feminine institutions.[10] In the home, growing boys are also primarily under the influence of a woman. This dominance of women in both school and in the home is a result of the imbalance in the sexual roles in this culture. Women are largely excluded from the male-dominated decision-making arenas. "Although the exclusion of women from 'man's work' has protected certain male privileges, it has also left some unintended marks on men." [11] The woman's resentment of this exclusion results in her resentment of the male in general. What is stressed and rewarded during the boy's education is not masculine but feminine behavior. "Many schools and academies are dehumanizing and unmanly places. Boys who succeed in them often do so by grossly violating many codes of honor and the norms of boy culture." [12] Their masculinity crisis, resulting from their earlier feminization, is expressed with rebellion and violence.

The quiet murderer, such as Oswald and Sirhan, the angry insistence by the young black male on a recognition of his manhood, the predominance of males among delinquents (at a ratio of 5 to 1) and among the population in state prisons (over 90 percent) are but a few of the indications of "rebellions [that] are alarms, alerting us to social forces that dangerously diminish manhood and spread alienation and violence." [13] Failure to adjust is not limited to the adult

---

[8] In Michael Kirkhorn, "Arthur Bremer: He was an Amateur at Everything," *Rolling Stone*, No. 111 (June 22, 1972), p. 51.

[9] Patricia Sexton, "How the American Boy is Feminized," *Psychology Today*, Vol. 3, No. 8 (January 1970), pp. 23–29, 66–67.

[10] Ibid., p. 25.

[11] Ibid., p. 66.

[12] Ibid.

[13] Ibid., p. 23. However, recent years have seen a growing equality between the rates of women's crimes and those of men. In seven of ten top categories, the female crime rate has been rising faster than that of males. From 1960 to 1969, property crime by men increased 59 percent, by women, 184 percent; forgery and counterfeiting rates for men increased 20 percent, for women, 92 percent; for embezzlement and fraud the comparative rate increases were 30 and 211 percent; for narcotic and drug crimes, the rates were up 487 and 516 percent respectively. ("Bonnie versus Clyde," *Science News*, Vol. 99, No. 25 [June 19, 1971], p. 416.) This comment would seem valid:

male; it begins early in life. Sexton studied the relationship of masculinity (as determined by psychological testing) to grades. Her results revealed that "more than half of the most masculine boys were failing, or close to it, in almost all academic subjects" and "the more masculine the boy, the lower his report card average tended to be."[14] "What we must do," she suggests, "is masculinize the school and feminize the power structure of the society—balancing out the sexes so they don't corrode any one spot where they concentrate."[15]

WHY UNDERSTAND VIOLENCE?

Mankind needs greatly to understand the roots of its own violence. The precipitating causes of violence are many and various. They range from racism and overpopulation to poverty and politics. Yet their origins lie within the personality of which sexuality is so central. Keniston's comparison between the sexual repressions of Victoria's day and the sexual expressions of today suggests a concept that is full of hope. And that hope is that today's youth may sense some of the reasons for the trend to violence. Fearing violence as their forebears feared sex, perhaps they can labor better to understand and forestall it.

Nor should one minimize the possible relationship between the early feminization of the male and his resentful violent eruptions. What Keniston, Sexton, and others suggest is that the survival of humankind may, at least in part, depend on a rational approach to sexuality. Knowing about sexuality is more than knowing about how to behave in bed. It is important to know about sexuality in order to better understand man's interpersonal behavior. A criminal may have an orgasm as he commits a robbery; a "fire-bug" may experience sexual satisfaction by viewing the flames he has lit; kleptomania is associated with a divergent form of sexual expression. Human sexuality must be explored not only as an expression of mutuality, but as an expression of alienation.

rock music and sexuality

In the last few decades popular song lyrics have acquired a new character. Lyrics of the mid-1960s have been compared with lyrics

---

"Men are not shaped so simply that more exposure to a male teacher in the early school grades would transfer them into healthy males, any more than girls become healthy females because of contact with same-sexed early teachers." (Max Sugar, commenting on an article by Arthur J. Rudy and Robert Peller, "Men's Liberation," *Medical Aspects of Human Sexuality,* Vol. 6, No. 9 [September 1972], pp. 84, 93-95, 96.) As Patricia Sexton knows, the causes of emotional distress, both individual and societal, are multifactorial.

[14] Ibid., p. 28.

[15] Ibid., p. 66.

of the mid-1950s.[16] In just one decade marked changes in their content and implications have become apparent. Since these changes may reflect new attitudes toward sexual behavior they are enumerated below. Compared to the lyrics of the mid-1950s the lyrics of the mid-1960s had (among other things): replaced personal commitment and prolonged attachment in the boy-girl relationship with temporary and easily terminated involvements; substituted sexual permissiveness based on affection with behavior in which sexual permissiveness without affection was acceptable (for example, in "Go Where You Wanna Go" by The Mamas and Papas); often reduced the girl to little more than an object of sexual gratification (for example, in "Wild Thing"); changed the boy-girl relationship controlled by fate to one in which the control is in the hands of the participants; and, as a corollary, changed the passive orientation of the boy-girl relationship (love is something that happens to them and is outside of their control) to an actively sought affair (they make it happen, and they control it.)

These observations surely demand further investigation. Among the questions that need answering is this: to what extent do the new attitudes expressed by the lyrics of popular music actually influence sexual behavior patterns? Or are the lyrics merely a reflection of changes in the sexual attitudes of society? Rock music is surely a valid and exciting means of musical expression. However, some aspects of it do merit thoughtful discussion.

better sexuality through chemistry?

SOME CAUSATIVE ASPECTS OF DRUG ABUSE

When I was sixteen, I was very ashamed that I was still a virgin. I was always shy with girls, and I hated to admit to other boys that I never slept with a girl. They boasted about the girls they had slept with. When I moved into Greenwich Village and

---

[16] James T. Carey, "Changing Courtship Patterns in the Popular Song," *The American Journal of Sociology,* Vol. 74, No. 6 (May 1969) pp. 720-31. Although hardly a characteristic of all rock concerts, the admixture of violence and sexuality at some of them has caused growing concern in recent years. One leader of a rock group, for example, comes to the front of the stage with a cute baby doll. As he sings a song called *Dead Babies,* he fondles the doll, rubs it across his body, and then slowly begins to undress it. With the quickening of the music, he rips off the doll's clothes. Then he raises a hatchet, and, as a baby's cries lament from a tape recorder backstage, he repeatedly chops the doll. Blood seeps onto the stage floor. "All the while he is singing. And the little girls in the audience are singing too; their eyes shine as they watch Alice kill the baby doll, and they sing along with him, 'Goodbye, little Betty . . . so long, little baby'." (Bob Greene, "Alice's New Restaurant," *Harper's Magazine,* Vol. 224, No. 1465 [June 1972], p. 18.) Numerous lyrics have no semblance of the subtle or gentler passions (*Jam up and Jelly Tight, Coca-Cola Douche*). And *Yesterday's Papers* equates woman, once used, as something "as valuable as an old newspaper, presumably good only for wrapping garbage." (Marion Meade, "Does Rock Degrade Women?" a commentary on an article by Herbert Goldberg, "Rock Music and Sex," *Sexual Behavior,* Vol. 1, No. 5 [August 1971], pp. 25-31.)

got on drugs, girls were easy. They're all in a state of total
rebellion, so they don't care who they sleep with. When I'm on
drugs, I forget about myself and my troubles and I'm not de-
pressed like I used to be.[17]

The drug approach to solving life's problems (sexual or otherwise)
is no longer uncommon among today's teen-agers. Nor is this approach limited to those living in disadvantaged areas. Not without
considerable justification a black man said, "We've had a drug problem for years. But nobody paid much attention to it until it spread
into the white neighborhoods."

the adult model for drug abuse

When it comes to drug abuse, the young have plenty of older people
to show them the way. Alcohol and tobacco are the two most destructive drugs abused in this culture, causing more serious sickness
and killing more people than all other drugs combined. Nevertheless,
the number of parents who completely forgo alcohol and tobacco
are in a distinct minority. Nor is drug abuse in the general population
limited to alcohol and tobacco.

Psychotropic drugs are the "mind-benders." They include the
sedatives and tranquilizers ("downers") and the stimulants ("up-
pers"). Evidence from two current national surveys suggests that
approximately one in four U.S. adults uses one or more kinds of
"upper" or "downer." Nearly one-half the U.S. adult population
reports the use of a psychotropic drug at some time.[18] How does this
widespread drug use affect the young? In one study, it was found
that 33 percent of young marijuana users had mothers who used
barbiturates. The mothers of 20 percent used stimulants. Thirty-six
percent had mothers taking tranquilizers. There is even a closer
association between parental drug use and youthful use of amphetamines ("speed"). Of the young "speed" users, 46 percent had mothers
who used tranquilizers; 32 percent, stimulants; and 43 percent, barbiturates. A recent study of 17,000 Toronto students revealed this
data: "Compared to the children of a mother who does not use
tranquilizers, the children of a mother who does will be twice as likely
to use marihuana or LSD, three times as likely to inhale glue or
solvents, four times as likely to use opiates, speed, stimulants, and
other hallucinogens, five times as likely to use tranquilizers." [19] Drug

[17] In Charles Clay Dahlberg, "Sexual Behavior in the Drug Culture," *Medical Aspects of Human Sexuality,* Vol. 5, No. 4 (April 1971), p. 64.
[18] Hugh J. Parry, "The Use of Psychotropic Drugs by U.S. Adults," *Public Health Reports,* Vol. 33, No. 10 (October 1968), p. 809.
[19] "Child Addiction Likelier if Mother is Pill Taker," *Internal Medicine and Diagnostic News,* Vol. 3, No. 23 (December 1, 1970), pp. 1, 14.

use seems to run in families. To reduce adolescent drug use, it appears that it will be necessary to reach both the parent and the child.[20]

To the educational influence of parents (and the other causes of youthful drug abuse) must be added the enormous impact of television. In this culture, the young person is exposed from toddlerhood on to countless hours of television advertising. What is being sold? It is the idea that the resolution of life's problems is to be found not in one's inner self, but in an external chemical. For every problem there is a drug. The search is not for the best way of life; it is for the best drug. No educational program against drug abuse can equal the educational program for it.

drugs and the alienated college student

In discussing the alienated college student Seymour Halleck has suggested that "alienation viewed as a sense of detachment from the values of one's society, family, and even from one's own feelings is fostered among susceptible college students by the exclusiveness of the university campus, isolated as it is from the adult world."[21] The tendency to live in the present, rejecting both past and future; the avoidance of commitment to causes or people; the inability to communicate with older persons; serious problems in concentration; and the abuse of drugs—particularly marijuana and amphetamines— are among the basic traits of the alienated college student. Promiscuity among these individuals is the rule and depression common.[22]

The most common symptom differentiating the person who experiments with drugs and the chronic drug abuser is a prolonged depression. Unrelieved boredom, intense sexual shyness, and a deep sense of inadequacy and frustration combine to produce an inner despair. Unable to communicate with those who care about him and would want to help him, the depressed youth turns to available drugs. Why? Because they make him feel better. The depressed drug abuser seeks not only an effective drug but an effective dose. He may begin with marijuana. Soon the initial dose of a drug loses its effectiveness, and a larger dose is needed. If that loses its effectiveness he may try another drug. It is true that the ordinary marijuana smoker will not necessarily be led to the abuse of more destructive drugs. But the person who is enduring a prolonged and severe depression is not ordinary. For him marijuana, for example, is no more a social drug than alcohol is to the alcoholic. And there is abundant evidence to

[20] "Research Indicates—Drug Use Runs in Families," *Canada's Mental Health*, Vol. 19, No. 2 (March-April 1971), pp. 28, 29.
[21] Seymour Halleck, "Psychiatric Treatment of the Alienated College Student," *American Journal of Psychiatry*, Vol. 124, No. 5 (November 1967), p. 642.
[22] It should not be assumed that the student who occasionally uses drugs is necessarily alienated.

show that the *frequency* of marijuana abuse is highly correlated to the frequency of the abuse of other drugs.[23]

HEROIN REPLACES SEXUALITY

When they are
in the street
they pass it
along to each
other but when
they see the
police they would
just stand still
and be beat
so pity ful
that they want
to cry.[24]

How do those who are dependent on heroin view themselves? Drug use provides them with identity. "You are a teacher," one heroin abuser said. "You are a cop. You are a parent, a man, a woman, a citizen, a voter, a landlord, a housewife. Me, I'm a junkie."[25] Long before their drug abuse began such individuals had failed to establish a true identity (see page 4). Disturbed parental relationships may be one cause. A study at Tufts University showed that of 100 heroin dependent persons, one-half had lost their fathers and one-fifth their mothers by the time they were sixteen. These data are three times the national average.

The confusion of sexual identity, the inability to relate sexually
to the female, pimping for the wife or girlfriend, all indicate an
early and pervasive disturbance in the mother-child rela-

[23] *The Use of Cannabis*, report of a WHO Scientific Group (Geneva, 1971), p. 12, citing R. H. Blum et al., *Drugs, II. Students and Drugs* (San Francisco, 1969); E. Goode, "Multiple Drug Use Among Marihuana Smokers," *Sociological Problems*, Vol. 17 (1969), pp. 48–64; and M. I. Soueif (unpublished data). Richard Colestock Pillard, "Marihuana," *The New England Journal of Medicine*, Vol. 283, No. 6 (August 6, 1970), p. 30, citing B. E. Leonard, "Cannabis: A Short Review of its Effects and the Possible Dangers of its Use," *Brit. J. Addict.*, Vol. 64 (1969), pp. 121-30; P. A. L. Chapple, "Cannabis: A Toxic and Dangerous Substance. A Study of Eighty Takers," *Brit. J. Addict.*, Vol. 61 (1966), pp. 269-82; D. Silberman and J. Levy, "A Preliminary Survey of Twenty-four Victorian Marijuana Users," *Med. J. Aust.*, Vol. 2 (1969), pp. 286-89; W. H. McGlothlin, D. O. Arnold, and P. K. Rowan, "Marihuana Use Among Adults," *Psychiatry* (in press); and L. N. Robins, H. S. Darvish, and G. E. Murphy, "The Long-term Outcome for Adolescent Drug Users: A Follow-up Study of 76 Users and 146 Non-users," in J. Zubin and A. Freedman, eds., *Psychopathology and Adolescence* (New York, in press). Leo F. Hollister, "Marihuana in Man: Three Years Later," *Science*, Vol. 172, No. 3978, p. 26, citing J. C. Ball, C. D. Chambers, and M. J. Ball, *J. Criminal Law Criminol. Police Science*, Vol. 59 (1968), p. 171. "The Marijuana Problem," *Annals of Internal Medicine*, Vol. 73, No. 3 (September 1970), p. 43.
[24] Marie Ford, "The Junkies," from Herbert Kohl, *36 Children* (New York, 1967), p. 147.
[25] In Oliver Gillie, "Drug Addiction—Facts and Folklore," *Science Journal*, Vol. 5, No. 12 (December 1969), pp. 75-80.

tionship. This is further evidenced by an unreal attitude to the actual mother. The addict usually is a staunch supporter of motherhood, and very verbal in his concern for his own mother's welfare, while simultaneously making life miserable for her in every possible way.[26]

Among ordinary young men there is usually a great deal of sexual talk and action. Among heroin dependent men this is not the case. Heroin is the primary interest. Heroin is a depressant, and the abuser, hovering on the border of withdrawn sleep, is completely uninvolved, sexually or otherwise. For the heroin abuser there is only one reality. Somehow more of the drug must be gotten, and it costs money. This is his dilemma. He takes the drug to escape, but he cannot escape from the constant need for money. Often he steals or pimps or becomes a male prostitute.

The female abuser steals or prostitutes. But usually her sexual activity is totally passive. The male heroin abuser whose behavior happens to be homosexual tends to assume the female-passive role. In any case, whether homosexual or heterosexual behavior is preferred, it is only the sexual organs that are involved. The heroin abuser does not give more of himself than his organs. "His acme of joy . . . is the thud of heroin against his nervous system."[27] To the heroin abuser being "on the nod" is like the sense of peace following an orgasm.

With blunt clarity one addict explained that he always ended up "screwing myself." He did not fail to see the significance of his remark. "When we're out hustling for a ball [of heroin]," he went on, "we're like a high school boy trying to round up a broad. We get that bag, cook it, get that needle stuck in the vein, shoot that white stuff into us, then what a climax!"[28]

For the heroin dependent the excitement involved in the search for heroin substitutes for the excitement of sex. The drug destroys the desire for sexual expression. Often, however, the ability to perform sexually remains. On a "mild high" the heroin dependent male is able to have an erection, but because of his absence of sexual desire, his wife must initiate the act. Interestingly, the drug delays ejaculation. If the man had had the problem of premature ejaculation, the

[26] James L. Mathis, "Sexual Aspects of Heroin Addiction," *Medical Aspects of Human Sexuality,* Vol. 4, No. 9 (September 1970), p. 104.

[27] Ibid. A recent study revealed that heroin-dependent men frequently reported a marked reduction of sexual desire and potency, as well as ejaculation difficulties. This had not been the case before their dependency. Following withdrawal from heroin, however, the men experienced a rapid return to their predependent sexual enjoyment. Most methadone-maintained patients experienced a level of sexual desire and performance that was superior to that during their heroin-dependent state. Since luteinizing hormone (LH) plays an important role in sexual behavior, it was also measured. The levels of blood plasma LH were normal for all the men who were studied. (Paul Cushman, Jr., "Sexual Behavior in Heroin Addiction and Methadone Maintenance," *New York State Journal of Medicine,* Vol. 72, No. 11 [June 1, 1972], pp. 1261-65.)

[28] Ibid.

wife, who may hate her husband's heroin dependence, often becomes ambivalent. She may suffer because of his dependence, but she enjoys the drug's effect on him.

In working with heroin dependents it is important to treat both husband and wife. This is particularly true if both partners abuse heroin. One partner may consciously or unconsciously encourage the other's drug dependence. The wife may have a deep need for a totally dependent husband. As long as he abuses the drug he is also dependent on her. Also, the husband may subtly encourage his wife's abuse of heroin in order to gain complete control of her.

ALCOHOL AND SEXUALITY

Speaking of alcohol, Ogden Nash commented that "two pints make one cavort." Although his observation may be true, alcohol is not a stimulant but a depressant. Most people who drink moderately do not seem depressed. On the contrary, they are relaxed, even gay. Why is this so? Alcohol does indeed depress and anesthetize the nervous system, but it also releases inhibitions. Carried by the blood stream to the brain, it courses through the cerebral cortex where it numbs the nerve connections of learning. If a person has learned to control his sexual impulses, for example, alcohol loosens the controls. If they slip enough, he may cavort. So although a few drinks of alcohol do not directly stimulate sexual behavior, they may do so indirectly by depressing inhibitions and fears about sex.

In *Macbeth* the porter makes this accurate observation about alcohol: "it provokes and unprovokes. It provokes the desire, but it takes away the performance." [29] Too much alcohol causes temporary impotence in the male. The action of smooth muscle, the nervous system, and blood pressure are involved in erection, and excessive drinking depresses them. An alcohol-induced temporary impotence may become semipermanent or even permanent. Anxiety-ridden because of one failure the male begins to doubt his potency. This may interfere with his further success in having an erection. Indeed, he may begin to abuse alcohol to handle his anxiety about the beginnings of an alcohol-induced impotence. In this way a relatively minor problem becomes major. Failing to understand that alcohol is at the root of the problem, the man may blame and berate his wife, and the entire relationship suffers.

A small amount of alcohol may help to relieve the tensions that can precipitate premature ejaculation in the young and relatively inexperienced male who feels that he is on trial to perform sexually. But under no circumstances should the use of alcohol become routine lest it become a crutch and then a trap. Some individuals, moreover, find drinking by a sexual partner offensive. Others feel that they are

[29] William Shakespeare, *Macbeth*, II.iii.33–35.

being replaced by alcohol as a sexual stimulant. "Why does she have to have a couple of drinks before sex?" one young husband asks his physician. "Aren't I enough? Does she have to drink to forget it's me?" Marriages complicated by a drinking problem are at great risk. Divorce in such cases is four times as common as in other marriages.

An occasional drink before sexual intercourse is certainly not contraindicated. However, if this practice becomes a dependency a perilous pattern may develop, and it is by no means rare. Eventually drinking may become as important as, or even more important than, sexual intercourse. It is known that premature ejaculation and excessive drinking are the most common causes of the preponderant type of impotence. How much is too much alcohol? This varies with the individual. But for the average person not more than one drink once or twice a week is a good rule. Two or three martinis a day is unwise, both physically and psychologically. The daily intake of that much alcohol is a sexual anesthetic. And there is increasing evidence that two to four martinis a day can harm vital organs.

MARIJUANA AND SEXUALITY

adolescent delusion

What effect has marijuana on the adolescent, who is seeking personal and sexual identity? Consider again the dependent infancy of the child on the mother (see page 5). Not only does the baby depend on her for material needs, but also for emotional support. She can dry his tears, bring a smile to his face, play games that help him to learn. Above all, she can bring him comfort and security. This has been aptly called the "magical effect." Slowly, as his self-esteem grows, the child separates himself from his parents. Approaching adolescence he has learned to depend on himself more and more.

He . . . has to relinquish his dependence on his parents for emotional support and learn to base his self-esteem on his own achievements. These achievements not only involve success in the path towards his profession, but also social and sexual success. He has to learn to get along with other people on his own and to develop confidence in his adult sexual functioning.

Before the adolescent reaches maturity he has to deal with many disappointments, frustrations, feelings of helplessness and wishes to escape . . . Conflicts such as dependence versus independence, or masturbation versus heterosexual relationships, have to be resolved. The question now is how are these inevitable conflicts of adolescence going to be settled? Is the adolescent going to tackle them by asking himself after a disappointment, "What did I do wrong?" "How can I do it differently?" Is he

*going to be able to base his self-esteem on his own achievements?
Or is he going to fall back on external "magic" [such as mari-
juana] that can elevate his self-esteem at command just as the
traditional objects that he used when he was a toddler did?*[30]

But although the adult may use alcohol and tobacco as blankets
and teddy bears there is a difference. Usually the adult has already
largely established a realistic life style. The adolescent has yet to do
so.

marijuana and sexual behavior

Reports about the effect of marijuana on sexual behavior, like so
many other reports about the drug, are largely anecdotal. It should
be reemphasized that, as with any drug, different doses of marijuana
affect different people differently at different places and at different
times. The individual who strongly opposes drug abuse, for example,
may find that marijuana interferes with sexual desire and pleasure.
However if a man and a woman find one another attractive they may
find that marijuana stimulates their sexual desire. That would not
necessarily be true in the case of a man and woman who are indifferent to one another. For some people, the conspiratorial aspect
of using an illegal drug seems to enhance sexual expression.

Marijuana causes varying degrees of distortion of hearing, taste,
touch, and sight. All of these senses are involved, in a complex way,
with sexual expression. It is, therefore, understandable that the drug
might heighten sexual sensitivity. Since the sense of time is distorted,
and time seems to pass very slowly, the sexual act, including orgasm,
may appear prolonged. Like a small amount of alcohol, a small dose
of marijuana also reduces inhibitions. Under its influence, therefore,
sexual activity may occur with diminished inhibition.

Does marijuana itself stimulate the physical ability to engage in
sexual activity? There is no evidence of an increased physical effect
on sexuality.

*Neither our random samplings nor my psychiatric interviews
with marijuana users have led us to conclude that marijuana
use is a significant precipitant of sexual behavior . . . Indeed,
one of the features . . . is the relative loneliness of the marijuana
user. Certainly he is a member of a group . . . each of whom is
desperately seeking an audience to whom he can pour out his
tale of expanded consciousness and global insights.*[31]

---

[30] Klaus Angel, "No Marihuana for Adolescents," *The New York Times Magazine* (November 30, 1969), p. 173.
[31] John A. Ewing, "Students, Sex, and Marihuana," *Medical Aspects of Human Sexuality*, Vol. 6, No. 2 (February 1972), p. 113

LSD: DISTORTED SEXUAL EXPRESSION

Most scientists agree that LSD (lysergic acid diethylamide) is a chemical excitant that acts on the central nervous system causing distortion of the senses. It is, however, thousands of times more powerful than any known marijuana extract. Two pounds, if equally distributed, "would mentally dissociate every man, woman, and child in greater New York for an eight-hour period." [32]

LSD also distorts the sexual experience. Time may seem to pass extraordinarily slowly; consequently, an orgasm and the orgasmic peak may seem to be very prolonged. Nevertheless, it has been observed that LSD intoxication may have disastrous effects on the sexual life. Episodes of panic are not uncommon during the LSD experience. The introduction of intense terror into the area of human sexuality is fraught with psychic danger. Not only will it destroy any single sexual experience, but it may inhibit future sexual encounters as well.

One psychologist reported the case of a

mature man of undoubted virility [who] became impotent with his newly married wife following one horrendous LSD trip. Under the influence of the drug he hallucinated her as a shark and thereafter this image was repeated whenever he attempted intercourse with her. Needless to say the effect upon his marriage was disastrous. His sexual relationships with other women were unaffected.[33]

MDA

MDA (alpha-methyl-3-4-methylenedioxyphenethylamine) is an amphetamine-related psychedelic drug that apparently stimulates sexual drive. Some of its abusers report prolonged intercourse, multiple orgasms, and sexual fantasies. Apparently it can also result in an episode of impotence. A case is reported in which a young male embraced and attempted sexual intercourse with a tree. He interpreted it as being "mother earth."[34]

AMPHETAMINES AND SEXUALITY

Amphetamines ("speed") are also stimulants, although amphetamine abusers have different reasons for taking the drug than do LSD abusers. The amphetamine abuser has primarily a sexual reason for

[32] Sidney Cohen, *Drugs of Hallucination* (London, 1964), pp. 34–35.
[33] Charles Clay Dahlberg, "Sexual Behavior in the Drug Culture," p. 70.
[34] George R. Gay and Charles W. Sheppard, "Sex in the Drug Culture," *Medical Aspects of Human Sexuality*, Vol. 6, No. 10 (October 1972), p. 44.

his drug abuse. The LSD abuser's reason is not basically sexual; he takes the drug for complex reasons, including self-psychoanalytic, pseudoreligious, and creative aspirations. However, the "speed freak" injects amphetamines into his veins in order to experience a "flash" or "rush." This he describes as a "full body orgasm." The acute anxiety, the hallucinations, the paranoia, and the severe depression associated with amphetamine abuse are all secondary experiences.

With large doses, the male amphetamine abuser can maintain an erection for hours and may thus engage in prolonged nonejaculatory sexual intercourse. Long-term abuse of amphetamines, however, destroys the male's sex drive as well as his ability to have an erection.[35] When use of the drug is discontinued this ability is regained. The effects on the sexuality of the female of the continuous use of large doses of amphetamines needs further investigation. There is some reason to believe that both menstrual disorders and inadequate sexual responses may result.

The "speed freak" usually injects massive doses of amphetamines into his veins. Do ordinary oral doses (similar to those used for the treatment of overweight persons) stimulate the average individual's sexual desire? For the shy or mildly depressed individual, small doses of amphetamines may provide a lift. This drug-induced confidence may make it easier to perform sexually. In this case, it may be the user's expectation that the drug will improve performance rather than the drug's actual action that is responsible for the result. Moderately larger doses have been known to enhance orgasmic feeling.

COCAINE

Injected intravenously or sniffed ("snorted"), this stimulant produces sexual effects that are similar to those caused by the amphetamines. Because of its rapid elimination from the body, a single intravenous dose has but a brief sexually stimulating effect. Street names for cocaine are "coke" and "girl." Intravenous injection causes intense excitement and, in many cases, spontaneous erection of the penis. Occasionally, the erection persists for a day or more. (Prolonged penile erection is called *priapism;* it also occurs with spinal cord tumors, injuries to the penis, and urinary bladder stones.) As is the case with the abuse of amphetamines, chronic cocaine abuse can lead to exhaustion, hallucination, delerium, and paranoia. Since cocaine is an anesthetic, some drug abusers also rub it on the head of the penis. This provides prolonged erection without orgasm—a desired sexual "ego trip" for these individuals. Occasionally, a woman who abuses cocaine, or whose male sexual partner has done so, must be

[35] A common complaint is this: "He used to shoot speed and then make love to me; now he only shoots speed." (Jared R. Tinklenberg, "Do Amphetamines Affect Sexual Function?" *Sexual Behavior,* Vol. 1, No. 5 [August 1971], p. 11.)

treated for spasm and a painfully raw and inflamed vaginal mucuous lining. (A similar condition is seen resulting from coitus under the influence of amphetamines. The amphetamines have a drying effect on the vaginal secretions; this plus the unusually prolonged coitus produces the symptoms.) Also reported among chronic cocaine sniffers is an inflammation of the nasal septum. Complicating this may be a perforation of this septum with eventual facial disfigurement caused by the depression of the bridge of the nose.

AMYL NITRITE

Amyl nitrite is a clear yellowish liquid, volatile at low temperatures, and used by physicians for inhalation as a vapor to relieve the pain of certain kinds of heart disease. When an artery to the heart is partially blocked, the involved heart muscle is deprived of blood and, therefore, of oxygen. Amyl nitrite relaxes the constricted artery, allowing oxygen-carrying blood to reach the heart muscle and thus relieve the pain.

Some "swinger" types of individuals inhale amyl nitrite vapors ("poppers" or "snappers") at insertion or just before orgasm. It is stated that this enhances sensation. This may be true. The smooth muscle fibers of the genital and urinary tracts are relaxed, and the blood supply to the area is increased. Orgasm may thus be heightened. But also heightened are the possibilities of dizziness, headache, low blood pressure, and fainting. Internal eye pressure may also be temporarily increased. For some people this may be hazardous. Nitrites may be associated with a rare blood disease, but reports of sudden death from this cause are infrequent. The drug's effect on the central nervous system is responsible for the combined "head and body trip" that is often described. Previously, amyl nitrite was most frequently abused by those whose orientation was homosexual. Its abuse is now reported in group sex situations.

IN SUMMARY

George R. Gay and Charles W. Sheppard have summarized the effects on sexual behavior of a variety of drugs.[36] It should be emphasized that their study included fifty patients at the San Francisco Haight-Ashbury Free Medical Clinic (twenty-five males and twenty-five females whose mean age was twenty-four). As confirmed members of the drug culture, the reactions of these patients may not be applicable to the general population. For example, some individuals who are inclined to abuse drugs may be inclined to certain kinds of sexual behavior. Thus, the relationships between the drug, as a specific cause, and the behavior, as the result, may be equivocal.

[36] George R. Gay and Charles W. Sheppard, "Sex in the Drug Culture," p. 47.

Moreover, it is of interest to note that most of the young people they studied almost invariably returned to sexual activity without drugs. For them, the use of drugs for sexual purposes was not of lasting importance.

Examples of drugs that *indirectly* stimulate sexual activity by releasing inhibitions are relatively small doses of alcohol and barbiturates. Those that *directly* stimulate sexual activity include the amphetamines and cocaine. Marijuana may fit into both groups. Difficult to categorize are the psychedelic drugs, particularly MDA.

Drugs that decrease sexual activity may do so either by diminishing desire or (with the male) by decreasing potency. Heroin and high doses of either barbiturates or alcohol are examples. Sometimes, however, a heroin-dependent male will experience a very temporary erection as he injects the drug. This may be due to sexual symbolism. The needle entering the vein symbolizes the penis entering a body orifice, or the pushing and withdrawal of the syringe's plunger may be symbolic of either sexual intercourse or masturbation. Withdrawal from heroin usually results in rapid reactivation of the dependent's former sexual expression. Jailed or hospitalized heroin-dependents often masturbate repeatedly.

By diminishing coordination and concentration, LSD may interfere with consummation of sexual intercourse.

OTHER SEXUAL STIMULANTS:
MUCH NONSENSE, LITTLE SENSE

Aphrodisiac refers to any and all agents (as a drug or food) used to excite sexual desire. The word is derived from the Greek *aphrodisia,* sexual pleasure (Aphrodite is the Greek goddess of love). Even the lowly potato was imagined to contain aphrodisiac powers when it was introduced into England. Like the oyster and the onion, also thought to contain compounds that stimulated sexual desire, the potato reminded people of a testicle.

The mandrake plant seems to have the longest history as an aphrodisiac. Again, the shape of this relative of the potato fired the imagination of the hopeful. Its stubby root divides into two parts so that it looks like a human trunk with two legs. The Elizabethan clergyman-poet John Donne (1573-1631) wrote:

> *Go and catch a falling star,*
> *Get with child a mandrake root,*
> *Tell me where all past years are,*
> *Or who cleft the Devil's foot.*[37]

[37] John Donne, "Song," lines 1-4.

It was understandable that the churchman Donne would think the mandrake plant an effective pregnancy promoter. The source of his belief was no less than the Bible. In Genesis one of mankind's earliest stories of human jealousy tells how mandrake was used by Leah to win back the love of Jacob (Genesis 30:14–16).

As the world's population increased so did its list of love potions. During the Middle Ages black dust from a tomb, scraps of human liver and donkey's lung, menstrual blood or blood from a blind baby, viper soup, and dried peacock bones moistened in mud were but a few of the fake philters. Elizabethan plays are full of reverent reference to love potions. In Shakespeare's *Merry Wives of Windsor*, the Host of the Garter Inn says to the French doctor Caius: "Shall I lose my doctor? no; he gives me the potions and the motions." [38] But the Roman philosopher Seneca knew the best aphrodisiac: in one of his *Epistles* he wrote: "I shall show you a philtre, without medicaments, without herbs, without a witch's incantations. It is this: If you want to be loved, love." [39] This advice has yet to be improved upon.

Any effectiveness of the philters of olden times was doubtless psychological. Successful sexual performance demands confidence in one's ability. The mere belief in potions could have produced a temporary beneficial result. One ancient compound (used by the Romans as well as by the mistress of Louis XV of France, Madame de Pompadour) is today popularly known as "Spanish Fly." This perilously irritating powder is neither from Spain nor made from flies. It is composed of the dried and powdered carcass of a beetle called the blister bug found in southern Europe, western Siberia, and parts of Africa. Applied to the skin the powder causes blistering. Taken internally in small doses it irritates both the urinary and gastrointestinal tracts. It has no direct effect on the genitalia. In large doses it can be fatal. Its irritating action on the urethra combined with blood vessel dilation may indeed cause penile erection. However, the erection is accompanied by too much pain to admit of any thoughts of sexual pleasure.

Yohimbine is yet another drug that is thought to be an aphrodisiac. Obtained from the bark of the West African yohimbine tree, its action depends on nerve center stimulation of the spinal cord. Its indiscriminate use is fraught with peril (it is a poisonous alkaloid), and its effectiveness remains unproved.

This pharmaceutical age has seen the production of a variety of drugs that seem to affect sexual sensitivity. Of these d-amphetamine (Dexedrine) and methylepinephrine (Methedrine) are among the most abused. Whether the sexual response is the result of a specific drug effect or is incidental to the diffuse cerebral stimulation is

[38] William Shakespeare, *The Merry Wives of Windsor*, III.i.104–05.
[39] In Harry A. Wedeck, *Love Potions Through the Ages* (New York, 1963), p. 302.

unknown. Ritalin and Preludin, more abused in Europe than in this country, may excite sexual desire; they may also cause intoxications that include psychoses. L-Dopa (L-dihydroxyphenylalanine) and PCPA (p-chlorphenylalanine) may also occasionally act as aphrodisiacs with some people. L-Dopa is used in the treatment of Parkinson's disease; because of serious side effects its dosage must be scrupulously controlled.[40] Moreover, that it is a chemical aphrodisiac is certainly open to question; more likely, the relief that L-Dopa provides from the depression and disability of Parkinson's disease makes sexual expression easier and more enjoyable. Cyclazocine, a drug being studied as a substitute for methadone in the maintenance treatment of heroin dependents, also has been reported to have aphrodisiac properties.

SEXUAL DEPRESSANTS

A safe and effective method of depressing sexual interest has yet to be found. This may be because research for anaphrodisiacs has been somewhat limited. A compound with an undeserved reputation as an anaphrodisiac is saltpeter (potassium nitrate). It does increase the secretion of urine and thus is a fairly effective diuretic, but as an anaphrodisiac saltpeter is utterly useless.

Ismelin (guanethidine sulphate) appears to affect male sexual potency. The drug has been used in the treatment of high blood pressure. However, in a high percentage of patients it produces a variety of disagreeable side effects that greatly limit its use. The prolonged use of a variety of tranquilizers has been reported to diminish sexual desire.

sexual vagabondage in some communes

In recent years two to three thousand communes have been established in the United States. A great number of these are sincere and honest attempts to find a richer meaning to life. Some early observations suggest that they may offer this to a considerable number of people who refuse to accept the emotional clutter of their lives and the utter confusion of cities. The communes vary from highly religious groups such as the Amish and Mennonites, whose sense of cohesion is very strong, to groups in which religious beliefs are either superficial or absent and whose membership is basically transient. There are many communes in which a sincere interest in spiritual development is an important aspect of daily living. Only time will

[40] Thomas G. Benedek, "Aphrodisiacs: Fact and Fable," *Medical Aspects of Human Sexuality,* Vol. 5, No. 12 (December 1971), pp. 62-63.

tell what the future of the groups that persist will be, and the eventual forms that they will take.

One serious shortcoming of some communes is the flagrant degradation of the woman. In these communes the young woman is relieved of society's sexual restrictions. But has she, at last, achieved freedom and equality? Noninvolved uncommitted sex has resulted in a girl with whom nobody is involved and to whom nobody is committed. She offers not a complex feminine personality but simply a convenient set of female sexual organs.

NOBODY GETS HURT?

This uncommitted life style has been described somewhat sanctimoniously by the statement, Nobody gets hurt. This is a cruel, even a hostile, appraisal. For in the response of the male to the female, in the context of this essentially alienated life style, she is indeed nobody.

> *Observers of life in communal pads have noticed certain patterns of male–female relatedness . . . A startling finding is that if one asks how many live in the pad the answer—be it 10, 15, or 20—will not include the women . . . there is no doubt that girls are considered as auxiliaries and not full members. This is true even though the men float in and out and are even less permanent residents than are the women. It is also noted that the women are, as a rule, sicker psychiatrically than the men. Their passivity is marked and the role they play is either as mothering the men or alternately as extremely babyish and dependent.*[41]

The nonperson status of the woman in these particular communes is singularly sad. For even with the first cry the newborn lets this be known: "I mean to be counted!"

A recent study of one group marriage commune is of particular interest. [42] Fourteen women and six men made up the membership; they ranged in age from approximately sixteen to thirty-five years. They worked on a ranch in return for condemned living quarters. Most of their food was garbage from the bins of grocery stores in a nearby town. The sexual practices among the members of the group were polygamous, that is, all members were expected to engage freely in sexual intercourse with one another. The members of the group considered conventional marriage psychologically destructive. Sexual relationships outside the group were forbidden. Another feature of

---

[41] Charles Clay Dahlberg, "Sexual Behavior in the Drug Culture," p. 70.
[42] David E. Smith and Alan J. Rose, "The Group Marriage Commune: A Case Study," *Journal of Psychedelic Drugs,* Vol. 3, No. 1 (September 1970), pp. 113-19.

the group was cooperative child-rearing. Moreover, birth certificates, immunizations, and prenatal and postnatal care were generally rejected by the group.

A thirty-five-year-old man called "Charlie" was the absolute ruler of the commune. Although he had a past history of criminal activity, at the time of the study Charlie had not been arrested or convicted for violent crimes, and "during the study expressed a philosophy of non-violence."[43] On occasion Charlie would refer to himself as "God" or "God and the Devil." In all matters, sexual or otherwise, his decision was final. He initiated all new female members into the group. If they refused mutual oral-genital contact, Charlie expelled them. In his opinion the woman's acceptance of mutual oral-genital stimulation indicated that she would be able to drop her sexual inhibitions. Stories of Charlie's sexual prowess helped him to maintain his position of leadership. They were related to all new members. One of these (never validated) was as follows:

> *Charlie would get up in the morning, make love, eat breakfast, make love, and go back to sleep. He would wake up later and make love, have lunch, make love, and go back to sleep. Waking up later, he would make love, eat dinner, make love, and go back to sleep—only to wake up in the middle of the night wanting intercourse again.*[44]

The major role of the women of the commune was to gratify the males. All the women wanted to bear Charlie's child. However, identification of the father of any child born to a female in the group could not be accurately made. Charlie believed that the child, untainted by society, was to be emulated by the adults. To prove his point, Charlie quoted Jesus: "He who is like a small child shall reap the rewards of heaven."

The authors of this study ask an as yet unanswered question: "Why . . . were these young girls so attracted and captivated by a disturbed mystic such as Charlie? What is happening within the framework of the dominant culture and its monogamous, nuclear family units, that so many youths must feel compelled not simply to rebel but to totally reject traditional living styles?"[45] This is indeed a question worth pondering. "There are no 'thems,' there is only us," these writers continued. "We cannot understand the group marriage commune and its societal implications unless we first understand ourselves and the more traditional ways in which the dominant

[43] Ibid, p. 116.
[44] Ibid. If this description is indeed accurate, Charlie may be an example of *satyriasis*—a condition in which there is an uncontrollable desire by a male for sexual intercourse. In the female this is known as *nymphomania*. Since people vary greatly in their sexual needs, both of these terms should be used with extreme caution. For example, men who are ignorant of the facts, or insecure, or both, have been known to label women who enjoy multiple orgasms as "nymphomaniacs."
[45] Ibid., p. 118.

culture has treated marriage and child-rearing."[46] Although the commune discussed above is not presented as typical of the majority of such groups, its members did exhibit symptoms of deep alienation.

Not long after the study of them was completed, Charlie Manson and some members of his family were convicted of a series of brutal murders.

women's lib for the sexes

Women are not all in the wrong when they reject the rules of life that have been introduced into the world, inasmuch as it is the men who have made them without consulting them.[47]

Recently several members of the Department of Psychiatry at the New York University School of Medicine reported their common experience that "(1) young men now appear more frequently with impotence, and (2) young women more frequently complain of initial impotence in their young lovers." They "suggest that this may be related to changed social attitudes towards premarital sexuality, particularly among women." Presenting several case studies, they found that "when we explored these sexual failures occurring early in a relationship, we found a common male complaint: These newly freed women demanded sexual performance. The male concern in the 1940's and 1950's was to satisfy the woman. In the late 1960's and early 1970's, it seems to be 'Will I have to maintain an erection to maintain a relationship.'" Although for some the new "sexual freedom may indeed be liberating, for others it merely induces different symptoms rather than improved mental health."[48] Still another psychiatrist has remarked that "the denial of differences between the sexes is one factor, an important one, in the prevalence of disappointment with sex and of actual sexual pathology."[49] Although there is considerable disagreement with these opinions, they do demand serious consideration.

Such observations must be viewed in the light of the past. When, for example, on June 17, 1815, Henry Cook of Effingham, Surrey, sold his wife to John Earl in the Croydon market for one shilling and received a receipt for her, he was aware of English law but not of woman's identity.[50] Some forty years later Ralph Waldo Emerson wrote of the English that "the right of the husband to sell the wife

---

[46] Ibid, citing J. L. Simmons, *Deviants* (New York, 1969).
[47] Michel de Montaigne, *Essays*, III, p. 62.
[48] George L. Ginsberg, William A. Frosch, and Theodore Shapiro, "The New Impotence," *Archives of General Psychiatry*, Vol. 26, No. 3 (March 1972), pp. 218-20.
[49] John L. Schimel, "The Fallacy of Equality in Sexual Relations," *Medical Aspects of Human Sexuality*, Vol. 3, No. 8 (August 1969), p. 24.
[50] Viola Klein, *The Feminine Character, History of an Ideology* (New York, 1948), pp. 7, 8.

has been retained down to our times."[51] In 1883, Sigmund Freud wrote to his fiancée: "My sweet princess: I dare say we agree that housekeeping and the care and education of children claim the whole person and practically rule out any profession . . . It seems a completely unrealistic notion to send women into the struggle for existence . . . Am I to think of my delicate, sweet girl as a competitor?"[52] He was deeply in love when he wrote these words. To sell his wife in a marketplace was unthinkable; to keep her in the home was quite natural.

It is almost ninety years since Freud wrote that letter. During that time millions of women have left their homes at least part of the time. Today women make up 37 percent of the labor force; one-half of all women between eighteen and sixty-four years of age are in that labor force; studies show that nine out of ten women work outside the home at some time in their lives. They do not work only because they want "pin money." Almost one-half of the 31 million working women in March 1970 were working because of pressing economic need. Their absentee rate from work due to illness and injury varies little from that of men. Can a woman do a man's work? With extremely rare exceptions, jobs today are sexless. In most occupations brain power has replaced muscle power. Women were found in all the 479 occupations listed in the 1960 census.[53] Despite all this, most women are assiduously excluded from the more attractive and responsible occupations. For example, only 2 percent are full professors in the nation's major universities; the annual doctorate production of women from those same universities is 12 percent.[54] And it was not until after sixty-five years of publication that, in 1972, the title of the prestigious biographical book *American Men of Science* was changed to *American Men and Women of Science*.

Such economic inequality has helped intensify the contemporary Women's Liberation movement. But the contemporary woman wants more than equal economic opportunity. She wants to achieve a sense of identity, to be an individual. This she cannot do without a redefinition of the term *femininity*. "Much of what is called femininity is actually a trait characteristic of the dependent personality; to the extent that the dependent person becomes neurotic, it causes much of the difficulty suffered by women in our culture."[55] It is this excessive dependency, expected during childhood but harmful during adulthood, from which the woman now seeks to be liberated. For to be so dependent breeds fears of loneliness, repressed hostility, and

---

[51] Ralph Waldo Emerson, "English Traits."

[52] In Ernst L. Freud, *Letters of Sigmund Freud* (New York, 1960), pp. 75-76.

[53] "The Myth and the Reality," U.S. Department of Labor, Employment Standards Administration, Women's Bureau (April 1971), pp. 1-3.

[54] Philip H. Abelson, "Women in Academia," *Science,* Vol. 175, No. 4018 (January 14, 1972), p. 127.

[55] Alexandra Symonds, "The Psychology of the Female Liberation Movement," *Medical Aspects of Human Sexuality,* Vol. 5, No. 4 (April 1971), p. 29.

many other emotional problems that are deleterious to sexual and other fulfillments.[56]

As the woman divests herself of her dependencies, the traditional definition of her femininity will change. She will remain feminine, but it will be a new kind of feminine personality. Why will this change bring problems? "Culture is the gatekeeper of sexual destiny," anthropologist Marvin Harris has written. "Subordination of females happens to occur with remarkable persistence in a great variety of cultures. When a human relationship occurs with great frequency across space and time, we must suppose that there are determinate reasons for it. Culture itself is a form of 'testing'."[57] A major change in the personality of the woman (and indeed in the culture) cannot help but precipitate new anxieties in both sexes. To weather the storm of so immense a social change will require considerable individual ego strength. Those whose sense of identity is strong will develop a better appreciation of the opposite sex. Inevitably, there will be some casualties such as those described above by the psychiatrists at the New York University School of Medicine. Moreover, every vital movement has its element of impatient rage demanding abrupt and revolutionary change. This even serves a purpose by bringing the movement to greater public attention. Nevertheless, the widely publicized and often extreme views of the Women's Liberation movement, such as living without men and dispensing with marriage and the family, are heard the most. In the minds of many, they have become a false stereotype of the movement. For a number of men this stereotype is an aggressive sexual threat. When this threat is added to other stresses it can foster impotence.[58]

The contemporary Women's Liberation movement need not result in a sexual impasse; the fulfillment of its goals need not make a battlefield of the marital bed. In today's world, a better sense of identity for one sex can bring a better sense of identity for the other. The woman is uniquely situated in guiding the early development of both sexes. In the adult world, each sex will have to work at

[56] Paul C. Weinberg, in "Has Women's Liberation Become a Cause of Marital and Sexual Strife," *Medical Aspects of Human Sexuality,* Vol. 5, No. 9 (September 1971), p. 12.

[57] Marvin Harris, "Women's Fib, The Human Strategy," *Natural History,* Vol. 81, No. 5 (May 1972), p. 20.

[58] Duane Hagen, in "Has Women's Liberation Become a Cause of Marital and Sexual Strife," p. 17.

The concept that there can be no women's liberation without men's liberation has a firm foothold in Sweden. Emphasizing that men who take on the entire burden of supporting the family are deprived of adequate emotional contact with their children, a 1968 Swedish report to the United Nations propounded the idea of men's emancipation. This attitude has reached into the Swedish educational system, where "boys have been taught such traditionally feminine role-dividing subjects as home economics, sewing, and child care. Girls learn modern manual handicraft and other once exclusively masculine skills." This and other social changes, it is held, have resulted in a togetherness in which, however, "each partner has his or her identity, and there is no need to place blame on one partner, as there tends to be in a superior-inferior relationship." (Birgitta Linnér, "What Does Equality Between the Sexes Imply?" *American Journal of Orthopsychiatry,* Vol. 41, No. 5 [October 1971], pp. 750-51.)

helping the other build a stronger sense of self-worth. This will require tolerance and patience. At its best, the Women's Liberation movement will also help to liberate men.

the fragile monogamous family

"Happy families are all alike; every unhappy family is unhappy in its own way," wrote Tolstoy at the beginning of his novel *Anna Karenina* more than seventy years ago.[59] It is a story of the destruction of a woman who loses her family because of her passion for a man other than her husband. In the eighteenth century William Blackstone, one of England's greatest jurists, set down the typical rule: "The husband and wife are one and that one is the husband."[60] Despite the publication (in 1792) of Mary Wollstonecraft's *Vindication of the Rights of Woman,* the rule held like iron. Indeed, there must have been many an "I told you so" uttered over English teacups when Mary Wollstonecraft's seventeen-year-old daughter ran off with the already married poet Percy Bysshe Shelley. In later years Queen Victoria could see nothing in the liberation of women but the ruination of the family. "The Queen is most anxious," she proclaimed in 1870, "to enlist everyone who can speak or write to join in checking this mad, wicked folly of Woman's Rights with all its attending horrors."[61] Today the family is in transition. But the family is not changing because of woman's persistent quest for equality and identity. During the founding years of this nation, the family was monogamous and tightly knit. Nevertheless, this hardly prevented Abigail Adams from writing a pointed letter to her politician husband John (approximately two years before he signed the Declaration of Independence) that read in part: "Do not put such unlimited power into the hands of husbands. Remember, all men would be tyrants if they could. If particular care and attention are not paid to the ladies, we are determined to foment a rebellion, and will not hold ourselves bound to obey any laws in which we have no voice nor representation."[62] Sentiments such as these did not weaken the family. Both the contemporary Women's Liberation movement and the

[59] Leo Tolstoy, *Anna Karenina* (New York, 1936), p. 3.
[60] Charles D. Aring, "Man Versus Woman," *Annals of Internal Medicine,* Vol. 73, No. 6 (December 1970), pp. 1028–29.
[61] Ibid., p. 1029. It is possible that Victoria carried the concept of the permanent family to extremes. After her beloved husband Albert died "every bed in which she slept had to be doubled, and above 'his' empty pillow had to be hung a framed photograph of his corpse, surrounded by immortelles [flowers that retain their form and color after having been dried]. Year after year, his night clothes were neatly laid out at the bedside, and the wash basin had water ready for his ghostly hands." (Lawrence Wright, *Warm and Snug* [London, 1962], p. 228.) On his deathbed, the great prime minister Benjamin Disraeli was told that Queen Victoria would like to visit him. "'What's the use?' he said. 'She would only want me to take a message to dear Albert.'" (W. H. Auden, *A Certain World* [New York, 1970], p. 404.)
[62] Donald Day, *The Evolution of Love,* p. 379.

changing family are the result of many changes in society, some of which reach back many years: the industrial, technological, and biological revolutions; wars; the typewriter; and the increased mobility provided first by the bicycle and then by the automobile. These changes had an impact on many aspects of life; one aspect that was greatly affected was the role of the father.

THE DIMINISHED FATHER

Perhaps the most famous diminished father in all of literature is Shakespeare's King Lear. Chiding his master, Lear's faithful Fool first speaks and then sings:

> *Ever since thou madest thy daughters thy mother. For when*
> *thou gavest them the rod and puttest down thine own breeches,*
> *Then they for sudden joy did weep,*
> *And I for sorrow sung,*
> *That such a king should play bopeep,*
> *And go the fools among.*[63]

It may be that the complex king was an exception during his time. But the notion of a diminished father persisted. Almost a century ago, Oscar Wilde prophetically wrote in his *An Ideal Husband:* "Fathers should be neither seen nor heard. That is the only proper basis for family living." Today, the father's position as the authoritarian head of the family is a thing of the past. According to sociologist E. E. Le Masters three events between 1900 and 1950 caused the transformation of the once powerful head of the family into "a family court jester."[64] First was the Great Depression of the 1930s, which took from him the role of principal breadwinner. Next came the Second World War, which wrenched him from the home and left the management of the family entirely to the mother. And the third was the successive crops of numerous and powerful adolescents and peer groups who challenged the father's values and authority. If, in more recent years, the media did not actually contribute to the diminution of the role of the father, with few exceptions they certainly reflected it. Dagwood Bumstead was the family fool of the 1940s, and growing children of the 1950s were taught to magnanimously "Make Room for Daddy." Today, the most visible father of the entertainment world is the ignorant bigot Archie Bunker. True, his wife is not much better than he, but it is she who seems to have the limited wisdom of the two.

If any kind of family is to endure, the father will have to be

---

[63] William Shakespeare, *King Lear,* I.iv.188-95.
[64] E. E. Le Masters, "The Passing of the Dominant Husband-Father," *Impact of Science on Society,* Vol. 21, No. 1 (January–March 1971), pp. 21-30.

reinstated in the family constellation, not as its tyrannical head but as a meaningful partner. His willingness to share will be no less important than the help he receives from the rest of the family and from society in general. Many young people are seeking ways of accomplishing this by means of sharing household chores and other responsibilities and in a new kind of mutuality.

THE MALE FEAR OF WOMAN

For the father to regain a significant role in the family, both sexes will have to find a new and better balance in their relationship. This, in turn, can only occur when they recognize and deal with man's fear of woman. This fear is hardly new, nor is it an isolated phenomenon. The notion of the castrating woman is as deeply rooted in this culture as are the tales of vaginal teeth in India.[65] Before praying, Moslems were instructed as follows: "if any of you cometh from the privy, or if you have touched woman, and ye find no water, take fine clean sand and rub your faces and your hands therewith." [66] And Paul's instruction to Timothy was that "Adam was not deceived, but the woman being deceived was in transgression" (I Timothy 2:14). "Nature," remarked Samuel Johnson, "has given women so much power that the law has wisely given them little." [67] It is neither wisdom nor logic that gives one-half of humanity the "right" to give or to take power from the other half. It is fear. Modern knowledge has led to a different vision of woman and her role in the family (see pages 351–54). As Judd Marmor has pointed out, Sigmund Freud's patriarchal notions about women are invalid (see page 352).[68] The idea that "anatomy is destiny" has been expanded to include and emphasize the pervasive influence of culture; "penis envy" (like "womb envy") is now understood to depend largely on environmental cues (see pages 82–84). In coitus, the male penetrator is now known to be quite capable of being passive, while the female receptor may be aggressive (there is a difference between behavior and motivation). And few still cling to the antiquated notion of a faulty female super-ego.[69]

[65] Wolfgang Lederer, *The Fear of Women* (New York, 1968), p. 45.
[66] B. Z. Goldberg, *The Sacred Fire* (New York, 1930), p. 214.
[67] Charles D. Aring, "Man Versus Woman," p. 1026.
[68] Judd Marmor, "Changing Patterns of Femininity," in Arlene S. Skolnick and Jerome H. Skolnick, eds., *Family in Transition* (Boston, 1971), pp. 210–21, and in S. Rosenbaum and S. Alger, eds., *The Marriage Relationship: Psychoanalytic Perspectives* (New York, 1968), pp. 31–44.
[69] The *superego* is Freud's term for that part of the psyche that acts to secure conformity of the ego to parental, social, and moral standards. It may be conscious or subconscious.

It has long been known that giving animals the male hormone testosterone increases their aggressiveness, resulting in a higher level of social dominance. Interestingly, recent research indicates that dosing male rats with the female hormone estrogen dramatically reduces both their aggressiveness and social dominance. Estrogen does "seem to have the opposite effect from testosterone on social dominance behavior patterns . . . The results seem to imply a direct effect on brain function." ("Do Hormones Make Females Submissive?" *New Scientist*, Vol. 55, No. 812 [September 21, 1972], p. 472.) It is well to remember that the application to human beings of results of animal experiments can be fallacious in some cases.

MARITAL EXPERIMENTS

As the sexes find their equilibrium in this rapidly changing society, the family will become more stable, but it may be a new kind of family. As it develops there will be, as there always have been, experiments. Some people will attempt the polygamy of the ancient Hebrews. There will be community group marriage with sexual sharing, as occurred in the Oneida community of religious zealots a century ago. There will be married couples who "swing," seeking only genital exchanges with other couples, as did ancients before them. As always, too, there will be couples who will try to raise a family without marriage; and as always there will be those who will try hard to get them married. One day a couple who horrified colonial New London, Connecticut, was met on the street by the town's outraged magistrate.

> *"John Rogers," the magistrate asked, "do you persist in calling this woman your wife?"*
>
> *"Yes, I do."*
>
> *"And do you, Mary, wish such an old man to be your husband?"*
>
> *"Indeed I do," was the reply.*
>
> *"Then, by the laws of God and this commonwealth," said the magistrate, "I pronounce you man and wife."* [70]

WHAT ARE MOST PEOPLE CHOOSING?

Of interest are the results of a recent investigation comparing eighteen unmarried couples living together and thirty-one couples who were going steady but not cohabiting. Three psychologists compared these couples from the viewpoint of a variety of factors considered important in a close, long-term relationship. These included childhood happiness, trust and respect, mutual need, involvement and happiness in the relationship, willingness to share personal feelings, commitment to marriage, and sexual satisfaction. To a striking degree, those couples living together out of wedlock failed to reciprocate those feelings considered significant to a good relationship between couples whose sexual orientation is heterosexual. Trust, happiness, and involvement were high in both groups. In addition, the men of both groups considered sexual relationships subordinate to mutual need and respect, trust, and involvement. However, the findings indicated that the couples who did not live together were more committed to marriage. Also, "men involved in living-together situations displayed a much lower degree of respect and need for their partners than males pursuing a conventional courtship . . . The woman who takes up

[70] Donald Day, *The Evolution of Love*, pp. 373-74.

housekeeping without a wedding ring is not likely to grab one on some marry-go-round of the future. More probably, she will be taken for a ride in the circular pattern more than familiar to common law wives." [71]

Despite apparent societal changes, the family based on monogamous marriage stubbornly prevails in this country. It has been repeatedly said that it is losing its popularity among the young, but in 1970 both the number and rate of marriages in the United States had increased for the twelfth consecutive year. In addition, approximately three-quarters of all marriages occurred in the eighteen- to twenty-four-year age group. [72] However, in 1970 the rate of divorce had also increased from approximately one in four marriages in 1960 to approximately one in three, although it did not reach the peak rate recorded after the Second World War between 1945 and 1947. [73] Despite the divorces, marriages in this country are far more prevalent today than they were at the turn of the century. In 1900 only 52.8 percent of men over fourteen years of age were married; in 1970 76 percent of men over eighteen years were married. In 1900 only 55 percent of women were married; in 1970 some 68 percent were married. [74] (The reason that the 1970 percentage for married women was lower than that for men is due to the greater number of women than men in this country.)

Today, then, the vast majority of people are still seeking the unique closeness that comes with monogamous marriage. Clearly, however, an increasing number are failing to find it on their first try. The result is a growing acceptance of serial marriage, that is, marriage, divorce, and remarriage. The futility of the hopeless marriage has long been recognized in this country. Although seventeenth-century Puritan moralists were scandalized by divorce, "they placed equal stress on the hypocrisy and misery of the many marriages that endured. One Puritan wrote: 'Yf it bee so, that they remayne styll together, what frowning . . . scolding, and chiding, is there between them, so that the whole house is filled up of those tragedies . . . unto the toppe.'" [75]

Anthropologist Margaret Mead has suggested two kinds of marriage, one a prerequisite for the other: the "student marriage" or "individual marriage," which would be licensed, require birth control,

[71] "Bed and Bored," *Human Behavior*, Vol. 1, No. 5 (September–October 1972), pp. 39–40, citing Judith L. Syness, Milton E. Lipetz, and Keith E. Davis, "Living Together: An Alternative to Marriage," *Journal of Marriage and the Family*, Vol. 34, No. 2 (May 1972), pp. 305–11.

[72] *Monthly Vital Statistics Report, Provisional Statistics, Annual Summary for the United States, 1970*, U.S. Department of Health, Education, and Welfare, Public Health Service, Health Services and Mental Health Administration, Vol. 19, No. 13 (September 21, 1971), pp. 8, 9.

[73] *Monthly Vital Statistics Report, Final Statistics*, Center for Health Statistics, U.S. Department of Health, Education, and Welfare, Public Health Service, Health Services and Mental Health Administration, Vol. 19, No. 19, Supplement (2), (January 26, 1971), p. 1.

[74] *U.S. Bureau of the Census, Statistical Abstract of the United States: 1971* (92nd edition), p. 33.

[75] In Ivy Pinchbeck and Margaret Hewitt, *Children in English Society*, Vol. I, *From Tudor Times to the Eighteenth Century* (London, 1969), p. 54.

and be dissoluble at will; and the "parental marriage." [76] Many people will doubtless disagree with this suggestion, but few will find fault with something she wrote a quarter of a century ago: "We can build a whole society only by using both the gifts special to each sex and those shared by both sexes—by using the gifts of the whole of humanity." [77]

[76] Ralph Hamil, "The Family in Search of a Future: Alternate Models for Moderns," *The Futurist,* Vol. 5, No. 4 (August 1971), p. 167.

[77] Margaret Mead, "Male and Female," in John Mason Brown and the editors of the *Ladies' Home Journal,* eds., *The Ladies' Home Journal Treasury* (New York, 1956), p. 345.

glossary

A

abortion—The premature expulsion (elimination) from the uterus of a fertilized ovum (egg), embryo, or nonviable fetus.

abstinence—The refraining from sexual intercourse or of the intake of food or drugs.

acid—Sour; sharp and biting to the taste. A compound that can react with a base to form a salt.

adolescence—The time of life beginning with puberty (when secondary sex characteristics appear) and ending with adulthood (when major body growth stops); generally culturally determined.

ADP (adenosine diphosphate)—A product of the breakdown of ATP (adenosine triphosphate) that results from the release of energy.

adrenal glands—Small ductless glands, one of which is situated on the upper part of each kidney.

adultery—Sexual intercourse between a married individual and a person other than his or her legal spouse.

afterbirth—The placenta and other fetal membranes expelled from the uterus following childbirth.

alkali—A base or hydroxide that is water soluble and capable of neutralizing acids.

allantois—A membranous pouch in the embryo that contributes to the formation of the placenta and umbilical cord.

amenorrhea—Absence of menstruation.

amino acids—A group of nitrogenous organic compounds that serve as the basic units of proteins, some of which are essential to human metabolism.

amniocentesis—A surgical procedure in which the uterus is perforated by a needle that has been passed through the abdomen of the pregnant woman; its purpose is to drain, for examination, some of the amniotic fluid surrounding the fetus.

amnion—The innermost membrane of the embryonic sac.

amphetamine—A synthetic substance used to stimulate the central nervous system; it increases blood pressure and reduces appetite.

anal intercourse—The insertion of the penis into the rectum via the anus.

anaphrodisiac—A drug or agent that decreases sexual desire.

androgen—A hormone that produces male sex characteristics and that influences body growth and the sex drive.

androsterone—A sex hormone (an androgen) excreted in the urine of both men and women.

anemia—A condition characterized by a lower than normal number of erythrocytes (red blood cells) in the blood.

antibiotic—A chemical or drug that has the ability to inhibit the growth of or destroy bacteria and other organisms.

antibody—A product of special cells in the lymphatic tissue of the body that is formed in response to a specific antigenic stimulus; it combines with and, in effect, neutralizes the antigen.

antigen—A substance, usually protein, that when foreign to the body stimulates the formation of a specific antibody.

anus—The opening of the lower end of the digestive tract or gut.

aphrodisiac—A drug or agent that stimulates sexual desire.

areola—The circular area of darkened tissue surrounding the nipple.

arteriole—A very small branch of an artery, especially one leading to a capillary.

artery—A tubular vessel through which the blood passes away from the heart to the parts of the body.

ATP (adenosine triphosphate)—A cellular compound that contains high-energy chemical bonds that when broken yield energy and ADP.

autosome—A chromosome that is not a sex chromosome; in humans there are forty-four autosomes (twenty-two pairs).

B

bacillus—Any rod-shaped bacterium.

bacterium (*plural* bacteria)—Any microorganism of the order *Eubacteriales;* a non-spore-forming microorganism.

barbiturate—A drug or agent used as a sedative; it is valuable in the treatment of sleeplessness.

Barr body—A dark area in the cells of normal females; sex chromatin.

Bartholin's gland—The two small bodies located on either side of the opening of the vagina that are imbedded in the labia minora; they produce a lubricating material during prolonged sexual intercourse.

benign—Not malignant; not recurrent.

bestiality—A form of sexual behavior in which a human engages in sexual relations with an animal.

birth control—Intentional limitation of the number or frequency of birth of children through such means as contraceptives, the rhythm method, tubal ligation, and vasectomy.

bisexual—Having gonads of both sexes. Also having either active or passive male and female characteristics or sexual interests.

bladder—The membranous sac that serves as a receptacle for the temporary retention of a body secretion, such as urine.

blastocyst—The modified spherical structure produced by the continued cleavage (division) of a fertilized ovum (zygote).

breech birth—The birth of a fetus (child) presenting itself with the buttocks at the head of the birth canal.

buggery—In some legal definitions this refers to any type of sexual intercourse considered "abnormal" by the writers of the law; both buggery and sodomy have been used to describe sexual relations between a human and an animal. Sodomy refers to the insertion of the penis into another male's rectum.

C

candidiasis—Urinary or reproductive tract infection by the fungus *Candida ablicans*. The mouth infection is called thrush. (Also known as moniliasis.)

capillary—One of the tiny blood vessels that connect an arteriole and a venule; their walls are semipermeable (allowing passage of only certain materials) membranes that exchange substances between the blood and tissues.

carbohydrate—Any of certain organic compounds made up of carbon, hydrogen, and oxygen and that include starches, sugars, and cellulose.

castration—The removal of the gonads—the testes in the male or the ovaries in the female.

catheter—A tubular surgical instrument used for removing fluids from a body cavity.

cautery—The application to dead or unwanted tissue of a caustic substance, an electric current, or a hot iron; in this way the tissue is destroyed.

celibacy—The state of being unmarried; generally inferred is the abstention from sexual activity.

cell—A minute bounded mass of protoplasm containing a nucleus, which is the basic unit of life and which makes up all tissue. Some lower forms of life, such as viruses and bacteria, may not have a nucleus, but do contain genetic material.

cervix—Neck. The lower, narrow necklike portion of the uterus that opens into the vagina.

Caesarean section—A not uncommon operation for delivery of a fetus done when birth by

natural means is dangerous or impossible; it is done by means of an incision through the walls of the abdomen and uterus.

chancre—The primary sore or ulcer that is the first sign of syphilis.

chancroid—A venereal disease caused by bacteria; it begins as a pustule on the genitalia and develops rapidly into a lesion that finally breaks down into an open sore discharging pus.

change of life—The period of life when a woman enters her postreproductive years; the menopause. Cessation of menstruation in the human female.

chorion—The outermost enveloping membrane of the developing embryo that serves as a protective and nutritive covering and in later development contributes to the placenta.

chromosome—One of the several, more or less rod-shaped bodies that appear in the nucleus of a cell. They are constant in number for each species and contain the genes or hereditary factors; the normal number in humans is forty-six: twenty-two pairs of autosomes, and two sex chromosomes.

chronic—Lasting or persisting over a long period of time.

circumcision—The surgical removal (usually several days after birth) of all or part of the foreskin, or prepuce, of the penis.

climacteric—The somatic (body), endocrine (glandular), and sometimes psychic (emotional) changes that occur at the end of the reproductive period in the woman and that usually result in some diminution of sexual activity in the man. In the woman menstruation ceases; in both sexes there is a reduction in the production of sex hormones.

climax—The period of greatest intensity in sexual response or excitement; the orgasm.

clitoris—A small, very sensitive, erectile body situated just above the urethral opening and in the upper angle of the vulva.

coccus—A type of bacterium that is spherical in shape.

codon—The groups of three nucleotides (compounds that make up a nucleic acid) that, when they occur in specific order, correspond to a particular amino acid in the genetic code.

coitus—Sexual union between individuals of the opposite sex in which the penis is inserted into the vagina.

coitus interruptus—The procedure in which the penis is withdrawn from the vagina before ejaculation occurs; often used as a method of birth control.

coitus reservatus—Sexual intercourse in which ejaculation is purposely delayed or suppressed.

colostrum—The thin, milky, yellowish-white liquid secreted by the mother's breast a few days before or after birth.

conception—The fertilization of an ovum (egg) by a spermatozoon.

condom—A male contraceptive made of thin rubber or gut that is placed over the erect penis before intercourse; it traps the semen and prevents it from being deposited in the vagina.

congenital—A condition existing at birth regardless of its cause; resulting from or developing in the prenatal environment.

contraception—The prevention of the fertilization of an ovum (egg) by a spermatozoon.

contraceptive—A device or method designed to prevent conception (fertilization).

copulation—Sexual intercourse; coitus.

corpus luteum—A yellow body on the ovary formed by an ovarian follicle that has matured and released its ovum; it secretes the hormone progesterone.

Cowper's glands—Two glands in the male, located on each side of the urethra close to the prostate, that secrete a material that is part of the seminal fluid.

cunnilinction—Using the mouth and tongue to stimulate the external female genitalia (sex organs).

curettage—The removal, by scraping, of material lining the walls of the uterus (or any body cavity) with a curette.

curette—A spoon-shaped medical instrument used for removing material from the walls of body cavities.

cytoplasm—The material contained within a cell excepting the nucleus.

D

defecate—To excrete waste matter from the bowels.

deletion—The loss of part of a chromosome.

depressant—A drug that depresses the central nervous system producing muscular relaxation.

dermatitis—Inflammation of the skin.

detumescence—The decline or subsidence of swelling of the body's erectile tissue following orgasm; it is due to the diminished congestion of the blood vessels.

diaphragm—A contraceptive used by women; it is a rubber hemisphere that fits like a cap over the opening of the cervix (neck) of the uterus. Also, the muscular-membranous partition separating the cavities of the chest and abdomen.

differentiation—The progressive specialization and modification of cells into tissues and organs.

dilation (dilatation)—The condition of being stretched beyond normal size or dimensions.

dilation and curettage ("D and C")—A procedure used to perform abortions; the opening of the cervix is slightly dilated and a curette is inserted into the uterus through the cervical opening; with manipulation of the curette, the pregnancy tissue is gently scraped from the surface wall of the uterus.

diploid—Having two sets of chromosomes, as is normal in the nucleus of the body cells of the human being.

DNA (deoxyribonucleic acid)—A chemical substance found in the nucleus of cells; it is the material of the gene and, thus, of heredity; along with proteins, it makes up the chromosomes.

douche—A stream of water or other liquid directed into the vagina for sanitary or medical purposes; a douche is a poor contraceptive.

"downer"—A term applied to barbiturates and other depressants.

Down's syndrome—Mongolism; a condition associated with a chromosomal abnormality; it is characterized by a somewhat flattened skull and nose, slanted eyes, and other physical abnormalities; there is usually moderate to severe mental retardation.

dysfunction—Disturbance, abnormality, or impairment of the functioning of an organ.

dysmenorrhea—Painful menstruation.

dyspareunia—Painful sexual intercourse.

dysuria—Difficult or painful urination.

E

ecosystem—The fundamental unit in ecology, made up of the living organisms and the nonliving elements all of which interact with each other in a defined area.

ectoderm—The outermost of the three germ layers of the embryo from which is formed the skin, nails, hair, glands of skin, nervous system, eyes and ears, and membranes of the mouth and anus.

ectopic pregnancy—A pregnancy in which the embryo develops outside the uterus, either in the abdominal cavity, in an ovary, or in a Fallopian tube.

ectoplasm—The outer layer of the cytoplasm of a cell.

ejaculation—The expulsion of semen that usually occurs at the climax of sexual stimulation; it is accomplished by peristaltic contractions of parts of the male genital system.

ejaculatory duct—The canal formed where the excretory duct of the testis (the vas deferens or ductus deferens) joins the seminal vesicle.

Electra complex—The conscious or unconscious tendency of excessive attachment of a daughter to her father. (See also **Oedipus complex.**)

embolus—A clot or plug in the blood vessel that leaves the site of its formation and plugs a smaller vessel.

embryo—The early developing stage of an organism in the uterus. In the human, the embryo is considered to be the period of development that lasts from one week after fertilization until the end of the second month.

endocrine glands—Ductless glands that secrete substances (hormones) directly into the circulatory system.

endoderm—The innermost of the three germ layers of the embryo from which is formed the linings of the pharynx, of the respiratory tract, and of the digestive and urinary tracts.

endometrium—The (internal) mucous lining of the uterine cavity.

endoplasm—The portion of the cytoplasm located at the central portion of a cell.

endoplasmic reticulum—A membranous transportation system of canals within the cytoplasm of cells, which are formed by inward folds of the plasma cell membrane that surrounds the cell. Materials needed by the cell move through these canals. The endoplasmic reticulum also connects with the nuclear membrane.

enema—A liquid medicine injected into the rectum as a purgative.

engorgement—Congestion, usually blood.

enzyme—An organic compound, usually a protein, that speeds up the reaction of other compounds.

epidemic—Attacking many individuals in an area at the same time, usually widely dispersed and spreading quickly; the occurrence in a community or region of illnesses of similar nature clearly in excess of normal expectancy and derived from a common or propagated source.

epididymis—The long cordlike structure located near the bottom of the testis in which the sperm are stored.

erogenous zone—An area of the body that is especially sensitive to sexual stimulation. Some of these are the mouth, lips, tongue, breasts and nipples, buttocks, and genitals.

estrogen—A hormone that produces female sex characteristics.

estrus—The recurrent cyclic period of physiologic changes in most female placental mammals that prepares the reproductive organs for the fertile period; during this time the sex drive is intense and the female is, of course, especially desirous of sexual gratification.

etiocholanolone—One of the chemicals produced in the urine when testosterone is broken down in the male's body.

exhibitionism—A type of behavior in which the individual derives sexual gratification from displaying his genitals.

F

Fallopian tube—The oviduct, or tube, that extends from the ovary to the uterus; through it the ovum (egg) travels. (Also known as the uterine tube.)

fecund—The ability to produce young; fertile.

fellatio—Oral stimulation of the penis. A fellator is a male who takes another male's penis into his mouth; however, fellatio is by no means limited to male homosexual behavior.

fertile—Capable of producing a new individual.

fetishism—The adoration of an inanimate (nonliving) object for purposes of sexual gratification.

fetus—In humans, the developing child in the uterus from the beginning of the third month until birth.

fimbria—The fingerlike projections at the end of the Fallopian tubes that lie close but not directly attached to the corresponding ovary.

follicle—The small sac or pouch close to the surface of the ovary that contains the developing ovum (egg cell).

follicle-stimulating hormone (FSH)—One of the gonadotropic (a substance that stimulates the gonads) hormones produced by the anterior lobe of the pituitary gland, which promotes the maturation of the Graafian follicle in the female and stimulates formation of spermatozoa in the male.

follicular fluid—The fluid secreted by the cells that surround the maturing ovum (egg) in the Graafian follicle; the fluid forms tiny pools that run together to form lakes within each follicle.

foreplay—Usually the preliminary stages of sexual relations, in which the individuals stimulate each other by kissing and caressing.

fornication—Voluntary sexual intercourse between two unmarried individuals.

frenulum—In this text, a delicate thin fold of skin on the lower surface of the head of the penis (glans); it connects the glans to the prepuce (foreskin).

G

gamete—Spermatozoon (mature sperm) or ovum (mature egg); the two cells the union of which is necessary for sexual reproduction.

gene—The basic unit of heredity and genetic information; it is self-reproducing and is located at a specific place on a chromosome.

genetic code—The hereditary instructions contained in DNA; structurally it is the arrangement of four chemicals (nitrogenous bases) that determines the formation of proteins.

genital—Pertaining to reproduction or the sexual organs.

genital herpes—A genital infection caused by a virus in which blisters form; these may become ulcers that, in turn, become infected.

genital lice—The "crab louse," a small parasitic insect, that is usually found in the pubic region but can spread to other hairy parts of the body.

genital wart—A benign viral tumor that may be transmitted by genital contact.

genitalia—The reproductive organs.

genotype—The particular assortment or combination of genes of an individual.

germ cell—A primary type of cell that is capable of participating in the development of an individual; sperm and ovum (egg).

gestation (pregnancy)—The period of time during which a female has a developing embryo or fetus in her uterus.

gland—A group of cells that separates elements from the blood and produces from them a specific substance for the body to use.

glycogen—The main carbohydrate stored by animals.

Golgi complex (body)—A system of canals found in a cell, the surface of which is always smooth and which has sacs; its purpose seems to be that of storage and transportation.

gonad—A gland that produces gametes; the ovary or testis.

gonadotropic hormone—Any hormone that influences a gonad.

gonadotropin—A hormone that stimulates or has an affinity for the gonads.

gonococcus (plural gonococci)—A single microorganism of the species *Neisseria gonorrhoeae;* the causative agent of gonorrhea.

gonorrhea—The most common of the venereal diseases; it is caused by the gonococcus.

Graafian follicle—A tiny sac or pouch in the ovary that contains the maturing ovum and from which it is released at ovulation.

granuloma inguinale—A venereal disease caused by a rod-shaped microorganism called the Donovan body and characterized by deep pus-filled ulcerations (sores) on the skin of the external sexual organs.

gynecologist—A physician who specializes in the treatment of diseases of the female reproductive and sexual organs.

H

hallucinogen—An agent or drug that produces hallucinations or the perception of things (sights and sounds) that are not actually present.

haploid—Having one set of unpaired chromosomes, as is normal in the gametes of the human being. The nucleus of a somatic (body) cell has double the haploid number of chromosomes.

hemophilia—A hereditary disease in which the blood cannot clot properly.

heredity—The transmission of physical and emotional traits and characteristics from parents to children.

hermaphrodite—An individual who possesses both male and female sex organs.

hermaphroditism—A condition in which both male and female sex organs exist in one individual. In the human it is characterized by the presence of both ovarian and testicular tissue and reproductive organs that are not typical of one gender.

heroin—A white, crystalline powder derived from morphine; it is a powerful narcotic.

herpes simplex—A virus disease characterized by blisters on the skin and mucous membranes. (Also known as cold sores.)

heterosexual behavior—Sexual interest or behavior that is directed toward individuals of the opposite sex.

homosexual behavior—Sexual interest or behavior that is directed toward individuals of the same sex.

hormone—A chemical substance secreted by the endocrine (ductless) glands into the circulatory system that has a specific effect on certain target organs.

hymen—The membrane that partly or entirely covers the external opening of the vagina in some females who have never had sexual intercourse. It may or may not be intact in virgins.

hypochondriasis—Undue and severe anxiety about health.

hypothalamus—A portion of the brain that regulates many basic body functions, such as water balance, temperature, and sleep. It also produces certain chemicals (factors) that stimulate the anterior lobe of the pituitary and other endocrine glands to produce and release hormones.

hysterectomy—The surgical removal of all or part of the uterus.

hysterotomy—Incision (cutting into) of the uterus (as in a Caesarean section).

I

imperforate hymen—A hymen that has no opening and that may completely cover the external opening of the vagina.

impotence—Inability of the male to have satisfactory sexual intercourse; usually the inability to achieve or maintain an erection.

incest—Sexual intercourse or relations between close relatives, such as mother and son, father and daughter, or sister and brother.

infanticide—The purposeful killing of an infant.

infection—Invasion of the body by a disease-causing organism. The reaction of the tissues to the presence of the organism and the toxins that it may generate.

inorganic—Chemical substances that are not derived from living organisms.

inpatient—A person who is housed and fed as well as treated in a hospital or clinic.

interfemoral—Between the thighs.

intersex—Varying degrees of intermingling in one individual of the structural characteristics of both sexes; there are both male and female intersexuals. True intersexuals show one or more contradictions of the structural criteria of gender and possess both male and female gonadal tissue.

intromission—Insertion of the penis into the vagina.

IUD (intrauterine device)—A contraceptive device (as a coil or loop of plastic) that is inserted in the uterus.

K

karyotype—A systematic arrangement on a chart of the chromosomes of a cell that is typical of an individual or species.

Kleinfelter's syndrome—A genetic disorder in which the mature sex cells of the individual have two X-chromosomes and one Y-chromosome (XXY). The individual may appear normal, but he is usually tall and has underdeveloped sexual structures. The individual is ordinarily sterile and is often mentally retarded.

L

labia majora—A pair of elongated folds that runs downward and backward from the mons pubis; it forms the outer, larger pair of lips of the external female genitalia (vulva).

labia minora—A pair of small folds of skin located between the labia majora and the vaginal opening that forms the smaller pair of lips of the female genitalia.

lactation—The secretion of milk by the breast.

lactiferous ducts—Channels in the breast that transport the milk to the nipples.

lanugo—The very fine, downy hairs covering the human fetus.

Lesbian—A woman whose behavior is homosexual.

lesion—An injury, damage, or other change of an organ or tissue that may result in loss or impairment of function.

libido—Sexual desire; the motivational force of sexuality.

ligation—The application of a thread or wire for tying (closing) a vessel or tube.

lobules—Small rounded projecting parts of an organ.

lumen—The channel or cavity within a tubular organ.

luteinizing hormone (LH)—A substance secreted and released by the anterior lobe of the pituitary gland that causes the mature Graafian follicle to rupture, releasing the ovum (egg). In the male, this hormone is involved in the production of testosterone.

luteinizing hormone-releasing hormone (factor) (LH-RH)—A substance that originates in the hypothalamus of the brain and that stimulates the anterior lobe of the pituitary gland to produce and release luteinizing hormone and follicle-stimulating hormone.

lymphogranuloma venereum—A viral venereal disease manifested by swelling of the lymph nodes in the groin.

lysosome—Tiny organelles found inside a cell that contain digestive enzymes capable of breaking down complex nutrients into simpler substances that the cell can use.

M

masochism—The obtaining of sexual pleasure and gratification from being cruelly treated or dominated by one's partner.

masturbation—Sexual self-stimulation; usually the achievement of orgasm by manipulation of one's own genitals. However, it is not uncommon for people to masturbate one another. A method of sexual expression almost universal in males and extremely common in females.

meconium—A dark green mucoid material in the intestine of a newly born infant.

meiosis—A special type of cell division that occurs in the maturation process of sex cells; each daughter nucleus receives one-half the number of chromosomes normally found in a somatic (body) cell.

membrane—A thin layer of tissue that divides a space or an organ or that covers a surface.

menarche—The beginning of menstruation.

meninges—The three membranes that enclose the brain and spinal cord.

menopause—The cessation of menstruation in the female, usually occurring between the ages of forty-five and fifty; there are, however, wide variations in age.

menorrhagia—Abnormally profuse menstrual flow.

menses—The monthly discharge of blood and tissue from the female genital tract.

menstruation—The premenopausal cyclic uterine bleeding, which recurs about every four weeks in the absence of pregnancy.

mesoderm—The middle layer of the three germ layers of an embryo; it lies between the ectoderm and the endoderm and from it are formed the bones and cartilage, muscles, blood vessels and blood, kidneys, and reproductive organs.

messenger RNA—A type of RNA (ribonucleic acid) that transfers information from a portion of the DNA to the ribosome, where proteins are formed.

metabolism—All of the chemical and physical processes by which living substance is produced and maintained. The process by which energy is made available to the cell.

metrorrhagia—Abnormal uterine bleeding between menstrual periods.

microbe—A microscopic organism.

miscarriage—A premature and spontaneous expulsion from the uterus of the products of conception; a spontaneous abortion. This term is generally used by the layman.

mite—A tiny, sometimes microscopic animal, related to spiders, that is often parasitic to man, other animals, insects, or plants.

mitosis—A type of cell division in which the daughter nuclei receive the exact number and complement of chromosomes that the parent cell has.

molecule—The smallest particle of a compound or element that has the characteristics of that compound or element.

Mongolism—A congenital disease characterized by (among other features) a somewhat flattened skull, short and flattened nose, epicanthic (slanted) eyes, and moderate to severe mental retardation. It is associated with a chromosomal abnormality. (Also known as Down's syndrome.)

moniliasis—An infection caused by a fungus, *Monilia albicans* (*Candida albicans*), which is also known as candidiasis. The mouth infection is called thrush.

monogamy—The practice of being married to one person at a time.

monosomy—The absence of a chromosome from the normal number of chromosomes of a diploid cell. (A *diploid* cell has two sets of chromosomes, as is normal in the body cells of higher organisms.)

mons—An elevation or eminence.

mons pubis—The fleshy, rounded elevation located at the lowest part of the abdomen; in the adult, it is covered with hair. (Also known as the mons veneris.)

Montgomery's glands—Glands that secrete a lubricating substance in the (mammary) areola.

mosaicism—The presence of cells with different chromosomal make-up within an individual.

mucosa—Mucous membrane; thin body tissue that has a moist surface.

mucus—The slimy, protective material of the mucous membranes that contains their secretions and various other materials, such as dead cells.

N

necrophilia—A kind of sexual behavior in which the individual has a sexual attraction to a corpse or desires sexual intercourse with a dead body.

Neisseria gonorrhoeae—The microorganism responsible for gonorrhea.

nocturnal emission—The involuntary ejaculation of semen during sleep; "wet dreams"; a common experience of young males.

nondisjunction—Failure of paired chromosomes to separate during cell division (usually meiosis) so that one daughter nucleus receives both members of the pair, and the other daughter nucleus lacks that particular chromosome.

nubile—The age and stage of physical development at which a girl becomes marriageable.

nucleolus—A round body found within the nucleus of a cell.

nucleus—A spherical body found within a cell and consisting of several characteristic organelles, such as a nuclear membrane, nucleoli, granules of chromatin (the easily stained portion of the nucleus), and diffuse protoplasm. Also within the nucleus are the chromosomes.

O

obstetrician—A physician who specializes in the treatment of women during pregnancy, labor, and the period after childbirth.

Oedipus complex—The conscious or unconscious tendency of emotional and psychological attachment of a son to his mother. The term also refers to a similar attachment of the daughter for the father.

oöcyte—A developing egg that has not finished its maturation process.

oögenesis—The origin and maturation of the ovum.

oögonium—The primordial (first or existing at the beginning) cell from which an ovum derives; its divisions produce oöcytes.

organelle—A particular type of organized living material, usually with a specific function, that is present in most cells; among these are the nucleus, ribosomes, mitochondria, endoplasmic reticulum, and Golgi complex.

organic—Derived from living organisms.

orgasm—The pleasurable peak of sexual excitement; climax; the culmination of sexual intercourse.

osmosis—The flow of a pure liquid from the lesser to the greater concentration when the solutions are separated by a semipermeable membrane that allows passage of only certain molecules in the liquid. It is usually by this method that nutrients are absorbed by cells and wastes are excreted.

outpatient—An individual who comes to a hospital, clinic, doctor's office, or other dispensary for diagnosis or treatment but does not occupy a bed there; an ambulatory patient.

ovarian follicle—The ovum and its enclosing envelope of cells at any stage in its development.

ovary—The female gonad; the reproductive gland of the female in which the ova (eggs) develop.

oviduct—The tube that extends from the ovary to the uterus and through which the ovum travels. (Also known as the Fallopian tube or the uterine tube.)

ovulation—The discharge of a mature ovum from the Graafian follicle (the sac in which the maturing ovum develops) of the ovary.

ovum—The mature female reproductive cell that after fertilization by a spermatozoon develops into a new individual of the same species.

P

parthenogenesis—Reproduction by development of an unfertilized ovum (egg).

partner surrogate—Surrogate means substitute; in this text it refers to the substitute for the wife in the Masters and Johnson treatment of sexual inadequacy in single males.

pectoral—Having to do with the chest or breast.

pederasty—Sexual relations (anal intercourse) by a man with a boy.

pedophilia—A type of sexual behavior in which an adult engages in or desires sexual relations with a child.

penicillin—A substance that has the ability to inhibit the growth of or destroy bacteria (an antibiotic); it is extracted from certain molds.

penis—The male organ of sexual intercourse and, in mammals, the external organ of urination.

perineal—Having to do with the perineum.

perineum—The area between the genital organs and the rectum. It is sometimes defined as the whole area at the pelvic outlet, including the anus and the internal genitals.

pessary—An instrument that is placed in the vagina to support the rectum or uterus.

petting—Sexual stimulation between partners that excludes sexual intercourse.

pH—The symbol for the degree of acidity or alkalinity in a solution; a pH of 7 is neutral (neither acid or alkaline); pH values from 0 to 7 indicate acidity; pH values from 7 to 14 indicate alkalinity.

pharyngitis—An inflammation or infection of the pharynx.

pharynx—The membranous and muscular sac leading from the back of the mouth and nostrils to the esophagus (the tube leading from the back of the mouth to the stomach).

phenotype—The visible expression of the hereditary or genetic makeup of an individual.

pheromones—Body odors that, as chemical messengers, may influence sexual and other responses among animals. The existence of human pheromones remains to be proved.

phimosis—Tightness of the prepuce (foreskin) of the penis so that it cannot be drawn back over the glans; an analogous condition can exist with the clitoris.

pituitary gland—This small gland of tremendous importance is located at the base of the brain; it has a profound effect on the function of certain other glands, especially the thyroid, adrenals, and sex glands.

placenta—The organ in the uterus that connects the fetus to the mother by means of the umbilical cord; through it, the fetus is nourished and wastes are removed; the afterbirth.

plasma membrane—The porous organelle that surrounds a cell and allows only certain kinds and amounts of materials to enter and leave the cell.

polygamy—The practice of having two or more spouses at the same time; plural marriage.

postnatal—Immediately after birth.

postpartum—After delivery or birth.

potency—The capability of the male to perform sexual intercourse; the ability of the male to have an erection.

pregnancy—The period of time during which a female has a developing embryo or fetus in her uterus.

prenatal—Before birth.

premature ejaculation—The expulsion of semen (ejaculation) prior to or immediately after insertion of the penis into the vagina.

prepuce (foreskin)—In the uncircumcised male, the fold of skin that covers the head of the penis (glans); in the female, the fold formed by the labia minora that covers the end of the clitoris.

primordial—Original; existing at the beginning; primitive.

primordial germ (sex) cells—The reproductive cells that have a diploid number of chromosomes (forty-six, in humans) and from which the gametes (secondary sex cells) arise by means of meiosis.

progeny—Offspring or children.

progesterone—The hormone secreted by the corpus luteum; its basic function is to ready the uterus for the reception and development of a fertilized ovum.

progestin—The name for certain brands of synthetic progesterone.

progonasyl—A drug used in the treatment of certain kinds of vaginitis that shows promise as a preventive against venereal disease.

promiscuous—Engaging in sexual intercourse indiscriminately or casually with many people; sexual activity without rules.

prophylactic—A device or agent that protects one from disease. May also refer to a device or agent that prevents pregnancy, such as a condom.

prostate gland—A gland that, in males, surrounds the neck of the bladder and upper urethra; it secretes an alkaline fluid that is discharged with the spermatozoa.

prostatitis—Inflammation of the prostate gland.

protein—A group of compounds made up mostly of amino acids that forms the principal part of protoplasm.

protoplasm—A semiliquid, translucent material that is the essential matter of all plant and animal cells.

psychoanalysis—A system of treatment, developed by Sigmund Freud and others, that tries to alleviate emotional disorders by means of the analysis of unconscious factors that are revealed in a variety of ways, such as dreams and free associations.

psychogenic—A symptom that has an emotional or psychological origin.

psychopathology—Emotional disorder.

psychosomatic—Having physical (bodily) symptoms of an emotional origin.

puberty—The period of time between the appearance of secondary sex characteristics and the end of body growth; the state of physical development when sexual reproduction first becomes possible.

pubes—The hair growing in the pubic area. Also, the plural of pubis, the pubic bone.

R

rape—Forcible sexual intercourse; intercourse with an individual who offers resistance or does not consent to it.

rectum—The lowest part of the large intestine, which is connected to the anus.

refractory period—A term used by Masters and Johnson to describe the temporary state of resistance to sexual stimulation immediately following orgasm.

"rhythm method"—A method of contraception that depends on abstinence from sexual intercourse during the time of the month when the woman is believed to be fertile.

ribosomal RNA—The RNA (ribonucleic acid) that is found in or that makes up the ribosome; it comprises 70 to 80 percent of the total RNA.

ribosome—A cellular organelle at which proteins are constructed or synthesized. It is not believed to be stationary and is thought to actively participate in protein formation.

RNA (ribonucleic acid)—A substance that is a template of portions of the DNA and functions in the cytoplasm; there are three types of RNA; messenger RNA (mRNA); ribosomal RNA (rRNA); and transfer RNA (tRNA).

S

sadism—A form of sexual behavior in which gratification is derived from cruelly dominating, mistreating, or hurting one's partner, physically or otherwise.

"safe period"—The time interval when it is believed that a woman is infertile or not capable of conception.

scabies—A contagious skin disease caused by a mite; the most prominent symptom is itching. (Also known as "the itch.")

scrotum—The male's external pouch or sac that contains the testes and related organs.

sebaceous glands—Skin glands that secrete a greasy lubricating substance.

secondary sex characteristics—The physical features, other than the genitalia, that distinguish the sexes.

semen—The thick, whitish secretion produced by the male that is ejaculated at orgasm and, in fertile men, contains spermatozoa.

seminal vesicles—The paired pouches attached to the urinary bladder that join the vas deferens to form the ejaculatory duct.

seminiferous tubules—Passages in the testis in which the sperm develop and through which they leave the testis.

sex drive—Desire for sexual expression.

sex flush—The skin response to sexual excitement; a temporary measleslike rash that may appear during the late excitement or early plateau phase and disappears after coitus.

sexual climax—Orgasm; the highest point of sexual excitement.

sexual foreplay—The preliminary stages of sexual relations, in which the individuals stimulate each other by kissing and caressing.

sexual intercourse—The joining of male and female sexual organs (the penis and vagina); coitus.

smegma—A thick, cheesy, ill-smelling collection of secretions found chiefly under the foreskin of the penis and around the clitoris, due to poor personal hygiene.

sodomy—According to some laws, may refer to any type of sexual intercourse regarded as "abnormal" by the writer of the law; anal intercourse.

somatic—Of the body; physical.

"speed"—A slang term for amphetamines (methamphetamines); drugs that stimulate the central nervous system.

sperm—A mature male reproductive cell that can fertilize an ovum.

spermatogenesis—The production and development of spermatozoa.

spermatogonium—A primordial male germ cell that originates in a seminal tubule; it divides into two primary spermatocytes.

spermatozoon (*plural* spermatozoa)—A mature male germ or sex cell that can fertilize an ovum (egg).

spermicide—A contraceptive substance designed to kill spermatozoa.

sphincter—A ringlike band of muscle fibers that surrounds a natural body opening and can open or close it by expanding or contracting.

spirochete—A bacterium that is spiral-shaped. The causative agent of syphilis, *Treponema pallidum,* is a type of spirochete.

staphylococcus (*plural* staphylococci)—A type of microorganism; as a group, staphylococci resemble a bunch of grapes.

sterile—Not fertile; not capable of producing a new individual.

stimulant—A drug or agent that temporarily increases the activity of some organ or vital process.

streptococcus (*plural* streptococci)—A type of microorganism that can occur in pairs but, as a group, usually resemble a twisted string of pearls.

subfertility—The state of being relatively sterile or less than normally fertile.

suppository—An easily melted medicated substance that is placed in a body opening such as the rectum or vagina.

sweating phenomenon—In this text, the appearance of small drops of a lubricating liquid on the walls of the vagina, usually early in the excitement phase of the female sexual response.

syphilis—A contagious venereal disease caused by the microorganism *Treponema pallidum* and usually transmitted by direct contact; the untreated disease can lead to many serious complications.

T

taboo—A social, religious, or traditional prohibition put on certain people, things, or acts.

tampon—A plug of absorbent material placed in a wound or cavity to stop bleeding or absorb secretions.

teratogen—An agent (as a chemical or disease) causing malformation of an embryo or fetus.

testis (*plural* testes)—The male gonad; an egg-shaped gland suspended in the scrotum that produces spermatozoa; testicle.

testoserone—The hormone produced by the testis that induces and maintains the male secondary sex characteristics.

thrombus—A plug or clot in a blood vessel or in the heart.

thrush—A disease caused by the fungus *Candida albicans* that is accompanied by whitish spots in the mouth; the spots are followed by small sores that can spread to the groin, buttocks, and other body parts.

thyroid gland—A large, ductless gland located on either side of the windpipe.

tissue—A group of cells that are organized and specialized to perform a similar particular function.

tranquilizer—A drug or agent used as a depressant in controlling and relieving various emotional disturbances.

transfer RNA—A type of RNA (ribonucleic acid) that, instructed by DNA, combines with a specific amino acid and transfers it to the ribosome in the process of protein synthesis.

transsexual—An individual who feels cross-sexed, that is, feels like a member of the opposite sex; the individual never obtains sexual pleasure from his own sex organs. Also a person who has undergone surgery and hormone injections to effect a change of sex.

transvestite—An individual who derives sexual satisfaction by dressing in the clothing of the opposite sex.

Treponema pallidum—The microorganism that is the causative agent of syphilis.

tribadism—A technique that may be used by some women whose behavior is homosexual; it involves mutual friction of the genitals.

trichomoniasis—A vaginal infection caused by *Trichomonas vaginalis,* a type of parasitic protozoa (a one-celled animal).

trisomy—The presence of an extra (third) chromosome of one type in a diploid cell.

Trisomy 21—The presence of chromosome 21 in triplicate; one of the causes of Mongolism, or Down's syndrome.

troilism—Sexual intercourse or relations that involve three persons.

trophoblast—A layer of nutritive tissue outside the embryo that attaches the blastocyst to the wall of the uterus and supplies nutrition to the embryo.

tubal ligation—The application of a thread or wire to close the Fallopian tube as a means of birth control.

tumescence—Swelling, usually with blood.

Turner's syndrome—A genetic abnormality that results from nondisjunction, in which the individual has only an X-chromosome (OX); it is characterized by retarded physical growth and sexual development.

U

umbilical cord—The flexible tube that connects the developing fetus to the placenta; it serves to convey nourishment to and remove waste from the fetus.

"ups"—A slang term for stimulants (an agent that increases the activity of an organ or vital function).

ureter—One of two tubes through which the urine passes from the kidney to the bladder.

urethra—The single tube through which the urine passes from the bladder to the outside of the body.

urine—The waste fluid (containing urea and certain salts) secreted by the kidneys and stored in the bladder; it is discharged by way of the urethra.

uterus—The, hollow muscular organ of female mammals in which the embryo and fetus develop and are nourished; the womb.

V

vacuum aspiration—A method of removing tissue or other material from the wall of the uterus by means of suction.

vagina—The canallike organ in the female that extends from the neck (lowest part) of the uterus to the vulva (external genital region) and that receives the penis in sexual intercourse.

vaginal barrel—The cavity of the vagina in the female.

vaginal lubrication—In this text, the material appearing on the vaginal walls within seconds of any effective sexual stimulation; it is the female's first functional response to sexual stimulation; the sweating phenomenon is an early phase of vaginal lubrication.

vaginismus—Painful spasm of the vagina; it usually prevents the insertion of the penis into the vagina.

vaginitis—Inflammation of the vagina, usually accompanied by a discharge.

vas deferens—The excretory duct of the testis, which forms part of the ejaculatory duct; ductus deferens. (Also known as the sperm duct.)

vasectomy—Surgical removal of all or (usually) part of the vas deferens; a type of birth control.

vasocongestion—Congestion of the blood vessels.

vein—A vessel through which blood passes from different organs and body parts back to the heart.

venereal disease—A contagious disease transmitted only or chiefly by sexual intercourse. Syphilis and gonorrhea are examples. Some diseases that may be sexually transmitted are not primarily venereal.

vernix caseosa—A cheesy substance that covers the skin of the fetus.

vestibule—The region surrounding and including the opening of the vagina.

virgin—A person who has not had sexual intercourse. Some writers seem to apply the term only to girls and women.

virus—A very small (usually ultramicroscopic) infective agent that is characterized by a lack of its own metabolism; it can multiply only within living cells.

voyeurism—A form of sexual behavior in which gratification is derived from looking at another person's sexual organs. (Also known as scoptophilia or scopophilia.)

vulva—The external genital organs of the female.

W

womb—The uterus; in the pregnant woman, the organ that contains the developing embryo and fetus.

X

X-chromosome—The sex chromosome carried by one-half of the male gametes and all of the female gametes. The male carries one X-chromosome; the female, two.

Y

Y-chromosome—The sex chromosome carried by one-half of the male gametes and none of the female gametes. The male carries one Y-chromosome; the female, none.

Z

zygote—The single-celled fertilized ovum (egg) that results from the union of the male and female gametes.

Nomura, "Ribosomes," *Scientific American,* Vol. 221, No. 14 (October 1969). Copyright © 1969 by Scientific American, Inc. All rights reserved.

DAVID BELAIS FRIEDMAN for Table 1-1, "Parent and Child Development," from his "Parent Development," *California Medicine,* Vol. 86, No. 1 (January 1957). Reprinted by permission.

JOHN H. GAGNON for excerpts from John H. Gagnon and William Simon, "Prospects for Changes in American Sexual Patterns," *Medical Aspects of Human Sexuality,* Vol. 4, No. 1 (January 1970).

HARCOURT BRACE JOVANOVICH, INC. for Table 7-1, "Marriage Stability: The Religious Factor," from Robert K. Kelley, *Courtship, Marriage, and the Family* (New York: Harcourt Brace Jovanovich, 1969), adapted from Judson T. Landis, "Marriages of Mixed and Non-Mixed Religious Faith," *American Sociological Review,* Vol. 14, No. 3 (June 1949). Reprinted by permission.

GERALD A. HEIDBREDER for Table 2-1, "Natural History of Acquired Syphilis," and Table 2-2, "Natural History of Acquired Gonorrhea." Reprinted by permission of Gerald A. Heidbreder, Deputy Director, County of Los Angeles Department of Health Services.

THE HOGARTH PRESS, LTD for an excerpt from Anna Freud, *The Ego and the Mechanisms of Defense,* rev. ed. (New York: International Universities Press, 1967). Reprinted by permission.

INTERNATIONAL UNIVERSITIES PRESS, INC. for an excerpt reprinted from *The Ego and the Mechanisms of Defense* by Anna Freud. By permission of International Universities Press, Inc. Copyright © 1967 by Anna Freud.

THE JOURNAL OF THE AMERICAN MEDICAL ASSOCIATION for an excerpt from Natalie Shainess, review of Masters and Johnson's *Human Sexual Inadequacy, The Journal of the American Medical Association,* Vol. 213, No. 12 (September 21, 1970). Reprinted by permission.

ALFRED A. KNOPF, INC. for an excerpt reprinted from *The Prophet,* by Kahlil Gibran, with permission of the publisher, Alfred A. Knopf, Inc. Copyright 1923 by Kahlil Gibran; renewal copyright 1951 by Administrators C.T.A. of Kahlil Gibran Estate, and Mary Gibran.

JUDSON T. LANDIS for Table 7-1, "Marriage Stability: The Religious Factor," adapted from his "Marriages of Mixed and Non-Mixed Religious Faith," *American Sociological Review,* Vol. 14, No. 3 (June 1949). Reprinted by permission.

J. B. LIPPINCOTT COMPANY for a poem excerpted from *Family Development,* 4th ed., by Evelyn Millis Duvall. Reprinted by permission of the publisher, J. B. Lippincott Company. Copyright © 1971.

LITTLE, BROWN AND COMPANY for an excerpt from "Tarkington, Thou Should'st Be Living in This Hour." Copyright, 1947, by Ogden Nash. This poem originally appeared in *The New Yorker.* For an excerpt from "Pediatric Reflection." Copyright, 1931, by Ogden Nash. For an excerpt from "The Kitten." Copyright, 1940, by The Curtis Publishing Company. For an excerpt from "A Child's Guide to Parents." Copyright, 1936, by Ogden Nash. For an excerpt from "The Parent." Copyright, 1933, by Ogden Nash. All reprinted from *Verses from 1929 On* by Ogden Nash, by permission of Little, Brown and Co. For excerpts from *Human Sexual Response* by William H. Masters and Virginia E. Johnson. Copyright © 1966 by William H. Masters and Virginia E. Johnson. By permission of Little, Brown and Co. And for excerpts from *Human Sexual Inadequacy* by William H. Masters and Virginia E. Johnson. Copyright © 1970 by William H. Masters and Virginia E. Johnson. By permission of Little, Brown and Co.

MCGRAW-HILL BOOK COMPANY for Figure 6-1, "The Development of Human Embryonic Membranes," adapted from *Human Embryology,* 3rd ed., by B. U. Patten. Copyright 1968 by B. U. Patten. Used with permission of McGraw-Hill Book Company.

MEDICAL ASPECTS OF HUMAN SEXUALITY for an excerpt from John Money, "Why Are Some Orgasms Better Than Others?" *Medical Aspects of Human Sexuality,* Vol. 5, No. 3 (March 1971), and for excerpts from Charles Clay Dahlberg, "Sexual Behavior in the Drug Culture," *Medical Aspects of Human Sexuality,* Vol. 5, No. 4 (April 1971). Reprinted by permission.

JOHN MONEY for an excerpt from his "Why Are Some Orgasms Better Than Others?"

Medical Aspects of Human Sexuality, Vol. 5, No. 3 (March 1971). Reprinted by permission.

THE NATIONAL FOUNDATION-MARCH OF DIMES for Table 5-5, "The More Common Birth Defects," adapted from a booklet published by The National Foundation-March of Dimes, White Plains, New York. Reprinted by permission.

NEW AMERICAN LIBRARY for Marie Ford, "The Junkies," from Herbert Kohl, *36 Children.* Copyright © 1967 by Herbert Kohl. Reprinted by permission.

THE NEW REPUBLIC for Paul Cummins, "Advice," *The New Republic,* Vol. 157, No. 21, Issue No. 2764 (November 18, 1967). Reprinted by permission of *The New Republic,* copyright © 1967, Harrison-Blaine of New Jersey, Inc.

THE NEW YORK TIMES for an excerpt from Klaus Angel, "No Marihuana for Adolescents," *The New York Times Magazine,* November 30, 1969. Copyright © 1969 by The New York Times Company. Reprinted by permission.

NUTRITION TODAY for Table 5-4, "Childbearing Children in the United States, 1965," from Lucille B. Hurley, "The Consequences of Fetal Impoverishment," *Nutrition Today,* Vol. 3, No. 4 (December 1968). Copyright © 1968 by *Nutrition Today.* Reprinted by permission.

PRINCETON UNIVERSITY PRESS for an excerpt from *George Seferis Collected Poems, 1924–1955,* translated, edited, and introduced by Edmund Keeley and Philip Sherrard. Copyright © 1967 by Princeton University Press; Supplemented Edn., 1969. Reprinted by permission.

SATURDAY REVIEW, INC. for an excerpt from John Lear, "Spinning the Thread of Life," *Saturday Review* (April 5, 1969). Copyright © 1969 by Saturday Review, Inc. Reprinted by permission.

W. B. SAUNDERS COMPANY for Table 6-1, "Stages of Labor," from M. Edward Davis and Reva Rubin, *De Lee's Obstetrics for Nurses,* 18th ed. (Philadelphia: Saunders, 1966). Reprinted by permission.

CHARLES SCRIBNER'S SONS for excerpts from *Sexuality and Man,* compiled and edited by the Sex Information and Education Council of the United States (New York: Scribner's, 1970). Copyright © 1970 by Sex Information and Education Council of the United States, Inc. Reprinted by permission.

SEARLE & CO. for Table 4-1, "A Summary of Birth Control Methods," adapted from "Contraceptive Methods Requiring Consultation with Physician," from *Your Future Family.* Reprinted by permission.

NATALIE SHAINESS for an excerpt from her review of Masters and Johnson's *Human Sexual Inadequacy, The Journal of the American Medical Association,* Vol. 213, No. 12 (September 21, 1970). Reprinted by permission.

THE STUDENT ASSOCIATION FOR THE STUDY OF HALLUCINOGENS, INC. for excerpts from David E. Smith and Alan J. Rose, "The Group Marriage Commune: A Case Study," *Journal of Psychedelic Drugs,* Vol. 13, No. 1 (September 1970). Reprinted by permission.

HARRY VON TILZER MUSIC PUBLISHING COMPANY for an excerpt from "I Want a Girl (Just Like the Girl That Married Dear Old Dad)," by Harry Von Tilzer and Will Dillon. Copyright © 1911 by Harry Von Tilzer Music Publishing Co., Inc. U.S. copyright renewed 1938 and assigned to Harry Von Tilzer Music Publishing Co. (a division of Teleklew Productions, Inc.). Reprinted by permission of the publisher, Harry Von Tilzer Music Publishing Company (a division of T. B. Harms Company).

JOHN WILEY AND SONS for Table 5-3, "Mean Birth Weights According to Socioeconomic Status," from World Health Organization, *Nutrition in Pregnancy and Lactation,* cited in Miriam E. Lowenberg et al., *Food and Man* (New York: Wiley, 1968). Reprinted by permission.

THE WILLIAMS & WILKINS CO. for Figure 2-2, "The Route of a Spermatozoon," adapted from Robert Latov Dickinson, *Atlas of Human Sex Anatomy,* 2nd ed., copyright 1949 by The Williams & Wilkins Co., Baltimore. Reprinted by permission.

WORLD HEALTH ORGANIZATION for Table 5-3, "Mean Birth Weights According to Socio-economic Status," from World Health Organization, *Nutrition in Pregnancy and Lactation,* cited in Miriam E. Lowenberg et al., *Food and Man* (New York: Wiley, 1968). Reprinted by permission.

index

(Page numbers in italics refer to illustrations; n refers to footnotes.)

A

Abortion, 129-36
  criminal, 129
  legal methods of, 133-34
  New York experience with, 131-33
  problems of, 135-36
  spontaneous (miscarriage), 129, 173
  therapeutic, 129
  trends in, 134-35
Abstinence, 241-42
Acne, and androgens, 35n
Acton, William, quoted, 287
Adenosine triphosphate (ATP), 139
Adolescence, defined, 16
Adolescent sterility, 91
Adoption, 219-21
Adrenal glands, and sexual desire, 82n
Adulthood, personality development during,
  21-25
Afterbirth (placenta), 202
Aggressiveness, and testosterone, 356n
Alcohol, and sexuality, 340-41
Alexander the Great, 271
Alienation, and sexuality, 330-31
Allantois, 193, *194*
Ambivalence, universality of, 26
Amenorrhea, 49, 204, 207
American Academy of Psychoanalysis, 242
American Association of Marriage
  Counselors, 269-70
American Endocrine Society, 31
American Law Institute, 130
American Medical Association Committee
  on Human Reproduction, 130
Amino acids, 143, 144, 145
Amniocentesis, 184, 186-87
Amnion, 193, *194*
Amniotic fluid, 193, *194*
  diagnosis of, 186-88
Amphetamines, and sexuality, 343-44
Amyl nitrite, sexuality and, 345-46
Androgens, 35n
  and acne, 35n
  and brain differentiation, 80-82
  and secondary sex characteristics, 35n
  and sexual differentiation, 80
Androsterone, 308
Anna Karenina (Tolstoy), quoted, 354
Antigens, Rh, 170
Anxiety, of new parents, 208-09
Aphrodisiacs, 346-48
Aquinas, Saint Thomas, quoted, 108-09
Aristotle, 271-72
Aschan, Roger, quoted, 3
Augustine, Saint, quoted, 107
Autonomy, of infant, 8

Autosomes, 140
Aveyron, "wild boy" of, 209

B

Balfour, Earl of, quoted, 24-25
Barr body, 184
Bartholin's glands, *40*, 51
Barzun, Jacques, quoted, 265
Basic trust versus basic mistrust (Erikson),
  4-5
Bell, Benjamin, 61-62
Bestiality, 325-27
Between Parent and Child (Ginott), quoted,
  19-20
Bieber, Irving, 305
Biological clock, 33
Birth control, 108-09
  female, 109, 113-19
  male, 119-29
  methods of, 110-14 (table)
  rhythm method of, 117-18
  temperature method of, 117-18
  by tubal ligation, 118-19
  by vasectomy, 119-22
  see also Contraception
Birth control pill, *see* Oral contraceptives
Birth defects, extent of, 176-82, 178-81
  (table)
Birth weights, and socioeconomic status, 164
  (table)
Birthmarks, 178 (table)
Bisexuality, 298
  of Lesbians, 314-15
Blackstone, William, quoted, 354
Bladder, control of in toddler, 8-9, 8n
Blastocyst, 191
Bowels, control of in toddler, 8-9
Brain, differentiation of, 80-82, 81n
Breast-feeding, 52-54, 204-05, 207-08
  and alcoholism, 52-54
  conception during, 207
  and drugs, 54
  see also Lactation
Breasts, 51, 52
  as erogenous zone, 59
Bremer, Arthur, 333
Browne, Sir Thomas, quoted, 292
Browning, Robert, quoted, 282
Burns, Robert, quoted, 75
Byron, Lord, quoted, 268

C

Castration, fear of, 13-14, 13n
Cato, quoted, 226

Catullus, quoted, 26
Cedergvist, Jane, 157
Cells, 138-40
  germ, 140
  hybridization of, 184-85
  kinds of, 140
  nucleus of, 138-39
  somatic, 140
  structure of, 138-40
Charles VIII, King of France, 61
Chaucer, Geoffrey, quoted, 254
Chemical pollution, and pregnancy, 167-68
Child
  and need for mothering, 209-10
  responsibility to, 28-29
Child and parent, development of, 28 (table)
Childbirth
  Lamaze method of (natural childbirth),
    203
  and love of child, 205-06, 206n
  pain of, 202-03
Child-rearing
  in Kibbutzin, 212
  and working mother, 210-12
Chorionic membrane, 192, *194*
Chorionic vesicle (body stalk), 192, *194*
Chorionic villi, 192, *194*
Chromosomal aberration, 151
  and radiation, 167
Chromosomal stripes, staining for, 185-86
Chromosomes
  and athletic competition, 157-58
  and crime, 155-56, 155-56n
  structure of, 138-39
Circumcision, 37
  and male dyspareunia, 291-92
Cleft lip (harelip), 178 (table)
Climacteric, 50
Clitoris, *40*, 51, 55-57
  as erogenous zone, 55-56
  retraction reaction of, 103
Clubfoot, 178 (table)
Cocaine, sexuality and, 344-45
Codon, 147, *148*, 149
Coitus interruptus, 108, 215-16
Colostrum, 51, 198
Columbus, Christopher, 61
Communal living, and sexuality, 348-51
Conception, 43
Condom, 112 (table)
  and venereal disease, 69
Congenital heart disease, 178 (table)
Congenital urinary tract defects, 178 (table)
Contact tracing, for venereal disease, 63-64
Contraception, 32, 32n
Contraceptives
  and clots, 109, 113-15
  oral, 109, 113-17, *116*
  research for, 122-26
  and venereal disease, 69, 70
Cooper's ligament, *52*, 52n

Coronary thrombosis, 113, 113n
Corpus luteum, 45, 46, 94
Courtship
  among animals, 224
  historical, 228-29
  importance of, 244-47
  modern, 229-30
  primitive, 228
Cowper's glands, *34,* 36
Cretinism, 165
Crib death, 213-14, 213n
Cross-dressing, among children, 321-22
Cummins, Paul, quoted, 330
Cunnilinction, 89-90, 325
  and venereal disease, 76, 77
Curiosity, of infant, 6
Cyanate, 163
Cyclazocaine, 348
Cystic fibrosis, 180 (table), 188
Cytomegalic inclusion disease, 166
Cytoplasm, 138, 139-40

D

Daphnis and Chloë (Longus), quoted, 225
Dark Ages, 19
Daughters of Bilitis, 304, 304n
  see also Lesbianism
David Copperfield (Dickens), quoted, 252
Day, Richard L., 182
Deaths
  causes of (by sex), 160 (table)
  male per 100 female, 159 (table)
de Graaf, Regner, 42
Deletion, of chromosomes, 152
Deoxyribonucleic acid (DNA), 138, 143, 145,
    146, 149
  and RNA synthesis, 144
Dexedrine, 347
Diabetes, 169, 179 (table)
Diaphragms, 111 (table)
Dickens, Charles, quoted, 252
Diethylstilbesterol, 124, 124-25n, 167
Dilation and curettage (D and C), 133
Discipline, of child, 26-27
Diseases, venereal, *see* Venereal disease
Divorce
  and age at marriage, 253-54
  in interfaith marriages, 248-50, 249 (table)
Domostroy, The, quoted, 262
Donne, John, quoted, 346
Down's syndrome, 138, 153, 153n, 180 (table),
    188
Drug abuse
  and alienated college student, 337-38
  among parents and their children, 336-37
  and sexuality, 335-40
  and unborn children, 172-73
Dual-sex treatment team, 279
Dysmenorrhea, 48-49, 308

Dyspareunia
  female, 284-87
  male, 291-92
  psychological causes of, 286-87

E

Eclampsia, 165-66
Ectoderm, 191
Ectopic pregnancy, 46n
Egg, differentiation of fertilized, 191-93
Ego, 22
Ego-identity, 4
Einstein, Albert, quoted, 25
Ejaculation, 87
  force of, 273, 273n
  mechanism of, 38-39
  premature, 87, 102, 293, 294-96
Ejaculatory demand, 273
Ejaculatory ducts, 34, 35
Ejaculatory incompetence, 296
Ejaculatory inevitability, 273, 295, 295n
Electroencephalogram (EEG), and sexual
  preferences, 93n
Electron microscope, 140
Embolus, 109
Embryo, 143, 143n
  see also Fetus
Embryology, 191
Emerson, Ralph Waldo, quoted, 351-52
Emotional ambivalence, 13
Emotions, and pregnancy, 172
Endocrine glands, 30-32
  and influence on homosexuality, 301-02
  and pregnancy, 169
Endoderm, 191
Endometrium, 41, 47
Endoplasmic reticulum, 139
Environment
  and effect on homosexuality, 302
  and sexuality, 3
Enzymes, 138
  and ribosomal structure, 144, 144n
Epididymis, 34, 35
Erasmus, quoted, 243
Erection
  according to Masters and Johnson, 1n
  in infancy, 1
  mechanism of, 37-38
Erikson, Erik, 3-4, 17
Erogenous zones, structure and function of,
  54-60
Erythroblastosis fetalis, 169-70, 179 (table)
Estrogen, 42, 44
Etiocholanolone, 308
Evolution, of man, 137
Excitement phase, of sexual response, 84
Exhibitionism, 322
Extra fingers and toes (polydactyly), 179
  (table)

F

Fallopian tubes, 39, 40, 44-45, *45*
  blockage of and sterility, 44, 44n
Fallopio, Gabriello, 39
Fallopius, 61
Family Service Association of America, 270
Father
  diminished, 355-56
  and effect of television on, 355
Father Tertullian, quoted, 245
Favorinus, quoted, 54
Fellatio, 89-90, 90n, 325
Females
  birth control methods of, 109, 113-19
  dyspareunia in, 284-87
  external genitalia of, *40*, 50-51
  frigidity of, 283-84, 283n
  increase of violence among, 333n
  orgasmic dysfunction of, 287-89, *289*
  orgasms of, 86
  periodicity of, 94-95
  primordial, 79-80
  reproductive system of, 39, *40,* 41-49
  sexual desire of, 94-95
  sexual inadequacy in, 283-91
  sexual response of, 85-86
  sexual satisfaction of, 98-99, 99n
  survival rates of, 159-61
  vaginismus in, 289-91, 291n
Feminization, of male children, 333
Fertility
  period of, 44
  problems of, 214-17
Fertility drugs, 216-17
"Fertility switch," 30-32
Fetus, 143n
  diagnosis of, 186-89
  monthly stages of development, 193,
    195-96
Fleming, Alexander, quoted, 66
Fluorescing compounds, and chromosomal
  bands, 186
Follicle-stimulating hormone (FSH), 31-32,
    41, 42, *42,* 94, 95, 127
  and fertility, 216
  and homosexuality, 309
Follicular fluid, 42
Food and Drug Administration, 113
Fracastorious, Girolamo, 61
Freud, Anna, quoted, 16-17
Freud, Sigmund, 2-3, 356
  and homosexuality, 310
  quoted, 352
Frigidity, 283-84, 283n
Fused fingers and toes (syndactyly), 179
  (table)

G

Gagnon, John H., 238-41

Galactosemia, 180 (table)
Gametes, 140
Gay, George R., 345
Gender identity, 10
  and learning, 82–84
Gender Identity Clinic (University of
    California, L. A.), 321–22
Gene, structure of, 139
Generativity versus stagnation (Erikson), 24
Genetic counseling, 183–84
Genetic disorders, 151–63
  research into, 184–89
Genetic predetermination, 150–51
Genetics
  and environment, 149–51
  and race, 161–63
Genital herpes, 74
Genital lice, 75
Genital ridges, 79
Genitals, size of, 105–06
Genital warts, 74
Genotype, 150
German measles (rubella), 166
Germ cells, 140
Gibran, Kahlil, quoted, 222, 276–77
Ginot, Haim, quoted, 19–20
Glans penis, *34*, 36–37, 292
Glycogen, 138
Golgi complex, 139–40
Gonadotropic hormone, 46
Gonadotropins, 127
  and fertility, 216
Gonads, development of, 79–80
Gonococcal amniotic infection syndrome, 71
Gonorrhea
  and birth control pill, 69
  disease process of, 63
  natural history of, 63 (table)
  percent increase and decrease, 65 (table)
  prevention of, 69–70
  reported cases of, 64 (table)
Graafian follicle, 42, 94
Grapes of Wrath (Steinbeck), 53
Group sex, 323

H

Halleck, Seymour L., quoted, 243
Hamlet (Shakespeare), quoted, 232
Hemoglobin, and sickle cell disease, 162–63,
    163n
Hemophilia, 152, 161
Heredity, importance of, 137–38
Hermaphrodite, 83, 83n, 224, 224n
Hermaphroditus, 298
Heroin
  and pregnancy, 175–76
  sexuality and, 338–40
Herpes, genital, 74
Heterosexuality, 298
  defined, 299

Homologue, defined, 55–56
Homosexuality, 11, 11n, 12n, 298
  and biochemistry, 307–10, 308–09n
  defined, 299
  as a disease, 310–12
  early indications of, 304–06
  and endocrine influence, 301–02, 302n
  and environment, 302
  expression of, 300–01
  extent of, 300–01
  and FSH, 309
  and LH, 309
  misconceptions about, 299–300
  parental factors and, 12n, 306–07
  roots of, 301–02
  and society, 312–14
  Spartan, 297–98
  and testosterone, 308, 308n
  tomboyishness and, 305
  treatment for, 314–16
  and venereal disease, 66–67
Horace, quoted, 71–72
Hormones, releasing, 30
Human Sexual Inadequacy (Masters and
    Johnson), 87, 278
  critics of, 280–81
  discussion of, 281ff.
Human Sexual Response (Masters and
    Johnson), 276, 278
  discussion of, 84–87
Hunter, John, 61
Hybridization, of cells, 185
Hydrocephaly (water on the brain), 180
  (table)
Hydrocortisone, 172
Hymen, *40*, 50
Hypothalamus, 30–31
Hysterotomy, 134

I

Identity versus self-diffusion (Erikson), 16
Implantation, of fertilized egg, 191, 191n
Impotence, 292–94, 292–93n
  causes of, 292–93
  treatment of, 293–94
Incest, 256, 256n
Independence, seeking of, 25–27
Industry versus inferiority (Erikson), 14
Infant
  autonomy of, 8
  characteristics of, 1–2
  curiosity of, 6
  erection in, 1, 1n, 6
  peripheral vision of, 1
  personality development of, 4–7
  pleasure in, 3, 6
  self-love in, 5
  sexuality of, 5–7
Infanticide, 108, 108n
Infection, and pregnancy, 166

Infectious hepatitis, 166
Initiative versus guilt (Erikson), 10-11
Inner cell mass, of fertilized egg, 192
Insulin, 169
Integrity versus despair and disgust
    (Erikson), 24-25
Interclass marriage, 251-52
Intercourse, *see* Sexual intercourse
International Directory of Genetic Services,
    The, 183
Intersexuality, 155, 155n
Intervillous spaces, 192
Intimacy versus isolation (Erikson), 22
Intrauterine devices (IUD), 110 (table)
Isaiah, quote from, 60-61
Islets of Langerhans, 169
Ismelin, 348
Ivan IV, Tsar of Russia, 262

J

Johnson, Samuel, quoted, 245
Johnson, Virginia E., 84
Jorgensen, Christine, 319
Journal of the American Medical
    Association, 280

K

Kelley, Robert L., 251
Keniston, Kenneth, 331, 332
Kibbutzim, and child-rearing, 212
King Henry the Fourth (Shakespeare),
    quoted, 270
King Lear (Shakespeare), quoted, 355
Kinsey, Alfred
    and heterosexuality, 299
    and homosexuality, 299
Kinsey Report, and masturbation, 93
Kissing, and erogenous zones, 59, 59n
Kleptomania, 334
Klinefelter's syndrome, 154-55, *154, 155*
Klobukowska, Ewa, 157
Krafft-Ebing, Richard von 307

L

Labia majora, *40,* 50-51, 57
Labia minora, *40,* 51, 57
Labor
    of pregnancy, 201
    stages of, 201 (table), 201-02
Lactation, 52-54, 204-05, 207-08
    and alcoholism, 54
    and drugs, 54
    see also Breast-feeding
Ladies Book, The, quoted, 262
Lamaze method, of childbirth (natural
    childbirth), 203

Lanugo, of fetus, 195
Latency period (Freud), 14
L-Dopa, 348
Lear, John, quoted, 144
Learning, and gender identity, 82-84
Lesbianism, 304
Lesbians, bisexuality of, 314-15, 314n
Liberation, male and female, 353-54, 353n
Lice, genital, 75
Longus, quoted, 225
"Look, The" (Teasdale), 231
Lucretius, quoted, 255
Luteinizing hormone (LH), 42, 43, 45, 94, 95,
    127
    and homosexuality, 309
Luteinizing hormone-releasing hormone
    (LH-RH), 31-32, 127
    as a contraceptive, 32n
    and fertility, 216
Lysergic acid diethylamide (LSD)
    and pregnancy, 175
    and sexuality, 343
Lysosomes, 139

M

Macbeth (Shakespeare), quoted, 340
Males
    birth-control methods of, 119-29
    dyspareunia of, 291-92
    and fear of woman, 356
    feminization of, 333
    orgasm in, 87
    reproductive system of, 33, *34,* 35-37
    sexual response of, 86-87
    survival rates of, 159-61
Mammary glands, 51, *52*
    and lactation, 52-54
    see also Breasts
Man, evolution of, 137
Man-mouse cell hybrids, 184-85
Manson, Charles, 350-51
Marcusis of Guyana, 228
Marijuana
    and pregnancy, 175
    sexuality and, 341-42
    use of, 337-38
Marital codes, establishment of, 225-28
Marital experiments, 351
Marmor, Judd, quoted, 325, 356
Marriage
    age at time of, 253-54
    campus, 258-61
    changes in, 357-59
    interclass, 251-52
    interfaith, 248-50, 249 (table)
    interracial, 250-51
    kinds of (Mead), 358-59
    masturbation and, 268-69
    and money problems, 252-53
    monotony of, 261-63

Marriage (*continued*)
  problems of, 247-54, 269-70
  reasons for, 244
  and sexual apathy, 263-70
  and war, 256-58
Marriage counselors, 269-70
Mary Tudor, Queen of England, 197n
Masochism, 327-28
Masters, E. E., quoted, 355
Masters and Johnson, 266
  critics of, 280-81
  Human Sexual Inadequacy, 87, 278, 280-81,
    281ff.
  Human Sexual Response, 84-87, 276, 278
  study of human sexual inadequacy, 278-96
  study of human sexual response, 84-87
  and treatment of sexual inadequacy,
    281-83
Masters, William H., 84
Masturbation, 18-21, 93
  and marriage, 268-69
  in toddlers, 9
May, Rollo, 243
MDA, sexuality and, 343
Mead, Margaret, quoted, 358-59
Meconium, 1
Medical Aspects of Human Sexuality, 281
Meditations of a Parish Priest (Roux),
    quoted, 15
Meiosis, 140-42, *141*
  disorders during, 153-58
Meiotic nondisjunction, 153
Melatonin, 33
Memoirs of the Prince of Talleyrand, quoted,
    15
Menopause, 49-50
Menorrhagia, 48
Menstruation, 41-45, *41, 42, 45*
  age of beginning (menarche), 237-38
  truths about, 48-49
  untruths about, 47-48
  variations in, 49
Merchant of Venice, The (Shakespeare),
    quoted, 2
Merry Wives of Windsor, The,
    (Shakespeare), quoted, 75, 347
Mesoderm, 191
Messenger RNA, 145-46, 146n
Methedrine, 347
Metrorrhagia, 48-49
Milton, John, quoted, 55
Miscarriage, 129
Missing limbs, 180 (table)
Mitochondria, 139
Mitosis, 140-42, *141*
  disorders during, 158-61
Molecular biology, 140
Money, and marriage problems, 252-53
Money, John, quoted, 100
Mongolism (Down's syndrome), 138, 153,
    153n, 180 (table), 188

Monilia albicans, 73
Moniliasis, 73
  and birth control pills, 73n
Monogamous family, fragility of, 354-59
Monogamy, 358
Monosomy, 153
Mons pubis, *40,* 50
Montaigne, Michel de, quoted, 351
Mosaicism, 159
Mothers
  unwed, 221-23
  working, 210-12
Mutations, spontaneous, 152

N

Nash, Ogden, quoted, 340
National Research Council Committee on
    Maternal Nutrition, 165
Necrophilism, 325
New London Letter Writer, quoted, 229
Noise, and effect on newborns, 168-69
Nondisjunction
  meiotic, 153
  mitotic, 158
Nubility, defined, 91
Nuclear sex, 157
Nucleolus, 138
Nucleus, of cell, 138-39
Nutrition, during pregnancy, 164-66
Nymphomania, 350n

O

Obesity, and sexual expression, 268, 268n
Obstetric Advisory Committee, 131
Odors, and sexual expression, 265, 265n, 283
Oedipus complex, 11
Oedipus Tyrannus (Sophocles), quoted, 11
Oneida community, 357
Oögenesis, 16
Open spine (spina bifida), 181 (table)
Opiates (heroin), and pregnancy, 175-76
Oral area, as erogenous zone, 59
Oral contraceptives, 47, 109, 110 (table),
    113-17, 116
  and clots, 109, 113-15
  and gonorrhea, 69
  male, 126-27
  and moniliasis, 73n
  and premarital sexual intercourse, 240n
  and thromboembolic disease, 114, 114-15n
  see also Contraceptives
Oral-genital contact, 89-90
Oral-genital transmission of venereal
    disease, 76-77
Oral phase, 6
Oral thrush, 77
Organelles, 138, 139-40

Orgasm, 60, 60n, 84, 100–02
  clitoral, 103–05
  defined, 22
  female, 86, 96–97
  male, 87
  pretended, 97
  quality of, 99–100
  simultaneous, 102
  and use of mechanical devices, 267
  vaginal, 103–05
Orgasmic dysfunction
  female, 287–89
  treatment of, 287–89, 289
Orgasmic expulsion, 273
Orgasmic phase, of sexual response, 84
Oswald, Lee Harvey, 151
Ovaries, 39, 39n, 40, 41
Ovid, quoted, 20
Ovulation, 31, 41–45, *41,* 42, 45
Ovum
  fertilization of, 46–47
  growth of, 150
  viability of, 46
Oxford English Dictionary, quoted, 55
Oxytocin stimulation method, of inducing
    abortion, 134

P

Packard, Vance, study of college coital rates,
    235–37, 242
Pancreas, 169
Papanicolaou test (Pap test), 49, 115
Parent, development of, 27–28, 28 (table)
Parkinson's disease, 348
Partner surrogates, 279
Pasteur, Louis, quoted, 185
Paternity blood tests, 223n
PCPA (p-chlorphenylalanine), 348
Pedigree chart, 184
Pedophilia, 328–29
Pelvic congestion, 86
Pelvic inflammatory disease (PID), 68
Pelvic pain
  and congestion, 77–78
  and petting, 77–78
Penicillin, resistance to, 66
Penis, *34,* 35–36
  as erogenous zone, 55
  glans of, *34,* 36–37, 292
  size of, 105–06
Penis envy, 13n, 356
Penn, William, quoted, 263
Pepys, Samuel, quoted, 234–35
Perineal area, 58
Periodicity, of female, 94–95
Peripheral vision, of infants, 1
Personality development, stages of
    (Erikson), 4–29
Personality, establishment of, 3

Pharmacogentics, 172–73
Pharyngitis, 76
Phenylketonuria (PKU), 152
Phimosis, 291
Physiology, of human sexual response,
    84–87
Pineal gland, 32–33
Pituitary gland, 30
PKU (Phenylketonuria), 152, 181 (table)
Place, Francis, 109
Placenta, 46, 202
  formation of, 192, 193, 194
Plasma membrane, 139
Plateau phase, of sexual response, 84
Plato, quoted, 298
Pliny, 47
Plutarch, quoted, 297
Pollution
  chemical, 167–68
  noise, 168–69
Polo, Marco, 203
Polychlorianted biphenyls (PCB), 168
Polygamy, 227
Population Council's International
    Committee for Contraceptive Research,
    127
Potency, differences in, 96–97
Pregnancy
  and age of mother, 171
  and age of parents, 182–83
  among children (ten to fourteen years of
      age), 172 (table)
  and chemical pollution, 167–68
  and direct radiation, 166–67
  duration of, 190–91
  ectopic, 46n
  and effect of drugs, 172–73
  and emotions of mother, 172, 197
  and endocrine glands, 169
  false, 197n, 203n (male)
  and the father, 203–04
  and infection, 166
  intervals of, 182
  laboratory tests for, 197–98
  and LSD, 175
  and marijuana smoking, 175
  and nutrition, 164–66
  and opiates (heroin), 175–76
  postnatal care, 205
  and Rh factor, 169–70
  and sexual intercourse, 199–201
  signs of, 197–99, 197n
  and smoking, 165, 173–74
  and venereal disease, 71
Preludin, 348
Premarital sexual behavior, patterns of,
    241–43
Premarital sexual intercourse, 232–35
  and birth control pills, 240n
  prevalence of, 238–41
Premarital sexual standards, 231–32

Premature ejaculation, 87, 102, 293, 294-96
  treatment of, 295-96
Premenstrual tension, 48
Prenatal care, 199
Prepuce (foreskin), of penis, 34, 36-37
Preschooler (three to six years), personality
  development of, 10-14
Primordial female, 79-80
Primordial sex cells, 140, 141, *141*
Progesterone, 46
Progestin, 123, 124
Progonasyl, 70
Prolactin, 204, 205n
Promiscuity, sexual, 240-241, 242-43
Prophet, The (Gibran), quoted, 222, 276-77
Prostaglandins, 125-26
Prostate gland, 34, 36
Protein synthesis, 145-49, *148*
Protoplasm, 138
Psychosomatic illness, and vaginismus,
  289-90, 289n
Psychotropic drugs, 336
Puberty
  defined, 16, 91
  personality development in, 16-18
Pubes, *40, 50*
Pulmonary embolism, 113, 113n

Q

Quintillian, quoted, 226

R

Racial amalgamation, 248
Radiation
  and chromosomal aberrations, 167
  and pregnancy, 166-67
Raleigh, Sir Walter, quoted, 244
Refractory period, of male, 87, 273
Reproductive Biology Research Foundation
  (St. Louis), 84, 281
Reproductive systems
  development of, 79-80
  female, 39, *40,* 41-49
  male, 33, *34,* 35-37
Research Committee on Female
  Homosexuality, 304
Resolution phase, of sexual response, 84
Retraction reaction, of clitoris, 103
Reverse transcriptase, 149n
Rh antigens, 170
Rh factor, and pregnancy, 169-70
Rhythm method, of contraception, 111
  (table), 117-18
Ribonucleic acid (RNA), 143
  functions of, 145-49, 148
  messenger, 145-46, 146n

ribosomal, 144
  synthesis of, 144
  transfer, 146-47
Ribosomal RNA, 144
Ribosomes, 139
  function of, 145-49, *148*
  structure of, 144-45
Ritalin, 348
Rock, John, 127-28
Rock music, sexuality and, 334-35, 335n
Roux, Joseph, quoted, 15
Rubáiyát of Omar Khayyám, quoted, 98
Rubeola, 166
Ruby, Jack, 151
Russel, William, quoted, 247

S

Sacher-Masoch, Ritter Leopold von, 327
Sade, Marquis de, quoted, 327
Sadism, 327-28
Saline injection method of inducing
  abortion, 133-34
Saltpeter (potassium nitrate), 348
Salpingitis, 68
Sanger, Margaret, 109
Satyriasis, 350n
Scabies, 74-75
Schally, Andrew V., 31, 32
School-age child (six to twelve years),
  personality development of, 14-16
Scrotum, 33, *34*
  as erogenous zone, 57
Secondary sex characteristics, and
  androgens, 35n
Seeman, Melvin, 330-31
Seferis, George, quoted, 1
Self-love, 23
  in infancy, 5
Semen, 38-39
Semen banks, 122
Seminal fluid, chemistry of, 128-29
Seminal vesicle, *34,* 35
Seminiferous tubules, 33, *34,* 35
Senior citizens, and sexuality, 270-77
Sensate focus exercises, 282
Sex
  group, 323
  planning of child's, 217-19
  premarital standards of, 231-32
Sex-change surgery, 320-21
Sex chromosomes, 141-43
Sex flush, 85
Sex Information and Education Council of
  U.S., 241
Sexton, Patricia, quoted, 333
Sexual activity, peak of, 93-94
Sexual apathy, in marriage, 263-70
Sexual arousal, psychological differences in,
  92-93

Sexual behavior
  adolescent, 304-05
  complexity of, 302, 302n
  early adolescent, 303-04
  preadolescent, 303
  roots of, 82-84
Sexual choices, 357-59
Sexual depressants, 348
Sexual desire, and female cycle, 94-95
Sexual differentiation, and androgens, 80
Sexual expression
  of aging female, 274
  of aging male, 272-73
  casualness of, 243
  "normalcy" of, 268
  and obesity, 268, 268n
  and odors, 265, 265n, 283
  surroundings for, 264-65
  techniques of, 265-67
  and use of mechanical devices, 267
Sexual inadequacy
  Masters and Johnson's treatment of,
    281-83
  in men, 291-96
  treatment of, 107
  in women, 283-91
Sexual intercourse
  abstinence from, 106-07
  anal, 67, 284
  and clitoral stimulation, 102-03
  following childbirth, 206-07
  frequency among older people, 274-76
  frequency of, 95-96
  and personal hygiene, 285, 285n
  positions during, 87, 88, 89, 288-89, 289
  and pregnancy, 199-201
  premarital, 232-35
Sexuality
  adolescent, 91-92
  and alcohol, 340-41
  and alienation, 330-31
  and amphetamines, 343-44
  and amyl nitrite, 345-46
  attitudes toward, 92
  and cocaine, 344-45
  and communal living, 348-51
  defined, 2-3
  and drug abuse, 335-40
  and environment, 3
  and heroin, 338-40
  in infancy, 5-7
  and LSD, 343
  and marijuana, 341-42
  and MDA, 343
  myths and misconceptions of, 100-07
  problems arising from differences in,
    97-98
  and rock music, 334-35, 335n
  senior citizens and, 270-77
  and society, 234-35, 235n
  of toddler, 9-10

and violence, 331-34
  women's liberation and, 351-54
Sexual preferences, and
    electroencephalogram (EEG), 73n
Sexual response
  differences in, 93-94
  of female, 85-86
  of male, 86-87
  phases of, 84
  physiology of, 84-87
  similarities of, 90
Shainess, Natalie, quoted, 280
Shakespeare, William, quoted, 2, 61, 75, 232,
    270, 340, 347, 355
Shaw, George Bernard, 264
Shelley, Percy Bysshe, 354
Sheppard, Charles W., 345
Shettles, Landrum B., 218
Sickle cell anemia, 161, 162-63, 181 (table)
Sickle cell disease 162-63
Sickle cell trait, 162
Sight, peripheral, 1
Simon, William, 238-41
Skene's ducts, 51
Smoking, and pregnancy, 165, 173-74
Society
  and homosexuality, 312-14
  and sexuality, 234-35, 235n
Society of Medical Psychoanalysts of N.Y.C.,
    304
Sodomy, and the law, 324-25
Somatic cells, 140
Sophocles, quoted, 11
Sparta, and homosexual behavior, 297-98
Sperm, see Spermatozoa
Spermatogenesis, 16, 31
Spermatozoa, 31, 33, 35, 37, 38-39
  impeding maturation of, 128
  impeding production of, 127-28
  impeding transportation of, 128
  route of, 36
  structure of, 37
Sperm banks, 217
Spinoza, Baruch, quoted, 13, 90
Spontaneous abortion, and smoking, 173
Steinbeck, John, 53
Sterility
  and blockage of Fallopian tubes, 44, 44n
  and venereal disease, 67-68
Stevenson, Robert Louïs, quoted, 100
Subfertility, 214-17
Sudden infant death syndrome (SIDS),
    213-14, 213n
Summa Theologica (Aquinas), quoted, 108-09
Superego, 356n
Super-female syndrome, 156-57
Sylvester, Pope, 262
Symposium (Plato), quoted, 298
Syphilis, 61
  deaths due to, 159, 160 (table)
  disease process of, 62

Syphilis (*continued*)
  natural history of, 62 (table)
  of the newborn, 166
  percent increase and decrease of cases, 65
    (table), 65n
  prevention of, 69-70
  reported cases of, 64 (table)
Syphilus, 61

T

Taming of the Shrew, The, (Shakespeare),
    quoted, 230
Taylor, Jeremy, quoted, 263
Tay-Sachs Disease, 189
Teasdale, Sara, quoted, 231
Television, and diminished father, 355
Temperature method of birth control, 117-18
Terence, quoted, 297
Testes, 33, 34
  descending of, 33
  as erogenous zone, 57
Testosterone, 35, 35n, 308, 308n
  and aggressiveness, 356n
  and homosexuality, 308, 308n
Thales of Miletus, quoted, 3
Thalidomide, 172-73
Thromboembolic disease, and oral
    contraceptives, 114, 114-15n
Thrombus, 109
Thumb-sucking, 14, 14n
Toddler
  masturbation in, 9
  personality development of, 7-10
  sexuality of, 9-10
  toilet-training, 8-9
Tolstoy, Leo, quoted, 354
Tomboyishness, and homosexuality, 305
Toxemia, 165
Transfer RNA, 146-47
Translocation, of chromosomes, 152
Transsexual behavior, 318-21
  development of, 319-20
  treatment of, 320-21
Transvestite behavior, 316-18, 316n
Treponema pallidum, 62
Trichomonas vaginalis, 72
Trichomoniasis, 72-73
Trisomy, 21, 153
Troilism, 323
Trophoblast, 192, 194
True genitality (Erikson), 22-23, 22n
Tubal ligation, 112 (table), 118-19
Tumescence, 85
Turner's syndrome, 154, *154, 156*

U

Ultracentrifuge, 140
Umbilical cord, 192, *194*

Unwed mothers, 221-23
Urethra, *34, 35*
  of female, *40,* 51
Urethral strictures, 291
U.S. Food and Drug Administration, 124
Uterus, 39, *40,* 41
  structure of, 47

V

Vacuum aspiration (suction) method of
    inducing abortion, 133
Vagina
  lubrication of in infant, 1, 1n
  size of, 106
  structure of, *40,* 50
  vestibule of, 57
Vaginal foams, 113 (table)
Vaginal jellies and creams, 113 (table)
Vaginal suppositories, 113 (table)
Vaginal tablets, 113 (table)
Vaginal thrush, 73
Vaginal infections, and dyspareunia, 284,
    285-86, 286-87n
Vaginismus, 289-91
  treatment of, 290-91, 291n
Vas deferens, *34,* 35
Vasectomy, 119-22
Venereal diseases (V.D.), 60-72
  and condom, 69
  and contact tracing, 63-64
  and contraceptives, 69, 70
  cunnilinction and, 77
  dangers of, 67-68
  extent and causes of, 63-66
  and fellatio, 76
  and homosexuality, 66-67
  oral-genital transmission of, 76-77
  nonspecific, 76
  and pelvic inflammatory disease (PID), 68
  and pregnancy, 71
  and sterility, 67-68
Vernix caseosa, of fetus, 196
Vestibule, vaginal, *40,* 51
Victoria, Queen of England, 202
Villi, 192
Violence
  increase of, among women, 333n
  and sexuality, 331-34
Vitamins, 138
Voyeurism (scoptophilia), 322-23
  as a national problem, 323-24

W

Wallace, William, 62
War, and marriage, 256-58
Warts, genital, 74
Weismuller, Johnny, 157

Wells, H. G., quoted, 245
Wet dreams, 20-21
Whipple, Dorothy V., quoted, 5
Whitman, Charles J., 151
Whitman, Walt, quoted, 21, 54, 137
Wilde, Oscar, quoted, 355
William the Conqueror, 227
Wolfe, Thomas, quoted, 244
Wollstonecraft, Mary, quoted, 354
Women's liberation, and sexuality, 351-54

X

X-chromosome, 141-43, *143,* 157
X-rays, during pregnancy, 166

XYY syndrome, 155-56, *156*

Y

Y-chromosome, 141-43, *143*
Yohimbine, 347
Yolk sac, 193, *194*

Z

Zeno the Stoic, quoted, 15
Zygote, 140
    cleavage of, 191
    division of, 142-43

A   3
B   4
C   5
D   6
E   7
F   8
G   9
H   0
I   1
J   2

7